Blood & Circulatory Disorders Sourcebook

Basic Information about Disorders Such As Anemia, Hemorrhage, Shock, Embolism, and Thrombosis, along with Facts Concerning Rh Factor, Blood Banks, Blood Donation Programs, and Transfusions

Edited by Linda M. Ross. 600 pages. 1998. 0-7808-0203-9. $75.

Burns Sourcebook

Basic Information about Heat, Chemical, Electrical, and Sun Burns, along with Facts about Burn Treatment and Recovery, and Reports on Current Research Initiatives

Edited by Allan R. Cook. 600 pages. 1998. 0-7808-0204-7. $75.

Cancer Sourcebook

Basic Information on Cancer Types, Symptoms, Diagnostic Methods, and Treatments, Including Statistics on Cancer Occurrences Worldwide and the Risks Associated with Known Carcinogens and Activities

Edited by Frank E. Bair. 932 pages. 1990. 1-55888-888-8. $75.

"This publication's nontechnical nature and very comprehensive format make it useful for both the general public and undergraduate students."
— *Choice, Oct '90*

"This compact collection of reliable information, written in a positive, hopeful tone, is an invaluable tool for helping patients and patients' families and friends to take the first steps in coping with the many difficulties of cancer."   — *Medical Reference Services Quarterly, Winter '91*

"An important resource for the general reader trying to understand the complexities of cancer."
— *American Reference Books Annual, '91*

Cancer Sourcebook for Women

Basic Information about Specific Forms of Cancer That Affect Women, Featuring Facts about Breast Cancer, Cervical Cancer, Ovarian Cancer, Cancer of the Uterus and Uterine Sarcoma, Cancer of the Vagina, and Cancer of the Vulva; Statistical and Demographic Data; Treatments, Self-Help Management Suggestions

Edited by Allan
pages. 1996. 0-78

"This timely bo
sumer health an
libraries."

The availability under one cover of all these pertinent publications, grouped under cohesive headings, makes this certainly a most useful sourcebook."
— *Choice, Jun '96*

"Laudably, the book portrays the feelings of the cancer victim, as well as her mate . . .both benefit from the gold mine of information nestled between the two covers of this book. It is hard to conceive of any library that would not want it as part of its collection. Recommended."
— *Academic Library Book Review, Summer '96*

". . . written in easily understandable, non-technical language. Recommended for public libraries or hospital and academic libraries that collect patient education or consumer health materials."
— *Medical Reference Services Quarterly, Spring '97*

New Cancer Sourcebook

Basic Information about Major Forms and Stages of Cancer, Featuring Facts about Primary and Secondary Tumors of the Respiratory, Nervous, Lymphatic, Circulatory, Skeletal, and Gastrointestinal Systems, and Specific Organs; Statistical and Demographic Data, Treatment Options, and Strategies for Coping

Edited by Allan R. Cook. 1,313 pages. 1996. 0-7808-0041-9. $75.

"This book is an excellent resource. The dialogue is simple, direct, and comprehensive."
— *Doody's Health Sciences Book Review, Nov '96*

"The amount of factual and useful information is extensive. The writing is very clear, geared to general readers. Recommended for all levels."
— *Choice, Jan '97*

Cardiovascular Diseases & Disorders Sourcebook

Basic Information about Cardiovascular Diseases and Disorders, Featuring Facts about the Cardiovascular System, Demographic and Statistical Data, Descriptions of Pharmacological and Surgical Interventions, Lifestyle Modifications, and a Special Section Focusing on Heart Disorders in Children

Edited by Karen Bellenir and Peter D. Dresser. 683 pages. 1995. 0-7808-0032-X. $75.

". . . comprehensive format provides an extensive overview on this subject."   — *Choice, Jun '96*

"Easily understood, complete, up-to-date resource. This well executed public health tool will make valuable information available to those that need it most, . The typeface, sturdy non-
binding add a feel of quali-
publications. Highly recom-
general libraries."
Book Review, Summer '96*

Continues next page

Communication Disorders Sourcebook

Basic Information about Deafness and Hearing Loss, Speech and Language Disorders, Voice Disorders, Balance and Vestibular Disorders, and Disorders of Smell, Taste, and Touch

Edited by Linda M. Ross. 533 pages. 1996. 0-7808-0077-X. $75.

"This is skillfully edited and is a welcome resource for the layperson. It should be found in every public and medical library."
— *Doody's Health Sciences Book Review, May '96*

Congenital Disorders Sourcebook

Basic Information about Disorders Acquired during Gestation, Including Spina Bifida, Hydrocephalus, Cerebral Palsy, Heart Defects, Craniofacial Abnormalities, Fetal Alcohol Syndrome, and More, along with Current Treatment Options and Statistical Data

Edited by Karen Bellenir. 607 pages. 1997. 0-7808-0205-5. $75.

Consumer Issues in Health Care Sourcebook

Basic Information about Consumer Health Concerns, Including an Explanation of Physician Specialties, How to Choose a Doctor, How to Prepare for a Hospital Visit, Ways to Avoid Fraudulent "Miracle" Cures, How to Use Medications Safely, What to Look for when Choosing a Nursing Home, and End-of-Life Planning

Edited by Wendy Wilcox. 600 pages. 1998. 0-7808-0221-7. $75.

Contagious & Non-Contagious Infectious Diseases Sourcebook

Basic Information about Contagious Diseases like Measles, Polio, Hepatitis B, and Infectious Mononucleosis, and Non-Contagious Infectious Diseases like Tetanus and Toxic Shock Syndrome, and Diseases Occurring as Secondary Infections Such As Shingles and Reye Syndrome, along with Vaccination, Prevention, and Treatment Information, and a Section Describing Emerging Infectious Disease Threats

Edited by Karen Bellenir and Peter D. Dresser. 566 pages. 1996. 0-7808-0075-3. $75.

Diabetes Sourcebook

Basic Information about Insulin-Dependent and Noninsulin-Dependent Diabetes Mellitus, Gestational Diabetes, and Diabetic Complications, Symptoms, Treatment, and Research Results, Including Statistics on Prevalence, Morbidity, and Mortality, along with Source Listings for Further Help and Information

Edited by Karen Bellenir and Peter D. Dresser. 827 pages. 1994. 1-55888-751-2. $75.

"Very informative and understandable for the layperson without being simplistic. It provides a comprehensive overview for laypersons who want a general understanding of the disease or who want to focus on various aspects of the disease."
— *Bulletin of the MLA, Jan '96*

Diet & Nutrition Sourcebook

Basic Information about Nutrition, Including the Dietary Guidelines for Americans, the Food Guide Pyramid, and Their Applications in Daily Diet, Nutritional Advice for Specific Age Groups, Current Nutritional Issues and Controversies, the New Food Label and How to Use It to Promote Healthy Eating, and Recent Developments in Nutritional Research

Edited by Dan R. Harris. 662 pages. 1996. 0-7808-0084-2. $75.

"It is so refreshing to find a reliable and factual reference book. Recommended to aspiring professionals, librarians, and others seeking and giving reliable dietary advice. An excellent compilation."
— *Choice, Feb '97*

"Recommended for public and medical libraries that receive general information requests on nutrition. It is readable and will appeal to those interested in learning more about healthy dietary practices."
— *Medical Reference Services Quarterly, Fall '97*

Ear, Nose & Throat Disorders Sourcebook

Basic Information about Disorders of the Ears, Nose, Sinus Cavities, Tonsils, Adenoids, Pharynx, and Larynx, along with Statistical and Demographic Data and Reports on Current Research Initiatives

Edited by Linda M. Ross. 600 pages. 1998. 0-7808-0206-3. $75.

Endocrine & Metabolic Diseases & Disorders Sourcebook

Basic Information for the Layperson about Disorders Such As Graves' Disease, Goiter, Cushing's Syndrome, and Hormonal Imbalances, along with Reports on Current Research Initiatives

Edited by Linda M. Ross. 600 pages. 1998. 0-7808-0207-1. $75.

Continues on back end sheets

Ear, Nose, and Throat
DISORDERS
SOURCEBOOK

Health Reference Series

Volume Thirty-seven

Ear, Nose, and Throat
DISORDERS
SOURCEBOOK

*Basic Information about Disorders of the Ears,
Nose, Sinus Cavities, Pharynx, and Larynx
Including Ear Infections, Tinnitus, Vestibular
Disorders, Allergic and Non-Allergic Rhinitis,
Sore Throats, Tonsillitis, and Cancers that Affect
the Ears, Nose, Sinuses, and Throat along with
Reports on Current Research Initiatives, a Glossary
of Related Medical Terms, and a Directory of
Sources for Further Help and Information*

Edited by
Linda M. Shin and Karen Bellenir

Omnigraphics, Inc.

Penobscot Building / Detroit, MI 48226

phic Note

accommodate all the copyright no-
tices, the Bibliographic Note portion of the Preface constitutes an
extension of the copyright notice.

Edited by Linda M. Shin and Karen Bellenir

Peter D. Dresser, Managing Editor, *Health Reference Series*
Karen Bellenir, Series Editor, *Health Reference Series*
Bettie Farnham, *Verification Assistant*

Omnigraphics, Inc.

Matthew P. Barbour, *Manager, Production and Fulfillment*
Laurie Lanzen Harris, *Vice President, Editorial Director*
Peter E. Ruffner, *Vice President, Administration*
James A. Sellgren, *Vice President, Operations and Finance*
Jane J. Steele, *Marketing Consultant*

Frederick G. Ruffner, Jr., Publisher

Library of Congress Cataloging-in-Publication Data

Ear, nose, and throat disorders sourcebook : basic information about disorders of the
    ears, nose, sinus cavities, pharynx, and larynx including ear infections, tinnitus,
    vestibular disorders, allergic and non-allergic rhinitis, sore throats, tonsillitis, and
    cancers that affect the ears, nose, sinuses, and throat along with reports on current
    research initiatives, a glossary of related medical terms, and a directory of further
    help and information / edited by Linda M. Shin and Karen Bellenir.
        p. cm. -- (Health reference series ; v. 48)
    Includes bibliographical references and index.
    ISBN 0-7808-0206-3 (lib. bdg. : alk. paper)
    1. Otolaryngology—Popular works. I. Shin, Linda M. II. Bellenir, Karen. III.
    Series.
    RF59.E18 1998   98-29719
    617.5' 1 -- dc21   CIP

∞

This book is printed on acid-free paper meeting the ANSI Z39.48 Standard. The infinity symbol that appears above indicates that the paper in this book meets that standard.

Printed in the United States

Table of Contents

Part III: Vestibular Disorders

Part IV: Disorders of the Nose and Sinuses

Part V: Disorders of the Throat

Part VI: Cancers Related to the Ears, Nose, and Throat

Preface

About This Book

The ears, nose, and throat play important roles in a person's ability to breathe, swallow, and communicate. The health of these structures, however, is frequently threatened by allergies, infectious diseases, trauma, and cancer. According to statistics compiled by the American Academy of Otolaryngology–Head and Neck Surgery, more than 50% of all physician office visits are for problems related to the ears, nose, or throat. For example:

- Otitis media (inflammation of the middle ear) is the most frequent primary diagnosis at visits to U.S. physician offices by children younger than 15 years. Otitis media particularly affects infants and preschoolers. Almost all children experience one or more episodes of otitis media before the age of six.

- Tinnitus, a poorly understood condition that creates the sound of ringing in the ears, effects an estimated 50 million American adults. According to the American Tinnitus Association, however, only about 12 million sufferers seek medical assistance. Many others mistakenly believe that nothing can be done to help alleviate their symptoms.

- Chronic sinusitis, frequent recurring inflammation of the sinuses, affects an estimated 32 million people in the United States, and Americans spend millions of dollars each year for medications that promise relief from their sinus symptoms.

- The various forms of rhinitis, including seasonal allergic rhinitis (also called hay fever), affect nearly 40 million people in the U.S.

- While close to 50% of normal adults snore occasionally, approximately 25 percent are habitual snorers. The seriousness of snoring can range from being a mild annoyance to being a sign of sleep apnea, a serious, potentially life-threatening condition. According to the National Heart, Lung, and Blood Institute as many as 18 million Americans have sleep apnea.

This book provides information about some of the most common disorders of the ears, nose, and throat. It offers disease descriptions, symptoms, treatment options, and reports on current research initiatives. The documents selected for inclusion were chosen on the basis of their ability to present accurate, timely information to the lay reader. The topic of hearing loss is covered only as a symptom or consequence of other ear disorders. Readers seeking more detailed information on hearing loss and deafness will find an in-depth treatment of these important subjects in *Communication Disorders Sourcebook*, Volume 11 of the *Health Reference Series*.

How to Use This Book

This book is divided into parts and chapters. Parts focus on broad areas of interest. Chapters are devoted to single topics within a part.

Part I: Introduction to the Ear, Nose, and Throat provides an overview of the many services performed by Ear, Nose, and Throat (ENT) specialists. A glossary of terms will help the reader to understand printed literature and to better communicate with his or her personal physician. Chapter three provides an annotated directory of organizational resources with addresses, phone numbers, e-mail addresses, and website locations.

Part II: Disorders of the Inner and Outer Ear offers descriptions of common outer, middle, and inner ear problems. Descriptions of the different types of ear infections and treatment suggestions are provided along with information about other ear disorders such as otosclerosis, acoustic neuromas, tinnitus, and sensorineural hearing loss. A chapter describing otoplasty, plastic surgery of the ear, is also included.

Part III: Vestibular Disorders describes disorders specifically related to the vestibular system. These include dizziness and vertigo, labyrinthitis, neuronitis, Meniere's disease, and perilymph fistula. A separate chapter outlining recent accomplishments in vestibular research is provided.

Part IV: Disorders of the Nose and Sinuses provides information about symptoms and treatment measures for a variety of common ailments including sinusitis, allergic and non-allergic rhinitis, post-nasal drip, smell and taste disorders, and nosebleeds. Information about rhinoplasty, plastic surgery of the nose, is also included.

Part V: Disorders of the Throat covers sore throats, coughs, hoarseness, tonsil and adenoid problems, swallowing and salivary gland disorders, snoring, sleep apnea, spasmodic dysphonia, and disorders of the larynx. One chapter provides current information about recovering speech after a laryngectomy. The importance of tobacco avoidance in throat care programs is also explained.

Part VI: Cancers Related to the Ears, Nose, and Throat offers information about the symptoms and current treatment options for head and neck cancer, cancers of the oral cavity and upper throat, paranasal sinus cancer, nasal cavity cancer, nasopharyngeal cancer, oropharyngeal cancer, hypopharyngeal cancer, and laryngeal cancer. Information about obtaining cancer updates from the National Cancer Institute is also given.

Bibliographic Note

This volume contains documents and excerpts from publications issued by the following government agencies: Agency on Health Care Policy and Research (AHCPR), National Cancer Institute (NCI), National Institute on Allergies and Infectious Diseases (NIAID), National Institute on Deafness and Other Communication Disorders (NIDCD), National Heart, Lung, and Blood Institute (NHLBI), and the U.S. Food and Drug Administration (FDA).

In addition, this volume contains copyrighted documents from the following organizations: American Academy of Facial Plastic and Reconstructive Surgery, American Academy of Otolaryngology–Head and Neck Surgery, Inc., American Tinnitus Association, House Ear Institute, Hyperacusis Network, National Jewish Medical Research Center,

Vestibular Disorders Association, and the Voice Center at Eastern Virginia Medical School. Copyrighted articles from the following journals are also included: *Audicibel, Health After 50, Indiana Medicine, Johns Hopkins Medical Letter, Mayo Clinic Health Letter,* and *Postgraduate Medicine.*

All copyrighted material is reprinted with permission. Document numbers where applicable and specific source citations are provided on the first page of each chapter. Every effort has been made to secure all necessary rights to reprint the copyrighted material. If any omissions have been made, contact Omnigraphics to make corrections for future editions.

Acknowledgements

Many organizations provided the useful material in this book. Special thanks go to the American Academy of Otolaryngology–Head and Neck Surgery, Inc. whose contributions helped bring clarification to many complex topics. Thanks are also due to the American Academy of Facial Plastic and Reconstructive Surgery, the American Tinnitus Association, the House Ear Institute, the Hyperacusis Network, the National Jewish Medical Research Center, the Vestibular Disorders Association and the Voice Center at Eastern Virginia Medical Center for granting permission to reproduce their publications. In addition, thanks go to researchers Margaret Mary Missar and Jenifer Swanson for their tireless efforts in obtaining the documents included in this volume.

Note from the Editor

This book is part of Omnigraphics' *Health Reference Series.* The series provides basic information about a broad range of medical concerns. It is not intended to serve as a tool for diagnosing illness, in prescribing treatments, or as a substitute for the physician/patient relationship. All persons concerned about medical symptoms or the possibility of disease are encouraged to seek professional care from an appropriate health care provider.

Part One

Introduction to the Ear, Nose, and Throat

Chapter 1

What Is an ENT (Ear, Nose, and Throat) Specialist?

An ear, nose, and throat specialist (ENT) is a physician trained in the medical and surgical treatment of the ears, nose, throat, and related structures of the head and neck. They have special expertise in managing diseases of the ears, nose and nasal passage, sinuses, larynx (voice box), oral cavity and upper pharynx (mouth and throat), as well as structures of the neck and face. ENT is the oldest medical specialty in the United States.

The Ear

The unique domain of the ear, nose, and throat specialist is treatment of ear disorders. This includes medical and surgical treatment for hearing disorders, ear infections, balance disorders, facial nerve or cranial nerve disorders, as well as management of congenital (birth) and cancerous disorders of the outer and inner ear.

The Nose

Care of the nasal cavity and sinuses is one of the primary skills of the ENT specialist. Management of disorders of the nasal cavity, paranasal sinuses, allergies, sense of smell, and nasal respiration (breathing), as well as the external appearance of the nose are part of an ENT's area of expertise.

©1996 American Academy of Otolaryngology–Head and Neck Surgery, Inc. One Prince Street, Alexandria, VA 22315-3357; reprinted with permission.

The Throat

Also specific to the ENT specialty is expertise in managing diseases of the larynx (voice box) and the upper aerodigestive tract or esophagus, including disorders of the voice, respiration (breathing), and swallowing.

The Head and Neck

In the head and neck area, an ENT specialist is trained to treat infectious diseases, tumors (both benign and malignant/cancerous), facial trauma, and deformities of the face. They perform both cosmetic plastic and reconstructive surgery.

An ENT specialist may work with a team of doctors in other medical and surgical specialties. Common ground is shared with neurosurgery in treating skull base disorders; plastic surgery in correcting cosmetic and traumatic deformities; ophthalmology in treating structural abnormalities near the eye; oral surgery in treating jaw and dental trauma; allergy in managing sinus disease; dermatology in caring for skin cancers; oncology in managing head and neck cancers; and pediatrics and family practice in caring for common infectious, congenital, traumatic, and malignant (cancerous) diseases and disorders in the pediatric and general population.

Training

An ENT specialist is ready to start practicing after up to 15 years of college and post-graduate training. To qualify for certification from the American Board of Otolaryngology, an applicant must first complete college, medical school (usually four years), and at least five years of specialty training. Next, the physician must pass the American Board of Otolaryngology examination to be certified. Some ENT specialists pursue a one- or two-year fellowship for more extensive training in one of the seven subspecialty areas. These include pediatric otolaryngology (children), otology/neurotology (ears and balance), allergy, facial plastic and reconstructive surgery, head and neck surgery, laryngology (throat) and rhinology (nose). Some ENT specialists limit their practices to one of these seven areas.

The well-trained ENT specialist has a thorough knowledge of all of the organs and physical structures in the head and neck region. Virtually all ear, nose, and throat specialists routinely handle adenoidectomies, tonsillectomies, nosebleeds, earaches, hearing loss, dizziness, hoarseness, and sinus disease. The physician's qualifications and inclinations, as well as the community's needs, will influence of an individual's practice. The broad challenges of the specialty allow a choice of direction, in addition to providing the best in patient care.

The Seven Areas of Expertise

Otolology/Neurotology. Medical and surgical treatment of diseases of the ear, including traumatic and cancerous disorders of the external, middle, and inner ear, as well as the nerve pathways which affect hearing and balance.

Pediatric Otolaryngology. Medical and surgical treatment of diseases of the ears, nose, and throat in children.

Head and Neck Area. Medical and surgical treatment of cancerous (and noncancerous) tumors in the head and neck, including thyroid and parathyroid surgery.

Facial Plastic and Reconstructive Surgery. Treatment of cosmetic, functional, and reconstructive abnormalities of the face and neck.

Rhinology. Medical and surgical treatment of disorders of the nose and sinuses.

Laryngology. Medical and surgical treatment of disorders of the throat, including the voice.

Allergy. Medical treatment of inhalant allergies affecting the upper respiratory system.

Chapter 2

Glossary of Ear, Nose, and Throat Terms

A

acoustic: Related to sound or hearing.

acoustic neuroma: A benign tumor of the auditory nerve, whose growth can cause gradual hearing loss, tinnitus or ringing in the ears, and dizziness.

active immunity: Immunity produced by the body as a result of previous exposure to an antigen, an allergen, or vaccination.

acute: A condition or illness which is brief and usually causes pain and discomfort.

acute phase proteins: Serum proteins whose levels increase during infection or inflammatory reactions.

adjuvant: A substance that non-specifically enhances the immune response to an antigen.

The terms in this glossary were excerpted from: "Glossary," NIDCD Information Clearinghouse, NIH, November 1994; NIH Publication Nos. 86-76, 95-1568, and 97-1574; *The New Cancer Sourcebook* (1996; Volume 12 of the *Health Reference Series*); and *Allergy Sourcebook* (1997; Volume 19 of the *Health Reference Series*).

airway obstruction: A narrowing, clogging, or blocking of the airways that carry air to the lungs; a major problem in an acute asthma attack.

allergen: A substance capable of causing an allergic reaction. Plant pollens, fungi spores, and animal danders are some of the common allergens.

allergic reaction: An adverse immune response following repeat contact with otherwise harmless substances such as pollens, molds, foods, cosmetics, and drugs.

allergic rhinitis: An inflammation of the membranes in the nose caused by an allergic reaction; seasonal allergic rhinitis is known as hay fever.

allergy: An inappropriate and harmful response of the immune system to normally harmless substances. A specific IgE antibody response to a specific antigen.

agammaglobulinemia: An almost total lack of immunoglobulins, or antibodies.

analgesic: Medicine used to relieve pain.

anaplastic: Cancer cells that divide rapidly and bear little or no resemblance to normal cells.

anesthesia: Loss of feeling or sensation resulting from the use of certain drugs or gases.

anesthetic: Drugs or gases given to cause a loss of feeling. A local anesthetic makes an area of the body numb. A general anesthetic puts the patient to sleep.

angiogram: An x-ray of blood vessels. A dye is injected into an artery to outline the blood vessels on the x-ray picture. Also called an arteriogram.

antibiotic: Medicine used to treat infection.

antibody: A protein in the bloodstream or other body fluids that is produced in response to foreign materials that enter the body; antibodies, also known as immunoglobulins, usually protect us.

antigen: Any substance that, when introduced into the body, is recognized and elicits a response by the immune system.

antihistamine: Medication used to treat the symptoms of allergies and often prescribed to relieve the discomfort caused by ear infections.

antimetabolites: Anticancer drugs that closely resemble substances needed by cells for normal growth. The tumor cell uses the drug instead and "starves" for lack of proper substance.

antimicrobial therapy: Treatment to kill microorganisms (such as bacteria or fungi) or to suppress their growth.

asymptomatic: Without symptoms.

atopic/atopy: A genetically determined clinical manifestation of type I hypersensitivity, which includes reactions such as eczema, asthma, and rhinitis.

audiogram: Standard graph that shows a person's hearing sensitivity.

audiologist: A professional who is trained to identify and measure hearing loss and help rehabilitate individuals with hearing impairments. Audiologists use a battery of tests to detect hearing loss, including audiometry, a measure of how well a patient hears pure tones, and tympanometry, a measure of how well the eardrum and middle ear bones conduct sound.

auditory nerve: The eighth cranial nerve that connects the ear to the brain stem.

autoantibody: An antibody that reacts against a person's own tissue.

B

balance system: The complex biological system that enables us to know where our body is in space and to keep the position we want. Proper balance depends on information from the inner ear, from other senses such as sight and touch, and from muscle movements.

Barrett's esophagus: A change in the cells of the tissue that lines the bottom of the esophagus. The esophagus may become irritated when the contents of the stomach back up (reflux). Reflux that happens often over a long period of time can lead to Barrett's esophagus.

benign: Not cancerous; does not invade nearby tissues or spread to other parts of the body.

benign positional vertigo: A condition in which moving the head to one side or to a certain position brings on vertigo.

biofeedback: Involves concentration and relaxation exercises designed to teach voluntary control of bodily functions, such as blood circulation to various parts of the body and relaxation of muscle groups throughout the body. When this type of control is accomplished, it may be effective in reducing the severity of tinnitus in some patients.

biological therapy: Treatment to stimulate or restore the ability of the immune (defense) system to fight infection and disease. Sometimes called immunotherapy.

biopsy: The removal and microscopic examination of tissue from the living body for purposes of diagnosis.

blood-brain barrier: A network of blood vessels located around the central nervous system with very closely spaced cells that make it difficult for potentially toxic substances—including anticancer drugs—to penetrate the blood vessel walls and enter the brain and spinal cord.

blood count: The number of red blood cells, white blood cells, and platelets in a sample of blood. This is also called complete blood count (CBC).

brain stem auditory evoked response (BAER): Diagnostic test in which electrodes are attached to the surface of the scalp to determine the time it takes inner ear electrical responses to sound to travel from the ear to the brain. The test helps locate the cause of some types of dizziness.

buccal mucosa: The inner lining of the cheeks and lips.

C

caloric test: Diagnostic test in which warm or cold water or air is put into the ear. If a person experiences certain eye movements (nystagmus) after this procedure, the labyrinth is working correctly.

cancer: A term for more than 100 diseases in which abnormal cells divide without control. Cancer cells can invade nearby tissues and can spread through the bloodstream and lymphatic system to other parts of the body.

carcinoma: Cancer that begins in the lining or covering of an organ.

cartilage: Firm, rubbery tissue that cushions bones at joints. A more flexible kind of cartilage connects muscles with bones and makes up other parts of the body such as the larynx and the outside parts of the ears.

CAT or CT scan: See computed tomography (CT) scan.

challenge test: A medical procedure also known as provocative testing used to identify those substances to which a person is sensitive by deliberately exposing a patient to dilute amounts of those substances until allergic symptoms are provoked.

chemotherapy: Treatment with anticancer drugs.

cholesteatoma: A tumor-like accumulation of dead cells in the middle ear. This growth is thought to result from repeated middle ear infections.

chondrosarcoma: A cancer that forms in cartilage.

chronic: A term that is used to describe a disease of long duration or one that is progressing slowly.

clinical trial: The systematic investigation of the effects of materials or methods, according to a formal study plan and generally in a human population with a particular disease or class of diseases. In cancer research, a clinical trial generally refers to the evaluation of treatment methods such as surgery, drugs or radiation techniques, although methods of prevention, detection or diagnosis also may be the subject of such studies.

cochlea: The hearing part of the inner ear.

computed tomography (CT) scan: Radiological examination; useful for examining the inside of the ear and head, and other parts of the body.

conductive hearing impairment: Hearing loss caused by dysfunction of the outer or middle ear.

congenital: Present at birth.

corticosteroids: A group of hormones produced by the adrenal glands that play key roles in many body functions, such as metabolism, muscle function and resistance to stress. Man-made corticosteroids are used as powerful anti-inflammatory drugs.

cytomegalovirus (CMV) infection: A virus, related to the herpesvirus, found in saliva, urine, and other body fluids, that is easily spread. Congenital CMV can cause hearing loss in young children.

D

dander: Small scales from animal skin. Dander is a common allergen.

decongestant: Medication used to reduce swelling and congestion.

diuretic: Drug that promotes water loss from the body through the urine. Used to treat hypertension, diuretics may bring on dizziness due to postural hypotension.

dizziness: A feeling of physical instability with regard to the outside world.

dysphagia: Difficulty in swallowing.

dysplasia: Abnormal tissue growth that may progress to cancer.

E

earache: Pain in one or both ears caused by inflammations, infections, or growths.

electrolarynx: A battery-operated instrument that makes a humming sound to help laryngectomees talk.

elimination diet: A restricted diet in which foods suspected of causing allergic reactions are introduced one at a time so that the blameworthy ones can be identified.

encapsulated: Confined to a specific area; the tumor remains in a compact form.

endolymph: Fluid filling part of the labyrinth.

endoscope: A flexible, lighted instrument used to examine organs such as the throat or esophagus.

epiglottis: The flap that covers the trachea during swallowing so that food does not enter the lungs.

erythroplakia: A reddened patch with a velvety surface found in the mouth.

esophageal speech: Speech produced with air trapped in the esophagus and forced out again.

esophagectomy: An operation to remove a portion of the esophagus.

esophagus: The tube through which food passes from the throat to the stomach.

eustachian tube: A narrow tube connecting the middle ear with the back of the nose.

external otitis: Inflammation of the external auditory-canal, the opening of the ear. It can be caused by the growth of bacteria or fungi.

external radiation therapy: Radiation therapy using a machine located outside the body to aim high-energy rays at a tumor.

G

glottis: The middle part of the larynx; the area where the vocal cords are located.

Group C status: A designation for investigational anticancer drugs that are effective against one or more forms of cancer but have not been approved for general marketing by the U.S. Food and Drug Administration. Doctors may obtain Group C drugs from the National Cancer Institute to treat patients who would benefit from their use.

H

hair cells: Specialized cells of the inner ear responsible for translating sound waves into nerve impulses which are sent to the brain.

hearing aid: Any electronic device whose function is to bring sound more effectively into the listener's ear. A hearing aid typically consists of a microphone, amplifier, and receiver.

histamine: A chemical released by mast cells and considered responsible for much of the swelling and itching characteristic of hay fever and other allergies.

histamine-release test: A method of measuring the amount of histamine released by certain cells in a sample of blood from an allergic patient when the cells are exposed to an allergen. It is used to gain some idea of a patient's reactivity to specific substances.

humidifier: A machine that puts moisture in the air.

hypersensitivity: The condition—existing in a person previously exposed to an antigen—in which tissue damage results from an immune reaction to a further dose of the antigen. Classically, four different types of hypersensitivity are recognized, but the term is often used to mean the type of allergy associated with hay fever and asthma.

hyperthermia: The use of heat in treating disease.

hyperventilation: Repetitive deep breathing that reduces the carbon dioxide content of the blood and brings on dizziness. Anxiety may cause hyperventilation and dizziness.

I

immune system: The complex system of cells and chemicals that reacts against foreign substances entering the body.

immune reaction or response: The activity of various specialized body cells and chemicals against foreign substances.

immunity: The overall capability of an individual to resist or overcome an infection.

immunoglobulin E (IgE): A class of antibody normally present in very low levels in humans, but found in larger quantities in people with allergies and certain infections. Its protective role is unknown, but evidence suggests it is the only antibody responsible for the classic allergy symptoms.

immunotherapy: Injections of gradually increasing amounts of allergens known to trigger a patient's allergic response. Also called desensitization, hyposensitization, injection therapy, and "allergy shots."

inner ear: The inside part of the ear that sends signals to the brain. The inner ear also sends signals to the brain that help a person with balance.

internal radiation: Radiation therapy in which radioactive material is placed in or near a tumor.

intraoperative radiation: A type of external radiation used to deliver a large dose of radiation therapy to the tumor bed and surrounding tissue at the time of surgery. Also called IORT.

intravenous (IV): Injected into a vein.

L

labyrinth: The organ of balance, which is located in the inner ear. The labyrinth consists of the three semicircular canals and the vestibule.

labyrinthitis: Inflammation of the intercommunicating cavities or canals within the inner ear.

laryngeal: Having to do with the larynx.

laryngectomee: A person who has had his or her voice box removed.

laryngectomy: An operation to remove all or part of the larynx.

laryugoscope: A flexible, lighted tube used to examine the larynx.

laryngoscopy: Examination of the larynx with a mirror (indirect laryngoscopy) or with a laryngoscope (direct laryngoscopy).

larynx: An organ in the throat used in breathing, swallowing, and talking. It is made of cartilage and muscle and is lined by a mucous membrane similar to the lining of the mouth. Also called the voice box. The larynx has three parts: the supraglottis, the glottis, and the subglottis.

laser: A powerful beam of light used in some types of surgery.

leuloplakia: A white spot or patch in the mouth.

local therapy: Treatment that affects cells in a tumor and the area near it.

local anesthetic: A drug that blocks nerve conduction in the region where it is applied.

lymph: The almost colorless fluid that travels through the lymphatic system and carries cells that help fight infection.

lymph nodes: Small, bean-shaped organs located along the lymphatic system. Nodes filter bacteria or cancer cells from lymph. Also called lymph glands.

lymphatic system: The tissues and organs that produce, store, and carry cells that fight infection. This system includes the bone marrow, spleen, thymus, lymph nodes, and vessels that carry lymph.

M

magnetic resonance imaging (MRI): A procedure in which a magnet linked to a computer is used to create detailed pictures of areas inside the body.

malignant: Cancerous; can invade nearby tissue and spread to other parts of the body.

mast cells: Tissue cells which contain packets of chemicals responsible for the symptoms of allergy. When allergens attach to IgE antibodies sitting on the surface of these cells, a signal is sent, causing them to release these chemical mediators of allergy.

mastoid: The rear portion of the temporal bone behind the ear. It contains air cells that resemble a honeycomb.

mastoiditis: Inflammation of the air cells of the mastoid.

mediastinum: An area in the chest that contains the heart, the esophagus, many large blood and lymph vessels, and other structures. It is located between the lungs behind the breast bone and extends back to the spine.

Meniere's disease: Condition that causes vertigo. The disease is believed to be caused by too much endolymph in the labyrinth. Persons with this illness also experience hearing problems and tinnitus.

metastasis: The spread of cancer from one part of the body to another. The cells in the metastatic (secondary) tumor are like those in the original (primary) tumor.

middle ear: That part of the ear which directs sound energy to the inner ear. The eardrum, or tympanic membrane, is in the middle ear. It is also called the tympanic cavity.

mixed hearing impairment: Impairment in hearing that has components of both conductive and sensorineural hearing impairment.

MRI: See magnetic resonance imaging (MRI).

mucous membranes: Thin layers of tissue that are kept moist by a sticky substance called mucus. These membranes line the nose and other parts of the respiratory tract, and are found in other parts of the body which have communication with air.

multiple sensory deficits: Condition associated with dizziness in which damage to nerves of the eye and arms or legs reduces information about balance to the brain.

myringotomy: An operation in which a small opening is made in the eardrum to allow fluid to drain and to relieve pain.

N

narcotic: Pain relieving drug related in action and structure to the opiates.

nasopharynx: The area of the upper throat behind the nose.

neck dissection: Surgery to remove lymph nodes and other tissues in the neck.

nystagmus: Rapid back-and-forth movements of the eyes. These reflex movements may occur during the caloric test and are used in the diagnosis of balance problems.

O

oncologist: A doctor who specializes in treating cancer.

oral surgeon: A dentist with special training in surgery of the mouth and jaw.

oropharynx: The area of the throat at the back of the mouth.

orthostatic hypotension: See postural hypotension.

otitis externa: Infection which occurs at the opening or outer part of the ear. It can be caused by the growth of bacteria or fungi. Otitis externa is sometimes called swimmer's ear.

otitis media: Inflammation of the middle ear.

otolaryngologist: A physician who specializes in diseases and disorders of the ear, nose, and throat.

otologist: A physician who specializes in diseases of the ear.

otosclerosis: A disease characterized by the formation of spongy bone in the bone surrounding the inner ear which results in a gradual loss of hearing.

otoscope: An instrument used to look inside the ears.

outer ear: The outer structure of the ear, consisting of the auricle or pinna, and the external acoustic meatus or opening. Sound waves are funneled through the external ear to the middle ear.

P

palate: The roof of the mouth. The front portion is bony (hard palate), and the back portion is muscular (soft palate).

pathologist: A doctor who identifies diseases by studying cells and tissues under a microscope.

pediatrician: A doctor who takes care of infants and children and who treats their diseases.

peripheral vestibulopathy: A vestibular disorder in which the vestibular nerve appears inflamed and paralyzed. Patients may have one or several attacks of vertigo.

pharynx: The hollow tube about 5 inches long that starts behind the nose and ends at the top of the trachea (windpipe) and esophagus (the tube that goes to the stomach).

pneumatic larynx: A device that uses air to produce sound to help a laryngectomee talk.

pollen: The tiny spores of flowering plants. Airborne pollen is a major allergen responsible for hay fever.

polyp: A mass of tissue that develops on the inside wall of a hollow organ.

postural hypotension (also called orthostatic hypotension): Sudden dramatic drop in blood pressure when a person rises from a sitting, kneeling, or lying position. The prime symptom of postural hypotension, which is sometimes due to low blood volume, is dizziness or faintness. The condition can be dangerous in older persons, who may faint and injure themselves.

precancerous: A term used to describe a condition that may become cancer.

presbyeusis: The progressive hearing loss that occurs with age.

prognosis: The probable outcome of a disease; the chance of recovery.

prosthesis: An artificial replacement of part of the body, such as a tooth, a facial bone, or the palate.

R

rad: Short form for "radiation absorbed dose," a measurement of the amount of radiation absorbed by tissues (100 rad = 1 Gray).

radiation therapy: Treatment with high-energy rays from x-rays or other sources to kill cancer cells. Also called radiotherapy.

radioallergosorbent test (RAST): A test for measuring the amount of specific IgE antibodies in a patient's blood. Along with a medical history, this test can help identify some allergens to which a person is allergic.

radio-sensitizers: Drugs being studied to try to boost the effect of radiation therapy.

reflux: The term used when liquid backs up into the esophagus from the stomach.

remission: Disappearance of the signs and symptoms of cancer. When this happens, the disease is said to be "in remission." A remission can be temporary or permanent.

rhinitis: An inflammation of the membrane lining the nose. Allergic rhinitis (misnamed hay fever) is an IgE-mediated reaction. Nonallergic forms of rhinitis may result from infections, hormonal changes, or certain drugs.

rhinitis medicamentosa: A form of rhinitis caused by the prolonged use of decongestant nose drops and sprays.

S

salivary glands: Glands in the mouth that produce saliva.

semicircular canals: Three curved hollow tubes in the inner ear that are part of the balance organ, the labyrinth. The canals are joined at their wide ends and are filled with endolymph.

sensorineural hearing impairment: Hearing loss caused by dysfunction of the inner ear or the auditory canal.

serous otitis media: An inflammation of the middle ear, commonly found in infants and children with allergic rhinitis.

sinusitis: An inflammation of the air spaces around the nose.

speech/language pathologist: A health professional who helps people with their speech, language, and voice problems.

sputum: Material often containing mucus, pus, and micro-organisms which is expelled from the chest by coughing or clearing the throat.

squamous cell carcinoma: Cancer that begins in the flat, scale-like cells in the skin and in tissues that line certain organs of the body, including the larynx.

staging: Doing exams and tests to learn the extent of the cancer, especially whether it has spread from its original site to other parts of the body.

stoma: An opening made by a surgeon (see also tracheostomy).

subglottis: The lowest part of the larynx; the area from just below the vocal cords down to the top of the trachea.

supraglottis: The upper part of the larynx, including the epiglottis; the area above the vocal cords.

swimmer's ear: A type of external otitis seen in persons who swim for a long period of time or who fail to completely dry their ear canals after swimming.

systemic therapy: Treatment that reaches and affects cells all over the body.

T

thorax: The part of the body between the neck and the abdomen; the chest.

tinnitus: Sensation of sound in the head which may be experienced in one or both ears. The sounds have been described as roaring, hissing, whistling, clicking, buzzing, etc. Although the cause of tinnitus is often unknown, tinnitus can be a symptom of wax building up in the outer ear, middle ear problems, acoustic trauma, the ingestion of excessive aspirin, Meniere's disease, hearing loss associated with aging, acoustic neuroma, and many other ear-related problems.

tinnitus masker: A small electronic instrument built into a hearing aid case combined with a hearing aid. It generates a competitive but pleasant sound, which masks the tinnitus for some individuals.

tissue: A group or layer of cells that performs a specific function.

tonsils and adenoids: Prominent oval masses of lymphoid tissues on either side of the throat.

trachea: The airway that leads from the larynx to the lungs. Also called the windpipe.

tracheoesophageal puncture: A small opening made by a surgeon between the esophagus and the trachea. A valve keeps food out of the trachea but lets air into the esophagus for esophageal speech.

tracheostomy: Surgery to create an opening (stoma) into the windpipe. The opening itself may also be called a tracheostomy.

tracheostomy button: A ½ to 1½-inch-long plastic tube placed in the stoma to keep it open.

tracheostomy tube: A 2- to 3-inch metal or plastic tube that keeps the stoma and trachea open. Also called a trach ("trake") tube.

tumor: An abnormal mass of tissue.

tympanic membrane: The membrane that separates the external ear from the middle ear; the eardrum.

tympanogram: A test used to measure the air pressure in the middle ear; this measures how well the eustachian tube is working.

types of allergic reactions: Four groups of allergic mechanisms which generally cover all allergic reactions.

- **Type I:** The most common type of allergic reaction. Immediate hypersensitivity or anaphalaxis. Occurs with hay fever, insect stings, or other allergic shocks.

- **Type II:** Cytotoxic or reaction with cell membrane. Occurs with incompatible blood transfusions.

- **Type III:** Arthus or deposition of immune complexes in walls of blood vessels or kidneys. Occurs in serum sickness and some drug reactions.

- **Type IV:** Delayed hypersensitivity or cell-mediated response. Occurs with poison ivy and graft rejections.

U

ultrasonography: A test in which sound waves (ultrasound) are bounced off tissues and the echoes are converted into a picture (sonogram).

V

vertigo: An illusion of movement; a sensation as if the external world were revolving around the person (objective vertigo) or as if the person were revolving in space (subjective vertigo).

vestibular disorders: Disorders of the inner ear, such as motion sickness and vertigo.

vestibular nerve: Nerve that carries messages about balance from the labyrinth in the inner ear to the brain.

vestibular neuronitis: Another name for peripheral vestibulopathy.

vestibule: Part of the labyrinth, located at the base of the semicircular canals. This structure contains the endolymph and patches of hair cells.

vocal cords: Two small bands of muscle within the larynx. They close to prevent food from getting into the lungs, and they vibrate to produce the voice.

X

X-ray: High-energy radiation. It is used in low doses to diagnose diseases and in high doses to treat cancer.

Chapter 3

Sources of Help for Ear, Nose, and Throat Patients

Acoustic Neuroma Association (ANA)
P.O. Box 12402
Atlanta, GA 30355
(404) 237-8023 voice
(404) 237-2704 fax

e-mail: anausa@aol.com
website: www.anausa.org

The Acoustic Neuroma Association (ANA) is a patient-organized and administered information and mutual aid group incorporated as a nonprofit organization. The ANA provides information and support to patients who have experienced an acoustic neuroma or other benign problems affecting the cranial nerves. It also educates the public regarding symptoms suggestive of acoustic neuroma and promotes early diagnosis and successful treatment.

Publications: *Notes* (quarterly newsletter).

American Academy of Audiology (AAA)
8201 Greensboro Dr., Suite 300
McLean, VA 22102

Information in this chapter was compiled from resource listings produced by the National Institute on Deafness and Other Communication Disorders (NIDCD) Information Clearinghouse; addresses, phone numbers, and websites were updated and verified current as of March 1998.

(800) AAA-2336 toll free
(703) 610-9022 voice/TTY
(703) 610-9005 fax

website: www.audiology.com

The AAA is a professional organization of individuals dedicated to providing high quality hearing care to the public. The AAA enhances the ability of its members to achieve career and practice objectives through professional development, education, research, and increased public awareness of hearing disorders and audiologic services.

American Academy of Facial Plastic and Reconstructive Surgery (AAFPRS)
310 S. Henry St.
Alexandria, VA 22314
(800) 332-FACE toll free
(703) 299-9291 voice/TTY
(703) 299-8898 fax

e-mail: info@facial-plastic-surgery.org
website: www.facial-plastic-surgery.org

The American Academy of Facial Plastic and Reconstructive Surgery (AAFPRS) is the world's largest association of facial plastic surgeons. AAFPRS members are physicians who specialize in cosmetic and reconstructive surgery of the face, head, and neck and perform most of the nasal plastic surgery in the nation.

Publications: *Facial Plastic Times* (monthly newsletter), *Facial Plastic Surgery Today* (quarterly consumer newsletter), *Media Matters* (quarterly media newsletter), *Facial Plastic Surgery Information Service* (consumer brochures), *AAFPRS Membership Directory* (annual guide and directory), *The Face Book* (consumer book), *The Teen Face Book* (teen consumer book).

American Academy of Otolaryngology–Head and Neck Surgery (AAO–HNS)
One Prince Street
Alexandria, VA 22314
(703) 836-4444 voice
(703) 683-5100 fax

e-mail: entnet@aol.com

website: www.entnet.org

AAO–HNS promotes the art and science of medicine related to oto-laryngology-head and neck surgery, including providing continuing medical education courses and publications. It distributes free patient leaflets related to problems of the ears, nose, throat, head, and neck region and makes referrals to physicians.

American Auditory Society (AAS)
512 E. Canterbury Ln.
Phoenix, AZ 85022
(602) 789-0755 voice
(602) 942-1486 fax

website: www.boystown.org/aas

The purpose of the American Auditory Society (AAS) is to increase the knowledge and understanding of the ear, hearing, and balance, their disorders and how these may be prevented, and habilitation and rehabilitation of individuals with hearing and balance dysfunction.
Publications: *Ear and Hearing* (bimonthly journal), *Bulletin of the American Auditory Society* (newsletter).

American Cleft Palate-Craniofacial Association (ACPA)
Cleft Palate Foundation (CPF)
1829 E. Franklin St., Suite 1022
Chapel Hill, NC 27514
(800) 24-CLEFT toll free
(919) 933-9044 voice
(919) 933-9604 fax

e-mail: cleftline@aol.com
website: www.cleft.com

The purpose of the American Cleft Palate-Craniofacial Association (ACPA) is to encourage the improvement of scientific clinical services to persons suffering from cleft lip/palate and associated deformities. The Cleft Palate Foundation is the public service arm of the ACPA. Its primary purpose is to educate and assist the public regarding cleft lip and palate and other craniofacial anomalies and to encourage re-search in the field.
Publications: *Cleft Palate-Craniofacial Journal*, informational materials.

American Deafness and Rehabilitation Association (ADARA)

P.O. Box 6956
San Mateo, CA 94403
(650) 372-0620 voice/TDD
(650) 372-0661 fax

e-mail: adaraorgn@aol.com

The American Deafness and Rehabilitation Association (ADARA) is a membership organization and network that promotes, develops, and expands services, research, and legislation to individuals who are deaf. The American Society of Deaf Social Workers has reorganized as the Social Work Section of ADARA. ADARA provides a referral service regarding careers, university programs, job opportunities, and general information.

Publications: *Journal of American Deafness and Rehabilitation Association, ADARA Update*.

American Laryngeal Papilloma Foundation (ALPF)

P.O. Box 6108
Spring Hill, FL 34611-6108
(352) 686-8583 voice and fax

e-mail: info@alpf.org
website: www.alpf.org/

The purpose of the American Laryngeal Papilloma Foundation (ALPF) (formerly the Christina Lazar Foundation) is to increase public awareness of laryngeal papillomatosis; raise funds to help defray costs associated with medical treatment; promote the health and welfare and form a national register of individuals with laryngeal papillomatosis; and provide funds to reputable organizations engaged in research for the prevention and cure of laryngeal papillomatosis. The foundation loans TTY equipment and helps those who are in need with emergency funds (stipends).

American Laryngological Association (ALA)

Vanderbilt University Medical Center S-2100 MCN
2305 West End Avenue
c/o R.H. Ossoff, MD, Sec.
Nashville, TN 37232-2559
(615) 322-7267 voice

(615) 343-7604 fax

website: http://commercial.visi.net/ala

The ALA is a professional medical society of otorhinolaryngologists to advance research, medicine and surgery with emphasis on the upper aerodigestive tract.

American Laryngological, Rhinological and Otological Society (TRIO)
Boys Town National Research Hospital
555 N. 30th St.
Omaha, NE 68131-2136
(402) 498-6666 voice
(402) 498-6662 fax

The purpose of this professional society is to advance the science and art of medicine relates to laryngology, head and neck surgery, rhinology, and otology.

American Physical Therapy Association (APIA)
1111 N. Fairfax Street
Alexandria, VA 22314
(800) 999-2782 toll free
(703) 684-2782, Ext. 3210 voice
(703) 684-7343 fax

website: www.apta.org

The American Physical Therapy Association (APTA) is a national professional organization representing more than 56,000 physical therapists, physical therapist assistants, and physical therapy students throughout the United States. Its goals are to serve its members and the public by increasing the understanding of the physical therapist's role in the health care system and by fostering improvements in physical therapy education, practice, and research. Physical therapists are involved in the evaluation and treatment of postural deficits and balance disorders.

Publications: *Physical Therapy Journal* (monthly), *PT Magazine* (monthly).

American Society for Deaf Children (ASDC)
1820 Tribute Rd., Suite A
Sacramento, CA 95815

(800) 942-2732 toll free/TDD
(916) 641-6084 voice
(916) 461-6085 fax

e-mail: ASDC1@aol.com
website: http://deafchildren.org

The American Society for Deaf Children (ASDC) is a membership organization that provides information and support to parents and families with children who are deaf or have a hearing impairment. The ASDC promotes parents' rights regarding communication choices for their child and promotes quality education to improve the life-long achievements and well being of the child.

Publications: *The Endeavor* (quarterly).

American Speech-Language-Hearing Association (ASHA)
10801 Rockville Pike
Rockville, MD 20852
(301) 897-5700 voice/TTY
(800) 638-TALK toll free
(301) 571-0457 fax

website: www.asha.org

This is a professional scientific organization for speech-language pathologists and audiologists. It has several publications and journals and provides information on communication disorders and referrals to audiologists and speech-language pathologists.

American Tinnitus Association (ATA)
1618 SW 1st Ave., Suite 417
Portland, OR 97201
(800) 634-8979 toll free
(503) 248-9985 voice
(503) 248-0024 fax

e-mail: tinnitus@ata.org
website: www.ata.org

The ATA provides education, information, and telephone counseling about tinnitus and self-help support. Provides regional referrals to patients seeking help.

Association for Chemoreception Sciences (AChemS)
c/o Panacea Associates
744 Duparc Circle
Tallahassee, FL 32312
(904) 531-0854 voice and fax

website: http://neuro.fsu.edu/achems
e-mail: mmered@neuro.fsu.edu

The Association for Chemoreception Sciences (AChemS) is an international organization of professionals in the field of taste, smell, and related chemoreception. Members come from academic institutions, health care facilities, industrial environments, and private research laboratories. It represents the interests of the chemosensory community in basic research, health and disease, flavor and fragrances, food and beverages, personal products, and product development.
Publications: *Chemical Senses* (six issues per year), *Newsletter* (biannual), *AChemS Membership Directory* 1993.

Association of Late-Deafened Adults (ALDA)
10301 Main St., Suite #274
Fairfax, VA 22030
(404) 289-1596 TTY hotline
(404) 284-6862 fax

website: www.alda.org

The Association of Late-Deafened Adults (ALDA) serves as a resource center providing information and referral for late-deafened people. ALDA works to increase public awareness of the special needs of late-deafened adults.
Publications: *ALDA News*, brochures.

Bell, Alexander Graham Association for the Deaf (A.G. BELL)
3417 Volta Place, NW
Washington, DC 20007
(202) 337-5220 voice/TDD
(202) 337-8314 fax

e-mail: Agbell2@aol.com
website: www.agbell.org

31

The Alexander Graham Bell Association for the Deaf (A.G. Bell) is an organization comprised of individuals who are hearing impaired, parents, professionals, and other interested persons. Its mission is to empower persons who are hearing impaired to function independently by enhancing their ability to use, maintain, and improve all aspects of their verbal communication, including their ability to speak, speechread, use residual hearing, and process both spoken and written language. A.G. Bell publishes texts, consumer-oriented books and brochures, and audiovisual materials, and conducts conferences and conventions.

Publications: *Volta Review* (journal), *Volta Voices* (newsletter)

Better Hearing Institute (BHI)

5021-B Backlick Rd.
Annandale, VA 22003
(703) 642-0580 voice
(800) EAR-WELL TTY/toll free
(703) 750-9302 fax

e-mail: mail@betterhearing.org
website: www.betterhearing.org

BHI is a nonprofit educational organization dedicated to informing people with hearing impairments, their friends and relatives, and the general public about hearing loss and available medical, surgical, and amplification assistance.

Boys Town National Research Hospital (BTNRH)

555 North 30 Street
Omaha, NE 68131
(402) 498-6511 voice
(402) 498-6543 TTY
(402) 498-6638 fax

e-mail: btnrh-info@boystown.org
website: www.boystown.org/btnrh

Boys Town National Research Hospital (BTNRH) is dedicated to research, diagnosis, and treatment of communication disorders, especially in children. Clinical services in speech and language, audiology, otolaryngology, genetics, and pediatrics are available. Staff scientists conduct research in many aspects of the sciences of human hearing, speech, and language, as well as in all clinical areas. Staff members work with educational agencies and professionals to provide placement, education, and rehabilitation for children with hearing loss, speech, and language disorders. This center is one of the National Multipurpose Research and Training Centers supported by the NIDCD.

Publications: *Hereditary Deafness Newsletter* (semiannual), informational materials.

Cochlear Implant Club International (CICI)
5335 Wisconsin Ave. NW, Suite 440
Washington, DC 20015
(202) 895-2781 voice
(202) 895-2782 fax

Cochlear Implant Club International (CICI) provides information and support to cochlear implant users and their families, professionals, and the general public.

Publications: *Contact* (quarterly journal).

Deafness Research Foundation (DRF)
15 W. 39th St.
New York, NY 10018
(800) 535-DEAF toll free
(212) 768-1181 voice/TTY
(212) 768-1782 fax

The Deafness Research Foundation (DRF) is a voluntary health organization that provides grants for fellowships, symposia, and research into causes, treatment, and prevention of all ear disorders. The DRF maintains a National Human Temporal Bone Registry that is supported by NIDCD. This registry has an extensive mailing list of all known voluntary organizations involved in hearing and balance disorders. It also disseminates information on a national scale about donorship of temporal bone and brain tissue, the registry and its services, and otopathology. The DRF's major focus is to support audio-vestibular research in its early phases and to increase the public's awareness of issues related to hearing loss.

Publications: *The Receiver* (newsletter).

Dogs for the Deaf, Inc. (DFD)
10175 Wheeler Road
Central Point, OR 97502

(541) 826-9220 voice/TDD
(541) 826-6696 fax

e-mail: info@dogsforthedeaf.org
website: www.dogsforthedeaf.org

The mission of Dogs for the Deaf (DFD) is to rescue dogs from shelters, train them to serve as the ears of people who are deaf or hard of hearing, and place the dogs with qualified applicants.

Publications: *Canine Listeners* (quarterly newsletter), informational materials.

Dystonia Medical Research Foundation
One East Wacker Drive, Suite 2430
Chicago, IL 60601-2001
(312) 755-0198 voice
(312) 803-0138 fax

e-mail: dystsndt@aol.com

The goals of the Dystonia Medical Research Foundation are to provide medical research grants and medical information and videos on all types of dystonias. The foundation is also involved in increasing awareness of dystonia, forming patient and family support groups, and involving members in symposiums and activities of children's advocacy, fund raising, public relations, and medical education.

Publications: *Dystonia Dialogue* (quarterly newsletter), Physician referral lists by state, informational materials.

The Ear Foundation
1817 Patterson St.
Nashville, TN 37203
(800) 545-HEAR toll free
(615) 329-7849 TTY
(615) 329-7935 fax

website: www.theearfound.org

The goal of The Ear Foundation is to integrate persons who are hearing impaired into the mainstream of society through public awareness and medical education. The Foundation administers the Meniere's Network, a national network of patient support groups that provides people with the opportunity to share experiences and coping strategies.

Publications: *Steady* (Meniere's Network newsletter), *The Otoscope* (Ear Foundation newsletter).

FACES: *National Cranio-Facial Handicapped Association*
P.O. Box 11082
Chattanooga, TN 37401
(423) 266-1632 voice
(423) 267-3124 fax

e-mail: faces@mindspring.com

This association is a voluntary nonprofit organization providing financial assistance to individuals with severe facial deformities resulting from congenital defects or accidents. It also provides a resource file of available treatment centers, support groups, and general information regarding facial deformities.

Friends of the NIDCD
c/o American Speech-Language Hearing Association
10801 Rockville Pike
Rockville, MD 20852
(800) 498-2071 toll free
(301) 897-5700 voice
(301) 897-0157 TTY
(301) 571-0457 fax

website: www.asha.org

Friends of the NIDCD is an organization that promotes public awareness of disorders of hearing, balance, smell, taste, voice, speech, and language as well as expanded development of research and training for the National Institute on Deafness and Other Communication Disorders. It provides public education about issues before Congress and promotes exchange of information among members. Contact groups include physicians, researchers, practitioners, parents, the elderly, schools for individuals with hearing impairments, educators, organizations, volunteers, professionals in the communication disorders field, and individuals with communication disorders.

Hear Now (HN)
9745 E. Hampden Avenue, Suite 300
Denver,CO 80231-4923
(800) 648-4327

(303) 695-7797 voice/TDD
(303) 695-7789 fax

Hear Now (HN) provides hearing aids and cochlear implants for individuals with limited financial resources. HN coordinates a nation hearing aid bank and accepts hearing aid donations from people all over the country. HN is also involved in increasing public awareness of the need for available and affordable assistive technology for persons with hearing impairments.

Publications: newsletter (annual).

Hearing Education and Awareness for Rockers (H.E.A.R.)
P.O. Box 460847
San Francisco, CA 94146
(415) 773-9590 24-Hour hotline
(41 5) 441-9081 voice
(415) 476-7600 TDD
(415) 552-4296 fax

e-mail: hear@hearnet.com
website: www.hearnet.com

H.E.A.R. is a nonprofit organization founded by musicians and physicians for musicians, music professionals, music lovers, and those concerned with hearing issues. H.E.A.R offers information about hearing loss and hearing protection, operates a 24-hour hotline information referral and support network service, and conducts a free hearing screening program. H.E.A.R. launches public hearing awareness campaigns and produces public service announcements and information for the mass media and public events. Other activities include hearing education programs for schools; distribution of earplugs to clubs and concert-goers, music conventions, and conferences; and establishment of H.E.A.R. affiliates worldwide.

Publications: H.E.A.R. (brochure), *"Can't Hear You Knocking"* (video), informational materials.

Hearing Health
P.O. Drawer V
Ingleside, TX 78362
(512) 776-7240 voice/TTD
(512) 776-3278 fax

e-mail: ears2u@hearinghealthmag.com

website: www.hearinghealthmag.com

Hearing Health publishes a bimonthly, independent consumer magazine that focuses on hearing loss and hearing issues. Magazine features include research, technology, legislation, and human interest articles.

Publications: *Hearing Health* (bimonthly magazine).

House Ear Institute (HEI)
2100 West Third Street, 5th Floor
Los Angeles, CA 90057
(213) 483-4431 voice
(213) 484-2642 TDD
(213) 483-8789 fax

website: www.hei.org

HEI is a nonprofit organization that conducts research and provides information on hearing and balance disorders. The Center for Deaf Children, a section of HEI, performs evaluations and therapy. HEI is also involved in outreach programs to further knowledge and understanding of hearing disorders.

The Hyperacusis Network
444 Edgewood Drive
Green Bay, WI 54302
(920) 468-4667 voice
(920) 432-3321 fax

e-mail: malcare@netnet.net

The Hyperacusis Network is an international support group established to care for individuals with collapsed tolerance to sound (hyperacusis and recruitment). The network helps educate the medical community and families about this rare auditory disorder by sharing ways to cope, providing advice on how to secure disability assistance, and reporting on current research and/or treatment options. Membership in the network is free.

International Association of Laryngectomies (IAL)
c/o American Cancer Society
7440 N. Shadeland Ave., Suite 100
Indianapolis, IN 46250
(800) 227-2345 toll free

IAL is an international association involved in the exchange of ideas and methods of training and teaching of laryngeal methods of laryngectomies. It holds an annual Voice Rehabilitation Institute for training teachers of esophageal voice.

International Hearing Society (IHS)
20361 Middlebelt Road
Livonia, MI 48152
(800) 521-5247 toll free
(248) 478-2610 voice
(248) 478-4520 fax

IHS, a professional association of hearing instrument specialists, tests hearing and selects, fits, and dispenses hearing instruments. IHS provides consumer information through the toll free Hearing Aid Helpline.

Monell Chemical Senses Center
3500 Market Street
Philadelphia, PA 19104
(215) 898-6666 voice
(215) 898-2084 fax

e-mail: info@monell.org
website: www.monell.org

The Monell Chemical Senses Center is a research center for smell and taste disorders.

National Center for Neurogenic Communication Disorders
Speech and Hearing Sciences
P.O. Box 210071
Building 71
The University of Arizona
Tucson, AZ 85721
(520) 621-1472 voice
(520) 621-2226 fax

e-mail: cnet@w3.arizona.edu
website: w3.arizona.edu/~cnet/homepage.html

The National Center for Neurogenic Communication Disorders focuses on speech and language disorders caused by diseases of the nervous system. The center conducts research and provides opportunities for research training in the areas of muscular control of speech and voice production, auditory and visual perception of speech, cognition, and the impairment of language function after stroke or as a result of other diseases. The center provides information dissemination to the public and continuing education for professionals. The center is one of the National Multipurpose Research and Training Centers supported by the NIDCD.

Publications: *Tres cosas lindas hay en la vida* (fotonovela concerning stroke, Spanish only), Telerounds videotapes.

National Center for Voice and Speech (NCVS)
The University of Iowa
330 Wendell Johnson Speech and Hearing Center
Iowa City, IA 52242
(319) 335-6600 voice
(319) 335-8851 fax

e-mail: ncvs@shc.uiowa.edu
website: www.shc.uiowa.edu

The National Center for Voice and Speech (NCVS) is a consortium of institutions focusing on voice and speech disorders. The members of this consortium are: the University of Iowa, the Denver Center for Performing Arts, the University of Wisconsin-Madison, and the University of Utah. The NCVS trains scientists interested in careers in voice and speech research, provides continuing education for professionals, provides public information about voice and speech problems, and conducts research on voice and speech production. The NCVS is one of the National Multipurpose Research and Training Centers supported by the NIDCD.

Publications: informational materials.

National Hearing Conservation Association (NHCA)
9101 E. Kenyon Ave., Suite 3000
Denver, CO 80237
(303) 224-9022 voice
(303) 770-1812 fax

e-mail: nhca@gwami.com
website: www.globaldialog.com/~nhca

The National Hearing Conservation Association (NHCA) is an association of hearing conservation professionals that encourages education

39

and information exchange and provides referral services for members. NHCA offers industry in-depth information on consultants and services.

Publications: *Spectrum* newsletter, brochure, and directory (quarterly), *Membership Directory* (annual), *Professional Service Organization Directory* (annual).

National Information Center on Deafness (NICD)
Gallaudet University
800 Florida Avenue, NE
Washington, DC 20002
(202) 651-5051 voice
(202) 651-5052 TDD
(202) 651-5054 fax

e-mail: nicd@gallux.gallaudet.edu
website: www.gallaudet.edu/~nicd

The National Information Center on Deafness (NICD) collects, develops, and disseminates information about all aspects of hearing loss and services offered to people who are deaf or hard of hearing across the nation. The NICD makes referrals to other organizations and provides information about Gallaudet University.

Publications: informational materials.

National Institute on Deafness and Other Communication Disorders (NIDCD) Information Clearinghouse
1 Communication Avenue
Bethesda, MD 20892-3456
(800) 241-1044 toll free
(800) 241-1055 TTY
(301) 907-8830 fax

e-mail: nidcd@aerie.com
website: www.nih.gov/nidcd

The NIDCD Information Clearinghouse is a service of the National Institute on Deafness and Other Communication Disorders, National Institutes of Health.

National Organization for Rare Disorders (NORD)
PO. Box 8923
New Fairfield, CT 06812-8923
(203) 746-6518 voice

(203) 746-6927 TTY
(800) 999-6673, 9:00 a.m. - 5:00 p.m., eastern time
(203) 746-6481 fax

e-mail: orphan@nord-rdb.com
website: www.nord-rdb.com/~orphan

The National Organization for Rare Disorders (NORD) is a nonprofit, voluntary health agency that acts as a clearinghouse for information on rare disorders. A rare disorder is a disease or condition that affects fewer that 200,000 Americans. Cumulatively, there are more than 5,000 rare diseases affecting more than 20 million Americans. NORD is committed to the identification, treatment, and cure of rare diseases through programs of education, advocacy, research, and service. NORD's "networking" program seeks to link individuals with the same or similar rare health conditions. Rare diseases include neurofibromatosis, Niemann-Pick disease, and Usher syndrome Type 2.

National Rehabilitation Information Center (NARIC)
8455 Colesville Road, Suite 935
Silver Spring, MD 20910
(800) 346-2742 toll free
(301) 495-5626 TTY
(301) 587-1967 fax

website: www.naric.com/naric

The National Rehabilitation Information Center (NARIC) is a rehabilitation information service and research library that provides reference, research, and referral services; conducts custom database searches; publishes a quarterly newsletter; and disseminates rehabilitation related information. NARIC's database, REHABDATA, contains a computerized listing of rehabilitation literature.

Publications: *NARIC Quarterly* (newsletter), *Directory of Librarians and Information Specialists in Disability and Rehabilitation*, *NARIC Guide to Disability and Rehabilitation Periodicals*, *Directory of National Information Sources on Disability*, brochures, resource guides.

National Spasmodic Dysphonia Association, Inc. (NSDA)
1 E. Wacker Dr.
Chicago, IL 60601-1905
(800) 795-6732 toll free

(312) 755-0198 voice
(312) 803-0138 fax

e-mail: nsda@aol.com

The primary purposes of the National Spasmodic Dysphonia Association (NSDA) are to promote public awareness of spasmodic dysphonia and to promote the care, welfare, and rehabilitation of those with spasmodic dysphonia through education and support of research.

Publications: Quarterly report, Information materials, *Our Voice* (newsletter).

National Technical Institute for the Deaf (NTID)

Lyndon Baines Johnson Building
52 Lomb Memorial Drive
Rochester, NY 14623-5604
(716) 475-2411 TDD
(716) 475-6500 fax

The primary mission of the National Technical Institute for the Deaf (NTID) is to provide deaf students with outstanding state-of-the-art technical and professional education programs, complemented by a strong arts and sciences curriculum, that prepare them to live and work in the mainstream of a rapidly changing global community and enhance their lifelong learning. NTID also prepares professionals to work in fields related to deafness; undertakes a program of applied research designed to enhance the social, economic, and educational accommodation of deaf people; and shares its knowledge and expertise through outreach and other information dissemination programs.

Publications: *NTID Focus* (three issues per year), *NTID Resources Catalog*, informational materials.

Partners In Sign

612N 601 Pennsylvania Ave. NW
Washington, DC 20004
(202) 638-5630 voice/TDD
(202) 638-5632 fax

e-mail: pinsdc@aol.com

Partners In Sign is a nonprofit organization that provides free message relay, bulletin board, and interpreting services for individuals who are deaf. Partners In Sign also provides information referrals regarding telecommunication devices for people who are deaf.

Recurrent Respiratory Papillomatosis Foundation (RRPF)
P.O. Box 6643
Lawrenceville, NJ 08648-0643
(609) 530-1493 voice
(609) 530-1912 fax

website: http://members.aol.com/rrpf/RRPF.html

The Recurrent Respiratory Papillomatosis Foundation (RRPF) was created to provide family support, promote public awareness, and aid in the prevention, cure, and treatment of recurrent respiratory papillomatosis. The organization focuses primarily on networking within the MP community, including patients, families, medical practitioners, and researchers. Its goal is to stimulate more RRP-related research that will, the Foundation hopes, lead to more effective treatments and, ultimately, a cure for this disease.

Publications: *RRP Newsletter* (semiannual), *RRP Medical Reference Service* (semiannual), fact sheets.

Rehabilitation Services Administration
Deafness and Communicative Disorders Branch (RSA-DCDB)
330 C Street SW
Room 3228
Washington, DC 20202-2736
(202) 205-9152 voice
(202) 205-8352 TTY
(202) 205-9340 fax

The Deafness and Communicative Disorders Branch (DCDB) of the Rehabilitation Services Administration (RSA) promotes improved and expanded rehabilitation services for individuals with hearing impairments, speech disorders, or language disorders; provides technical assistance to RSA staff, state rehabilitation agencies, other public and private agencies, and individuals; and oversees national interpreter training grants, demonstration grants for the provision of rehabilitation services to traditionally underserved persons who are deaf, and a Hearing Research Center. The DCDB also provides interpreter referrals for U.S. Department of Education-sponsored activities nationwide (202-205-8694 voice, 202-205-5896 TTY). RSA is an agency of the U.S. Department of Education.

Publications: *American Rehabilitatian* (quarterly), *RSA Annual Report, Pocket Guide to Federal Help for Individuals with Disabilities* (brochure).

Research and Training Center for Hearing and Balance

Johns Hopkins University School of Medicine
720 Rutland Ave.
505 Traylor Bldg.
Baltimore, MD 21205
(410) 955-3162 voice
(410) 955-1299 fax

e-mail: jhuchb@bme.jhu.edu
website: www.bme.jhu.edu/labs/chb

The Center for Hearing and Balance focuses on the mechanisms of hearing and balance and on developing better ways to diagnose and treat hearing and balance disorders. Studies range from the physiology of the inner ear and auditory system to the design of rehabilitation programs for patients with balance problems. The center is one of the National Multipurpose Research and Training Centers supported by the NIDCD.

Publications: Informational materials.

Rocky Mountain Taste and Smell Center

Box B205
University of Colorado
Health Sciences Center
4200 East 9th Avenue
Denver, CO 80262
(303) 315-6600 voice
(303) 315-8787 fax

The Rocky Mountain Taste and Smell Center is a research center for smell and taste disorders.

Self Help for Hard of Hearing People, Inc. (SHHH)

7910 Woodmont Avenue, Suite 1200
Bethesda, MD 20814
(301) 657-2248 voice
(301) 657-2249 TDD
(301) 913-9413 fax

e-mail: national@shhh.org
website: www.shhh.org

Self Help for Hard of Hearing (SHHH) is a volunteer, international organization composed of people who are hard of hearing and their relatives and friends. It is a nonprofit, nonsectarian, educational organization devoted to the welfare and interests of those who cannot hear well but are committed to participating in the hearing world.

Publications: *SHHH Journal* (bimonthly magazine), informational materials.

SUNY Health Sciences Center at Syracuse
Clinical Olfactory Research Center
766 Irving Avenue
Syracuse, NY 13210
(315) 464-4538 voice
(315) 464-4544 fax

The SUNY (State University of New York) Health Sciences Center at Syracuse conducts research in smell and taste disorders.

Taste and Smell Center
Connecticut Chemosensory
Clinical Research Center
University of Connecticut Health Center
263 Farmington Ave.
Farmington, CT 06032
(860) 679-2459 voice
(860) 679-2910 fax

e-mail: taste@cortex.uchc.edu
website: http://cortex.uchc.edu/~taste/

The Taste and Smell Center is a research center for taste and smell disorders.

Telecommunications for the Deaf, Inc. (TDI)
8630 Fenton St., Suite 604
Silver Spring, MD 20910-3803
(301) 589-3786 voice
(301) 589- 3006 TDD
(301) 589-3797 fax

e-mail: TdiExDir@aol.com

Telecommunications for the Deaf (TDI) is a consumer-oriented organization that is constantly working to improve technology and accessibility for all who rely on visual telecommunications. TDI sells caption decoders and directories to people who are deaf; supports legislation; and advocates the use of TDDs, ASCII code, Emergency

Access (911), telecaptioning, and visual-alerting systems in the public, private, and government sectors.

Publications: *GA-SK* (quarterly newsletter), *National Directory of TDD: Numbers Users* (annual).

UCLA Balance and Dizziness Research Program
Vincente Honrubia, MD
Center for Health and Sciences 62-129
UCLA School of Medicine
Los Angeles, CA 90024-1624
(310) 825-5241 voice
(310) 206-8712 fax

e-mail: vh@ucla.com

The UCLA Balance and Dizziness Research Program integrates the disciplines of neurology, otolaryngology, and ophthalmology. The laboratories are involved in research and training in both basic and clinical sciences. The program specializes in the diagnosis and treatment of disorders of the inner ear and eye movement control and provides information to the public about dizziness and balance disorders as well as continuing education to professionals The program is a National Multipurpose Research and Training Center supported by the NIDCD.

Publications: Patient information materials.

United States Society for Augmentative and Alternative Communication (USSAAC)
c/o James Neils, Association Manager
P.O. Box 5271
Evanston, IL 60204-5271
(847) 869-2122 voice
(847) 869-2161 fax

e-mail: ussaac@northshore.net

The purposes of the United States Society for Augmentative and Alternative Communication (USSAAC) are to enhance the communication effectiveness of persons who can benefit from augmentative and alternative communication and to support the goals of the International Society for Augmentative and Alternative Communication (ISAAC). The specific purposes of USSAAC are to assist individuals in their right to communicate, allowing full participation in society; promote public awareness; influence national and state public policy and legislation; disseminate legislative, regulatory, and funding information; facilitate high quality service delivery; and promote transdisciplinary professional education.

Publications: *The USSAAC Newsletter* (Quarterly), informational materials.

University of Pennsylvania Smell and Taste Research Center
Hospital of the University of Pennsylvania
3400 Spruce Street
Philadelphia, PA 19104-4283
(215) 662-6580 voice
(215) 349-5266 fax

The Smell and Taste Research Center at the University of Pennsylvania conducts research in smell and taste disorders.

Vestibular Disorders Association (VEDA)
P.O. Box 4467
Portland, OR 97208-4467
(800) 837-8428 toll free
(503) 229-7705 voice
(503) 229-8064 fax

e-mail: veda@teleport.com
website: www.teleport.com/~veda

The Vestibular Disorders Association (VEDA) is a nonprofit organization established to provide information and support for people with vestibular disorders and to develop awareness of the issues surrounding these disorders.

Publications: Informational materials, quarterly newsletter.

Veterans Administration (VA)/Audiology and Speech Pathology Services
Audiology and Speech Pathology Service
50 Irving Street NW
Washington, DC 20422
(202) 745-8270 voice
(202) 745-8276 TTY
(202) 745-8579 fax

The Veterans Administration (VA) provides services for veterans who have hearing, speech, language, or balance problems.

Publications: *Hearing Aid Measurement* (annual publication).

The Voice Foundation
1721 Pine Street
Philadelphia, PA 19103-6771
(215) 735-7999 voice
(215) 735-9293 fax

e-mail: tvf@uscom.com

The goal of the Voice Foundation, a not-for-profit-corporation organized in 1969, is to understand the human voice, thereby improving its quality and care This understanding is achieved through funding research, enhancing education with respect to the human voice, and disseminating this knowledge internationally.

Publications: *Journal of Voice* (quarterly), newsletter (three to four issues per year).

Part Two

Disorders of the
Inner and Outer Ear

Chapter 4

Seven Signs of Serious Ear Disease

Primary care providers are asked to evaluate and treat an ever increasing number of both routine and complex medical problems. It is critical that the primary care provider be knowledgeable in a broad spectrum of routine medical problems, yet also recognize when the consultation of a specialist is indicated.

Seven signs of serious otologic (ear) disease that indicate the need for evaluation by a specialist are:

1. Ear pain or fullness
2. Discharge or bleeding from the ear
3. Sudden or progressive hearing loss, even with recovery
4. Unequal hearing between ears or noise in the ear
5. Hearing loss after an injury, loud sound, or air travel
6. Slow or abnormal speech development in children
7. Balance Disturbance or dizziness

Ear Pain or Fullness

Ear pain (otalgia) may arise as a result of ear diseases or as a result of an illness elsewhere in the head and neck. Otitis externa, or swimmer's ear, is often a benign infection that responds well to topical therapy; but in cases of immunocompromise or diabetes, otitis externa may be the first sign of and eventually lead to skull base osteomyelitis. Acute otitis media is a frequent cause of otalgia and is usually effectively treated with antibiotics, but a middle ear infection can become complicated and lead to facial paralysis, intracranial abscess or meningitis. Referred otalgia, or pain referred to the ear from another source, may be due to temporomandibular joint dysfunction (TMJ) as well as cancers of the upper aerodigestive tract. Tumors in the pharynx and base of tongue have a particular tendency to cause referred otalgia through a neural network that innervates both the source of the cancer as well as the ear.

Discharge or Bleeding from the Ear

Discharge or bleeding from the ear commonly results from infection or tumor. Otitis externa may lead to purulent discharge (otorrhea) or bleeding and is accompanied by severe otalgia. More diffuse disorders of the temporal bone include chronic otitis media and cholesteatoma. These are often associated with multiple episodes of ear drainage. Cholesteatoma is a slow growing lesion that erodes bone so that critical anatomy becomes vulnerable to erosion and infection over time. Complications of cholesteatoma include facial paralysis, labyrinthitis, meningitis, and brain abscess. Tumors of the external auditory canal, middle ear, and other regions of the temporal bone may present with bleeding from the ear. Bleeding from the ear may also be a result of trauma and can be a harbinger of more serious medical problems.

Sudden or Progressive Hearing Loss: Even with Recovery

Sudden sensorineural hearing loss is often ascribed to a viral infection or an ischemic event but may be a symptom of a far more ominous pathology. Up to one-third of patients with acoustic neuromas experience a hearing loss at some point during their illness. These tumors most commonly present as a unilateral or asymmetric sensorineural hearing loss, often with tinnitus. Hearing loss with recovery or fluctuating sensorineural hearing loss is also frequently noted in patients with Meniere's disease along with whirling vertigo, aural fullness, and tinnitus. Progressive losses may also be caused by immune disorders, syphilis or infections at other sights in the body. Conductive hearing losses should be evaluated medically because of the risks of cholesteatoma and because most causes of conductive hearing loss can be readily treated.

Unequal Hearing between Ears or Noise in the Ear

Progressive asymmetric hearing loss or unilateral noise in the ear may be associated with acoustic neuroma or other tumors.

Hearing Loss after an Injury, Loud Sound, or Air Travel

Hearing loss after an injury may be conductive or sensorineural. Conductive hearing losses are due to a disruption of the free movement of the vibrating tympanic membrane and ossicular unit. Both blunt and penetrating trauma may lead to tympanic membrane perforation or ossicular discontinuity. Noise-induced sensorineural hearing loss may occur after a single extremely loud noise or after repeated exposures to loud sounds. Air travel is one cause of otologic barotrauma and scuba diving is another. Hearing loss again may be either conductive, as in the case of hemorrhage behind an intact tympanic membrane (hemotympanum), or sensorineural, as in the case of an inner ear membrane tear. The membranes that are most vulnerable to this type of injury are the oval and round window membranes.

Slow or Abnormal Speech Development in Children

Abnormal speech development in children very frequently is a result of the child's inability to hear speech, recognize it, mimic it, and learn to use it appropriately. A common reason for hearing loss in young children may be otitis media with effusion that does not clear with treatment and that leads to a significant conductive hearing loss. However, significant delays in speech acquisition are usually due to more serious, permanent sensorineural losses. Abnormal speech development in children requires immediate action because speech and language are most efficiently acquired in early years of life.

Balance Disturbance or Vertigo

Balance disturbance or vertigo may originate from an otologic or a neurologic source. A variety of specific otologic etiologies for vertigo are amenable to either medical or surgical treatment, as in Meniere's disease, or perilymphatic fistula. It is particularly important to exclude some specific potentially dangerous etiologies for vertigo including: acoustic neuroma and other intracranial tumors, stroke, or demyelinating disease.

Conclusion

Primary care providers must be familiar with many types of diseases and decide which are to be treated in the primary care environment and which are to be referred to a specialist. The seven warning signs of serious ear disease were created to help in that decision. Each warning sign should be a "red flag" and could indicate a potentially serious condition. When these warning signs appear, the patient should be referred to an otolaryngologist–head and neck surgeon to rule out serious disease of the ear, nose or throat. The American Academy of Otolaryngology head and Neck Surgery is a resource that can be contacted and can supply a list of Academy members in a given region that may be of help.

What Is Otolaryngology–Head and Neck Surgery

Otolaryngology–head and neck surgery is a specialty concerned with the medical and surgical treatment of the ears, nose, throat and related structures of the head and neck. The specialty encompasses cosmetic facial reconstruction, surgery of benign and malignant tumors of the head and neck, management of patients with loss of hearing and balance, endoscopic examination of air and food passages, and treatment of allergic, sinus, laryngeal, thyroid and esophageal disorders.

To qualify for the American Board of Otolaryngology certification examination, a physician must complete five or more years of post-M.D. (or D.O.) specialty training.

Chapter 5

Otitis Externa and Bullous Myringitis

Eczematous Otitis Externa

The main symptom of eczematous otitis externa is continual itching of one or both ears. There is no particular pattern to the itching, although it is most common in winter. On clinical examination, the skin of the ear canal is devoid of wax. The skin overlying the bone and cartilage of the external auditory canal is shiny and thin, almost transparent. Some scaling of the surface epithelium may be noted. Generally, the ear canal is not red unless the patient has been manipulating the skin with a cotton swab or similar object. Careful examination of the surrounding scalp often reveals flaking from seborrhea or psoriasis.

Patients are often treated with ear drops that contain hydrocortisone and a broad-spectrum antibiotic, such as neomycin sulfate. The ear drops may be helpful initially, but with prolonged use secondary fungal infections may develop. Some patients may have a skin reaction to the broad-spectrum antibiotic, which intensifies the itching.

The first step in treatment of eczematous otitis externa is educating patients about the condition and about avoiding recurrence. If the scalp is involved, a debriding shampoo such as Sebulex helps remove the scaling skin around the ear. Once before initial treatment, the

From "Two Ear Problems You May Not Need to Refer: Otitis Externa and Bullous Myringitis," *Postgraduate Medicine*, October 1994, Vol. 96, No. 5; reprinted with permission.

patient should apply some of the shampoo to a washcloth and then wash the outer ear to help debride the skin.

Initial treatment involves application of a topical hydrocortisone cream and a hydrocortisone-containing acetic acid solution such as VöSoL HC Otic. The cream is necessary because the outer skin of the ear, especially the concha, is often involved. The cream should be applied directly to this region. Since creams cannot easily be applied in the ear canal, drops containing hydrocortisone are also necessary to completely eradicate symptoms. The cream and drops should be used three times a day for 3 to 5 days, depending on symptoms. If symptoms persist, irrigation of the ear canal with hydrogen peroxide and suctioning may be required.

Patients with eczematous otitis externa should receive instructions about future treatment, since this problem is never fully cured and often recurs on a seasonal basis. They should be advised to limit skin exposure to such irritants as soap, shampoos, cosmetics, and perfumes, which tend to precipitate or aggravate the condition. They should keep the drops and the cream after initial treatment in case symptoms recur.

Fungal Otitis Externa

Symptoms of fungal otitis externa include itching, soreness, and moisture or drainage from the ear. Patients often have a history of frequent water exposure, such as swimming, but previous use of broad-spectrum antibiotic drops containing hydrocortisone is even more common.

On physical examination, a fluffy white to off-white exudate that may contain gray or black specks is noted in the external auditory canal. The secretions clear easily with irrigation and cleansing, leaving the external auditory canal and tympanic membrane looking rather erythematous. In some patients, the tympanic membrane and skin of the ear canal may be red and thickened and may bleed easily if manipulated.

Initial treatment involves thorough cleansing of the ear canal by irrigation with full-strength hydrogen peroxide and then with rubbing alcohol, which helps to evaporate the moisture and kill the fungus on contact. The ear is then suctioned clean of debris and moisture.

Fungal otitis externa is usually caused by *Aspergillus*, which accounts for the gray to black specks within the secretions. *Aspergillus* tends to multiply and adhere to instruments used for examination, so all instruments should be carefully handled and sterilized to avoid contamination of other equipment or surfaces.

Successful treatment depends on thorough cleaning of the ear and does not require use of oral antifungal agents. After cleansing, several drops of an acetic acid solution such as Otic Domeboro are instilled into the ear canal. Patients should use several drops of the solution three times a day for 5 to 7 days, depending on symptoms. A follow-up visit for cleansing and reevaluation should be scheduled. By the second visit, patients are usually symptom-free and the drops can be discontinued. If the fugal infection has not cleared, three to four drops of clotrimazole solution (Lotrimin, Mycelex) should be used twice a day for 7 days.

Acute Otitis Externa

Acute otitis externa is a painful infection of the skin of the outer ear canal. In severe cases, the entire pinna is involved. Patients often have a history of exposure to pool or ocean water, which explains the term "swimmer's ear." Characteristic symptoms are intense pain upon manipulation or chewing and increased intensity of pain when patients lie flat. The condition may compromise hearing because the ear canal begins to swell shut, interfering with sound transmission.

On physical examination, mild temperature elevation (less than 101°F [38.3°C]), redness of the concha, and extensive swelling and redness of the external auditory canal may be noted. Examination of the canal or visualization of the eardrum may be difficult, if not impossible. Any manipulation of the ear causes extreme pain. Pressure applied near the tragus causes pain. Scattered nodes anterior to the tragus may be noted in the periparotid area.

Treatment of acute otitis externa is based on knowledge of its etiology. The normal pH of the skin of the external auditory canal is about 5.5, which is unsuitable for bacterial growth. The external auditory canal is sterile in only about 30% of patients. *Staphylococcus albus* and *Pseudomonas* are the bacteria that are most commonly isolated from the ear canal. The pH of soap and pool water is quite alkaline, which raises the pH of the external auditory canal skin, creating an ideal environment for surface bacterial growth and infection.

If acute otitis externa is precipitated by a change in pH, a simple solution is to return the skin surface pH to an acidic level, which kills the bacteria. First, the external auditory canal should be thoroughly

57

cleansed to remove the squamous debris and the superficial bacteria. This is difficult in a patient who has severe pain, but an attempt should be made to clean the auditory canal either by gentle irrigation or with an alcohol-saturated cotton swab. If the auditory canal is swollen, it is difficult for the drops to penetrate and kill all the bacteria. This problem can be solved by use of a sponge wick, which is easily inserted in the dry state into the canal. Saturating the wick with a solution of acetic acid such as Otic Domeboro makes the sponge expand and continually saturate the skin. Patients should be instructed to soak the wick every 2 to 3 hours while they are awake and to saturate a large cotton ball with the solution and place it in the concha to continually bathe the external skin. A heating pad may relieve pain (especially at night), and a strong analgesic such as codeine sulfate might be required. In 3 to 5 days, the wick can be removed, the ear cleaned, and a new wick inserted, if necessary.

Since *Pseudomonas* is the primary causative agent in acute otitis externa, oral fluoroquinolones have not been approved for use in children and should be avoided in patients with known sensitivity or systemic disease. Caution should be exercised when broad-spectrum antibiotic drops containing hydrocortisone are used, because the inflamed skin of the external auditory canal and pinna may react negatively to the antibiotic. This reaction can actually aggravate the conditions, causing multiple raised vesicles on the pinna and neck where the drops have touched the inflamed skin.

Patients should call immediately if pain, temperature, or swelling increase despite treatment. These may be symptoms of malignant otitis externa, a spread of the infection in the temporal bone and skull base. This conditions should always be suspected when symptoms persist, especially in immuno-compromised patients, such as those who have diabetes or AIDS or are receiving chemotherapy. Malignant otitis externa can be fatal if it is not recognized promptly and treated aggressively with intravenous therapy and surgical debridement. It requires immediate referral to an otolaryngologist.

Once acute otitis externa has resolved, avoiding future episodes is the goal. Since alkaline water is often the offending agent, patients should avoid water exposure by wearing earplugs when bathing or swimming. If long-term exposure to pool water occurs, especially in children, a few drops of acetic acid solution should be placed in the ear canal after swimming. This neutralizes the alkaline effect of the pool water and significantly reduces the likelihood of recurrent acute otitis externa.

Clinical Features of Otitis Externa and Bullous Myringitis

Eczematous otitis externa

- Continual itching of ear
- Shiny, thin skin in external auditory canal
- Scaling of surface epithelium
- Flaking of surrounding scalp

Fungal otitis externa

- Itching and soreness of ear
- Moisture or drainage from ear
- Fluffy white to off-white exudate in external auditory canal (may contain gray to black specks)
- Erythematous external auditory canal and tympanic membrane

Acute otitis externa

- Intense pain with manipulation of ear or chewing
- Increased intensity of pain when patient lies flat
- Compromised hearing
- Redness of concha
- Extensive swelling and redness of external auditory canal

Bullous myringitis

- Sudden onset of ear pain
- Bloody serosanguineous drainage
- Blistering of tympanic membrane

Bullous Myringitis

Bullous myringitis causes blisters on both the outer and inner surface of the tympanic membrane. Typically, patients have had an upper respiratory illness with a dry, nonproductive cough that is worse at night. Ear pain comes on very suddenly and is followed by bloody serosanguineous drainage.

Physical examination reveals an inflamed tympanic membrane with multiple small vesicles. The middle ear may be filled with a bloody, yellowish fluid. The blistering of the tympanic membrane and the bloody drainage are often confused with a tympanic membrane perforation.

In some cases, *Mycoplasma pneumoniae* is thought to be the cause of the respiratory illness that precipitates the ear infection. However, treatment should be directed at the most common causative organisms of bullous myringitis, *Haemophilus influenzae* and *Streptococcus pneumoniae*. The large collection of middle ear fluid slowly resolves in 2 to 3 weeks; the patient should be told that hearing may be diminished for several weeks. Oral decongestants, such as pseudoephedrine hydrochloride (e.g., Sudafed), are helpful in relieving pressure and fullness and may speed resolution of the serous fluid.

—by John F. Biedlingmaier, MD

Dr. Biedlingmaier is assistant professor of surgery, division of otolaryngology, University of Maryland School of Medicine, Baltimore, and director, head and neck services, Maryland General Hospital, Baltimore.

References

1. Feinmesser R, Wissel YM, Argaman M, et al. Otitis externa— bacteriological survey. ORL *J Otorhinolaryngol Relat Spec* 1982; 44(3):121-5.

2. Meyerhoff WL, Caruso VG, Trauma and infections of the external ear. In: Meyerhoff WL, Caruso VG, eds. *Otolaryngology*. Vol 2. Philadelphia: Saunders, 1992:1227-35.

3. Klein JO, Teele DW. Isolation of viruses and mycoplasmas from middle ear effusions: a review. *Ann Otol Rhinol Laryngol* 1976; 85(2 Suppl 25 Pt 2):140-4.

Chapter 6

Swimmer's Ear and Other Disorders of the Outer Ear

Causes

When water gets into the ear, it may bring in bacterial or fungal particles. Usually the water runs back out; the ear dries out; and the bacteria and fungi don't cause any problems. But sometimes water remains trapped in the ear canal, and the skin gets soggy. Then bacteria and fungi grow, flourish, and can infect the outer ear.

Symptoms

If you experience any of the following symptoms or if glands in your neck become swollen, see your doctor.

- The ear feels blocked and may itch;
- the ear canal becomes swollen, sometimes swelling shut;
- the ear starts draining a runny milky liquid; or
- the ear becomes very painful and very tender to touch, especially on the cartilage in front of the ear canal.

Prevention

If your ear feels moist or blocked after swimming, hairwashing, or showering, tilt your head sideways with that ear up, pull the ear upward and backward to put in eardrops to dry out the ear. Wiggle your ear to get the drops all the way down in the ear canal, and then turn your head to let them drain out. These eardrops are sold without prescription; check with your pharmacist.

WARNING: If you have an ear infection, have had a perforated or otherwise injured eardrum, or ear surgery, you should consult an ear, nose, and throat specialist before swimming or using any type of ear drops. If you don't know if you have ever had a perforated, punctured, ruptured, or otherwise injured eardrum, ask your doctor.

If your doctor says it is safe, make up your own ear drops to use after swimming. Many doctors recommend rubbing alcohol as part of the mixture. As the alcohol evaporates, it absorbs the water, helps dry out the ear, and may even kill the bacteria and fungi that cause swimmer's ear. Another effective ingredient is boric acid powder (2 tsp/pint) or white vinegar (mixed 50/50 with alcohol). A weak acid environment discourages the growth of bacteria and fungi.

A dry ear is least likely to get infected. Efforts to remove water from your ear should be limited to the drying effects of alcohol or, if you have a perforated eardrum, a hair dryer. You should not use cotton swabs (Q-tips®) because they pack material deeper in the narrow ear canal, irritate the thin skin of the ear canal, and make it "weep" or bleed.

If yours is a frequently recurring problem, your otolaryngologist (ENT doctor) may recommend placing oily (or lanolin) ear drops in your ears before swimming to protect them from the effects of the water.

People with itchy, flaky ears or ears that have wax build up are very likely to develop swimmer's ear. They should be especially conscientious about using the alcohol ear drops as described whenever water gets trapped into the ears. It may also help to have ears cleaned out each year before the swimming season starts.

Why Do Ears Itch?

An itchy ear is maddening. Sometimes it is caused by fungus, or allergies, but more often it is a chronic dermatitis (skin inflammation) of the ear canal. One type is seborrheic dermatitis, a condition similar to dandruff; the wax is dry, flaky, and abundant. Patients should avoid foods that aggravate it, such as greasy foods, sugars and starches, carbohydrates and chocolate. Doctors often prescribe a cortisone eardrop at bedtime when ears itch. There is no long-term cure, but it can be controlled.

What about Gnats or Other Insects?

Many types of insects get into the ears. Gnats get tangled in the wax and can't fly out. Bigger insects can't turn around; neither can crawl back out. They keep on struggling though, and their motion can be painful and frightening.

Wash out gnats with warm water from a rubber bulb syringe. (Remember to dry the ear afterwards with alcohol drops.) For a bigger insect, the first step is to fill the ear with mineral oil, which plugs off the breathing pores of the insect and kills it. It may take 5-to-10 minutes. See your doctor to have the insect removed; don't try to do it yourself.

What about Other Foreign Objects?

Beads, pencil lead, erasers, bits of plastic toys and dried beans are common objects that children put into their ears. Removal is a delicate task that **must** be performed by a doctor.

Chapter 7

Earwax:
What to Do about It

Never put anything smaller than your elbow in your ear! Cotton tips are for cleaning out bellybuttons—not ears. You have probably heard these admonitions from relatives and doctors ever since your childhood. What do they mean?

The Outer Ear and Canal

The outer ear is the funnel-like part of the ear you can see on the side of the head, plus the ear canal (the hole which leads down to the eardrum).

The ear canal is shaped somewhat like an hourglass—narrowing part way down. The skin of the outer part of the canal has special glands that produce earwax. This wax is supposed to trap dust and sand particles to keep them from reaching the eardrum. Usually the wax accumulates a bit, and then dries up and comes tumbling out of the ear, carrying sand and dust with it. Or it may slowly migrate to the outside where it is wiped off.

Should You Clean Your Ears?

Wax is not formed in the deep part of the ear canal near the eardrum, but only in the outer part of the canal. So when a patient has wax blocked up against the eardrum it is often because he has been probing his ear with such things as cotton-tipped applicators, bobby pins or twisted napkin corners. Such objects only serve as ramrods to push the wax in deeper. Also, the skin of the ear canal and the eardrum is very thin and fragile and is easily injured.

Earwax is healthy in normal amounts and serves to coat the skin of the ear canal where it acts as a temporary water repellent. The absence of earwax may result in dry, itchy ears.

Most of the time the ear canals are self-cleaning, that is, there is a slow and orderly migration of ear canal skin from the ear drum to the ear opening. Old earwax is constantly being transported from the ear canal to the ear opening where it usually dries, flakes, and falls out.

Under ideal circumstances, you should never have to clean your ear canals. However, we all know that this isn't always so. When wax has accumulated so much that it blocks the ear canal (and hearing), your physician may have to wash it out, vacuum it, or remove it with special instruments. Or he may prescribe ear drops which are designed to soften the wax. If so, you may first wish to try over-the-counter products such as Debrox® or Murine® Ear Drops. These are not as strong as the prescription wax softeners but are effective for

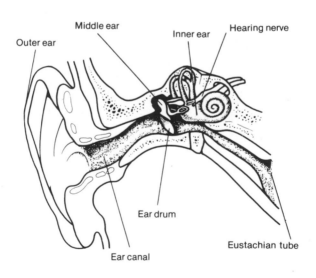

Figure 7.1. *The ear canal leads from the outer ear to the eardrum. Ear wax is formed only in the outer part of the canal.*

many patients. In the event that the nonprescription product is not satisfactory, a physician should be consulted.

You must know that you do not have a hole (perforation or puncture) in your eardrum. Putting the above eardrop products in your ear in the presence of an eardrum perforation may cause an infection. Certainly, washing water through such a hole would surely start up an infection. If you are uncertain whether you have a hole in your eardrum, consult your physician.

You may soften the wax for a few days by instilling several drops of an earwax softener into the ear canal twice a day. This can be purchased in your drugstore without a prescription. If your ear still feels blocked after using the ear drops, you should consult your physician, who may elect to wash it out.

Chapter 8

Otitis Media

What is otitis media?

Otitis media is an infection or inflammation of the middle ear. This inflammation often begins when infections that cause sore throats, colds, or other respiratory or breathing problems spread to the middle ear. Seventy-five percent of children experience at least one episode of otitis media by their third birthday. Almost half of these children will have three or more ear infections during their first three years. It is estimated that medical costs and lost wages because of otitis media amount to $5 billion a year in the United States. Although otitis media is primarily a disease of infants and young children, it can also affect adults.

How do we hear?

The ear consists of three major parts: the outer ear, the middle ear and the inner ear. The outer ear includes the pinna, the visible part of the ear and the ear canal. The outer ear extends to the tympanic membrane or eardrum, which separates the outer ear from the middle ear. The middle ear is an air-filled space that is located deep to the eardrum. The middle ear contains three tiny bones, the malleus, incus and stapes, which transmit sound from the eardrum to the inner

National Institute on Deafness and Other Communication Disorders, NIH Pub. No. 97-4216, May 1997.

ear. The inner ear contains the hearing and balance organs. The cochlea contains the hearing organ which converts sound into electrical signals which are associated with the origin of impulses carried by nerves to the brain where their meanings are appreciated.

What causes otitis media?

Otitis media usually results from a bacterial or viral infection secondary to a cold, sore throat or other respiratory problem.

Why are more children affected by otitis media than are adults?

There are many reasons why children are more likely to suffer from otitis media than adults. First, children have more trouble fighting infections. This is because their immune systems are still developing. Another reason has to do with the child's eustachian tube. The eustachian tube is a small passageway that connects the upper part of the throat to the middle ear. It is shorter and straighter in the child than in the adult. It can contribute to otitis media in several ways.

The eustachian tube is usually closed but opens regularly to ventilate or replenish the air in the middle ear. This tube also equalizes middle ear air pressure in the environment. However, a eustachian tube that is blocked by swelling of its lining or plugged with mucus from a cold or for some other reason cannot open to ventilate the middle ear. The lack of ventilation may allow fluid from the tissue that lines the middle ear to accumulate. If the eustachian tube remains plugged, the fluid cannot drain and begins to collect in the normally air-filled middle ear.

One more factor that makes children more susceptible to otitis media is that adenoids in children are larger than they are in adults. Adenoids are composed largely of cells (lymphocytes) that help fight infections. They are positioned in the back of the upper part of the throat near the eustachian tubes. Enlarged adenoids can, because of their size, interfere with the eustachian tube opening. In addition, adenoids may themselves become infected, and the infection may spread into the eustachian tubes.

Bacteria reach the middle ear through the lining or the passageway of the eustachian tube and can then produce infection which causes swelling of the lining of the middle ear, blocking of the eustachian tube and the migration of white cells from the bloodstream to help fight the infection. In this process the white cells accumulate, often killing bacteria and dying themselves, leading to the formation of pus, a thick yellowish-white fluid in the middle ear. As the fluid increases, the child may have trouble hearing because the eardrum and middle ear bones are unable to move as freely as they should. As the infection worsens, many children also experience severe ear pain. Too much fluid in the ear can put pressure on the eardrum and eventually tear it.

What are the effects of otitis media?

Otitis media not only causes severe pain but may result in serious complications if it is not treated. An untreated infection can travel from the middle ear to the nearby parts of the head, including the brain. Although the hearing loss caused by otitis media is usually temporary, untreated otitis media may lead to permanent hearing impairment. Persistent fluid in the middle ear and chronic otitis media can reduce a child's hearing at a time that is critical for speech and language development. Children who have early hearing impairment from frequent ear infections are likely to have speech and language disabilities.

How can someone tell if a child has otitis media?

Otitis media is often difficult to detect because most children affected by this disorder do not yet have sufficient speech and language skills to tell someone what is bothering them. Common signs to look for are:

- unusual irritability
- difficulty sleeping
- tugging or pulling at one or both ears
- fever
- fluid draining from the ear
- loss of balance
- unresponsiveness to quiet sounds or other signs of hearing difficulty such as sitting too close to the television or being inattentive

Can anything be done to prevent otitis media?

Specific prevention strategies applicable to all infants and children such as immunization against viral respiratory infections or specifically against the bacteria that cause otitis media are not currently available. Nevertheless it is known that children who are cared for in group care settings as well as children who live with adults who smoke cigarettes have more ear infections. Therefore a child who is prone to otitis media should avoid contact with sick playmates and environmental tobacco smoke. Infants who nurse from a bottle while lying down also appear to develop otitis media more frequently. Children who have been breast fed often have fewer episodes of otitis media. Research has shown that cold and allergy medications such as antihistamines and decongestants are not helpful in preventing ear infections. The best hope for avoiding ear infections is the development of vaccines against the bacteria that most often cause otitis media. Scientists are currently developing vaccines that show promise in preventing otitis media. Additional clinical research must be completed to assure their effectiveness and safety.

How does a child's physician diagnose otitis media?

The simplest way to detect an active infection in the middle ear is to look in the child's ear with an otoscope, a light instrument that allows the physician to examine the outer ear and the eardrum. Inflammation of the eardrum indicates an infection. There are several ways that a physician checks for middle ear fluid. The use of a special type of otoscope called a pneumatic otoscope allows the physician to blow a puff of air onto the eardrum to test eardrum movement. (An eardrum with fluid deep to it does not move as well as an eardrum with air deep to it.)

A useful test of middle ear function is called tympanometry. This test requires insertion of a small soft plug into the opening of the child's ear canal. The plug contains a speaker, microphone and a device that is able to change the air pressure in the ear canal, allowing for several measures of the middle ear. The child feels air pressure changes in the ear or hears a few brief tones. While this test provides information on the condition of the middle ear, it does not determine how well the child hears. A physician may suggest a hearing test for a child who has frequent ear infections to determine the extent of hearing loss. The hearing test is usually performed by an audiologist, a person who is specially trained to measure hearing.

How is otitis media treated?

Most physicians recommend the use of an antibiotic (a drug that kills bacteria) when there is an active middle-ear infection. If a child is experiencing pain, the physician may also recommend a pain reliever. Once started, the antibiotic usually must be given to the child regularly for 10 to 14 days. Most physicians have the child return for a follow up examination 10 to 14 days after the start of the antibiotic to see if the infection has cleared. Unfortunately, there are many bacteria that can cause otitis media and some have become resistant to some antibiotics so several different antibiotics may have to be tried before an ear infection clears. Antibiotics may also produce unwanted side effects such as nausea, diarrhea and rashes.

Once the infections clears, fluid may remain in the middle ear for several months. Middle-ear fluid that is not infected often disappears after three to six weeks. Neither antihistamines nor decongestants are recommended as helpful in the treatment of otitis media at any stage in the disease process. Sometimes physicians will treat the child with an antibiotic to hasten the elimination of the fluid. If the fluid persists for more than three months and is associated with a loss of hearing, many physicians suggest the insertion of "tubes" in the affected ears. This operation, called a myringotomy, can usually be done on an outpatient basis by a surgeon, who is usually an otolaryngologist (a physician who specializes in the ears, nose and throat). While the child is asleep under general anesthesia, the surgeon makes a small opening in the child's eardrum. A small metal or plastic tube is placed into the opening in the eardrum. The tube ventilates the middle ear and helps keep the air pressure in the middle ear equal to the air pressure in the environment. The tube normally stays in the eardrum for six to twelve months after which time it usually comes out spontaneously. If a child has enlarged or infected adenoids, the surgeon may recommend removal of the adenoids at the same time the ear tubes are inserted. Removal of the adenoids has been shown to reduce episodes of otitis media in some children but not those who are under four years of age. Research, however, has shown that removal of a child's tonsils does not reduce occurrences of otitis media. Tonsillotomy and adnoidectomy may be appropriate for reasons other than middle-ear fluid.

Hearing should be fully restored once the fluid is removed. Some children may need to have the operation again if the otitis media returns after the tubes come out. While the tubes are in place, water should be kept out of the ears. Many physicians recommend that a child with tubes wear special ear plugs while swimming or bathing so that water does not enter the middle ear.

What research is being done on otitis media?

Several avenues of research are being explored to further improve the prevention, diagnosis and treatment of otitis media. For example, research is better defining those children who are at high risk for developing otitis media and conditions that predispose certain individuals to middle ear infections. Emphasis is being placed on discovering the reasons why some children have more ear infections than other children. The effects of otitis media on children's speech and language development are important areas of study as well as research to develop more accurate methods to help physicians detect middle-ear infections. How the defense molecules and cells involved with immunity respond to bacteria and viruses that often lead to otitis media is also under investigation. Scientists are evaluating the success of certain drugs currently being used for the treatment of otitis media and are examining new drugs that may be more effective, easier to administer and more adequately prevent new infections. Most importantly, research is leading to the availability of vaccines that will prevent otitis media.

Where can I get additional information?

Agency for Health Care Policy and Research
Publications Clearinghouse
P.O. Box 8547
Silver Spring, MD 20907
1-800-358-9295 (toll free)

American Academy of Otolaryngology–Head and Neck Surgery
One Prince Street
Alexandria, VA 22314
(703-836-4444 (voice)
(703) 519-1585 (TTY)
(703) 683-5100 (fax)

American Academy of Pediatrics
141 Northwest Point Boulevard
Elk Grove Village, IL 60007-1098 USA
(847) 228-5005 (voice)
(847) 228-5097 (fax)

American Speech-Language-Hearing Association
10801 Rockville Pike
Rockville, MD 20852
(301) 987-5700 (voice/TTY)
(800) 638-8255 (toll free)
(301) 571-0457 (fax)

NIDCD Information Clearinghouse
1 Communication Avenue
Bethesda, Maryland 20892-3456
1-800-241-1044 (voice)
1-800-241-1055 (TTY)
Send e-mail to nidcd@aerie.com

Chapter 9

Otitis Media in Children

Eavesdrop among parents at any playground and you'll hear them swapping tales about one of the most common maladies of toddlerhood—ear infections. The sleepless nights, endless trips to the pediatrician, and repeated rounds of expensive antibiotics are so common they're something of a preschool rite of passage. Ninety percent of American children will have had at least one ear infection before age 6.

Collectively called otitis media (inflammation of the middle ear), ear infections and middle ear fluid accounted for 24.5 million doctors' visits in 1990, a 150 percent increase since 1975, according to the national Centers for Disease Control and Prevention. Americans spend $3.5 billion each year to treat them.

Physicians have traditionally taken an aggressive approach to fight various types of otitis media, maintaining that a young child's hearing needs to be at its best during language development.

Yet recently, doctors and researchers have begun to debate traditional approaches to treating otitis media, especially otitis media with effusion (OME), which is chronic and can cause mild hearing loss. Although FDA doesn't have authority over how doctors treat ear infections, the agency does regulate all drugs and devices used in the process and is interested in the outcome of recent OME research.

OME occurs when the middle ear doesn't drain properly and fills with a sticky fluid, but causes no symptoms of infection such as pain

---

FDA Consumer, December 1994.

or fever. Sometimes called "glue ear," OME often appears after a cold or acute ear infection. Children are more prone to the condition than adults because their eustachian tubes, which drain fluid from the ear to the nose, are short and horizontal and often don't function properly.

An acute ear infection, called acute otitis media (AOM), is caused by bacteria or viruses. This condition is very painful and makes a child feverish and fretful (often in the middle of the night).

While most American doctors agree about how to treat acute otitis media, much debate has risen recently in the United States about the best remedy for otitis media with effusion.

Ironically perhaps, the latest consensus among researchers reveals that the best treatment is an easy one—"watch and wait."

A Frustrating Earful

As parents and doctors can attest, getting rid of middle ear fluid is tricky. Antibiotics don't always work, while surgical remedies are costly, often frightening, and may not solve the problem once and for all.

Last July, the Agency for Health Care Policy and Research (AHCPR), a component of the Public Health Service, issued new guidelines for treating otitis media with effusion.

A panel of independent experts recommended changing the traditional approach for treating OME in children ages 1 to 3, which has involved initially prescribing antibiotics. If that didn't clear it up, doctors inserted tympanostomy tubes, small tubes in the eardrum to drain the fluid behind it.

The panel found, however, that rushing into either treatment is not necessary. Middle ear fluid goes away on its own within three months in about 60 percent of cases and within six months in 85 percent of cases.

The panel recommended that when a child has ear fluid and no signs of infection, physicians should take a "watch and wait" attitude for three months. After that, if the fluid is still present, the child's hearing should be tested. If hearing is normal, the doctor should either continue watchful waiting or begin antibiotic treatment.

In the event of hearing loss, however, the physician should begin antibiotic treatment or try tympanostomy tubes. FDA has approved a number of tubes for the procedure. The panel recommends them only if the OME lasts four to six months and there's hearing loss in both ears.

Procedures such as taking out the child's adenoids or tonsils, or administering steroids, decongestants and antihistamines, are ineffective and should not be done, the panel said.

"If all doctors followed these guidelines, there would be fewer antibiotics prescribed and fewer surgeries as well," says Alfred Berg, M.D., co-chairman of the panel and professor of family medicine at the University of Washington School of Medicine in Seattle.

Although the panel limited its recommendations to OME, some researchers have begun to question the way American doctors use antibiotics for acute otitis media as well. AOM is treated with a 7- to 10-day round of antibiotics in more than 90 percent of cases. For children with recurrent infections, physicians sometimes prescribe a daily low dose of antibiotics for weeks as a preventative measure. While this approach can be effective, it may also encourage resistant strains of bacteria to develop. Physicians aware of this possibility can adjust medications if necessary.

"Treatment of acute otitis media is basically by tradition, a tradition that has not been adequately investigated," says Larry Culpepper, M.D., a professor of family medicine at Brown University and member of the AHCPR panel.

"I think the real answer is that we don't know for sure if there's a significant benefit for treating kids with antibiotics [for acute otitis media]," he says.

European doctors don't treat AOM the way American doctors do, Culpepper says. Overseas, doctors commonly take a "watch and wait" attitude. When they do order antibiotics, it's for a shorter period and at lower doses.

Culpepper is conducting a study comparing treatment of AOM in the Netherlands, the United Kingdom, and the United States. By examining the results of treating 4,500 children, he hopes to see which country's approach produces the best results.

Two Treatments

For now in the United States, antibiotics and tympanostomy tubes remain the most common and accepted tools for treating acute otitis media and otitis media with effusion.

Both approaches have benefits. Many oral antibiotics are inexpensive and can relieve a child's pain and fever from an acute ear infection in a few hours. For chronic fluid, tympanostomy tubes instantly drain the middle ear and restore hearing. According to the National Center for Health Statistics, there were about 670,000 surgeries in

1988 to insert ear tubes, making it the most common surgical procedure for children.

But there are drawbacks to both approaches as well. Antibiotics don't always work completely, leaving some infected fluid. Other times, the bacteria are resistant to the drug. Some researchers believe resistant bacteria are on the rise because our country overuses many antibiotics.

Antibiotics have side effects, too—the most troubling one being diarrhea. Others include thrush (an oral yeast infection) and vaginal yeast infections in girls.

If antibiotics are used, parents must be vigilant in giving each dose on time. Skipping or getting off schedule with doses will only make the infection worse, allowing bacteria that are resistant to the drug to grow.

"The child gets better, and the parents get lax," says Michael Blum, M.D., a medical officer at FDA. "If you skip a day here or there, there's more potential for resistant bacteria to develop."

When antibiotics fail, surgery is the next option. Most tympanostomies are done by ear, nose and throat specialists in an outpatient setting at a hospital. A general anesthesia is used for most children, not because it's very painful, but because the child needs to lie perfectly still.

During surgery, the physician cleans the ear canal, makes a small incision in the eardrum, suctions out the fluid behind it (a procedure called myringotomy), and places a tiny tube in the incision. The procedure is done under a microscope with an instrument that resembles a small pair of tweezers. It lasts about 15 to 30 minutes.

The AHCPR panel estimated the cost of tubes at about $2,174 (including a parent's lost time in work). Unfortunately, the tubes can easily fall out within weeks or months, and must be replaced. One-third of children with tubes have them replaced within five years of the first operation.

Other drawbacks of tubes include the risk of complications from anesthesia and the need for children to protect their ears with earplugs while swimming or bathing. It's a good idea to wait until autumn to put in tubes so that they won't interfere with beach and pool trips.

A child's hearing should always be tested before inserting tubes, the panel said. A loss of 20 decibels in each ear (as loud as a humming refrigerator) warrants treatment, the panel said. Although that's not a large hearing loss, experts are quick to point out that no one knows just how much loss might impede a child's language development.

Accurate Diagnosis

Before a child undergoes any treatment, it's crucial to get an accurate diagnosis, the panel advised.

A magnifying instrument called a pneumatic otoscope enables the doctor to see the eardrum while pumping a puff of air against it. If the eardrum is red and inflamed, it's probably infected. If it's not inflamed, but still doesn't move properly when the air hits it, it probably has uninfected fluid behind it.

"Many doctors do not use the pneumatic otoscope," says Cynthia Carney, a journalist and consumer representative on the AHCPR panel. "We say very clearly in the guidelines that that's the only way to be sure."

Many doctors either don't know how to use the pneumatic otoscope properly, or they can't get an accurate reading on a squirming, screaming 2-year-old. But experts say the results with a pneumatic otoscope are worth the extra time and effort.

The diagnosis can be confirmed by a specialist with another test called a tympanogram. Using a soft plug fitted snugly into the ear canal, the tympanometer emits a low noise and records how the eardrum reacts. If it doesn't move well, that's an indication that there's fluid behind the drum.

Prevention

Although the causes of otitis media aren't fully known, several factors increase a child's risk for developing ear infections:

Bottle-feeding. Bottle-fed babies are two to three times more likely to develop otitis media in the first year of life than are breast-fed babies. Breast milk may have antibodies that ward off the infections.

Second-hand smoke. Studies have shown that children whose parents smoke are nearly three times more likely to develop middle ear fluid than children whose parents don't smoke. They also take longer to recover.

Group childcare. Because they're exposed to a wide variety of cold viruses, children in group child-care facilities have a greater chance of developing ear infections than children cared for at home.

Allergies. Allergies can increase a child's likelihood of ear infections because watery mucus from the nose can clog the eustachian

81

tube and prevent it from draining properly. That's why doctors some-times prescribe antihistamines to help clear up middle ear fluid. The AHCPR panel did not find enough scientific evidence to support that treatment, however, and did not recommend it.

Birth defects. Certain conditions such as cleft palate, Down syn-drome, and nervous system abnormalities can increase a child's chances of developing ear infections. The panel's recommendations don't apply to these children, who should be evaluated individually by their doctors.

Ear Fluid and Hearing

The ear has three parts—the outer ear, the middle ear, and the inner ear. The outer ear includes the part outside the head and the ear canal. The eardrum is a small circle of tissue about the size of a fingertip at the end of the ear canal. The middle ear is the space, usu-ally filled with air, behind the eardrum. When a child has middle ear fluid, this is where it is found. A small tube—the eustachian tube—connects the middle ear to the back of the nose. Three tiny bones (the malleus, incus and stapes) connect the eardrum through the middle ear to the inner ear. The inner ear is farther inside the head and is important for hearing and balance.

In a healthy ear, sound waves travel through the ear canal and make the eardrum move back and forth. This makes the three bones in the middle ear move. The movement of these bones sends sound waves across the middle ear to the inner ear. The inner ear sends the sound messages to the brain. If the middle ear has fluid in it, then the eardrum and the bones cannot move well, and hearing problems may result (Source: Agency for Health Care Policy and Research).

Common Antibiotics for Ear Infections

Many antibiotics are approved by FDA to fight otitis media, al-though most doctors rely on a few favorites. Drug manufacturers have made a number of drugs in liquid fruity flavors palatable to kids. Most antibiotics fall under four families: penicillins, cephalosporins, sul-fonamides, and erythromycins. Here are some common brand names.

Amoxicillin. A generic name for the most common antibiotic used to treat ear infections. This is a synthetic penicillin. Physicians like it because it causes less diarrhea than some other antibiotics, it's absorbed well, and it's only given three times a day. It's also inexpensive. Side effects may include mild diarrhea and rashes. If the rash itches, the child might be allergic to the drug.

Pediazole. A brand-name combination of erythromycin and sulfisoxazole. Can be used if a child is allergic to penicillin. Side effects may include some abdominal cramping and discomfort and, infrequently, nausea, vomiting and diarrhea. If any rash develops, the drug should be discontinued.

Bactrim and Septra. Two brand names of a sulfonamide drug combined with trimethoprim. They can be used in children who are allergic to penicillin. Side effects may include mild nausea, vomiting, diarrhea, rashes, an increased sensitivity to sunlight, and a reductions in white blood cells.

Ceclor. A brand name of a cephalosporin antibiotic that is effective, but expensive. Side effects may include diarrhea and a rash. Children may be allergic to penicillin. Some newer cephalosporins include Ceftin, Cefzil, Vantin, Suprax, and Lorabid.

Gantrisin. In its liquid forms, Gantrisin is a brand name for acetyl sulfisoxazole and is often used as a preventative drug for children with recurrent infections, because it's given only once a day. It's approved for acute otitis media when used in combination with penicillin or erythromycin.

Augmentin. An amoxicillin drug with extra ingredients to inhibit bacterial resistance. May clear up infections when other drugs have failed.

Despite the number of antibiotics available to treat ear infections, FDA is concerned about the growth of increasing numbers of bacteria resistant to antibiotics.

"The agency is actively pursuing the establishment of a surveillance program for all antimicrobial products," says Albert Sheldon, Ph.D., a microbiologist in FDA's division of anti-infective drug products.

Last year, FDA asked manufacturers of new drugs seeking FDA approval to track their effect on certain strains of bacteria. FDA officials also participate in professional organizations that track bacterial resistance both in this country and around the world.

One way for parents to combat bacterial resistance is to be vigilant in giving each dose on schedule. Skipping or delaying doses can encourage resistant bacteria to develop.

—by Rebecca D. Williams

Rebecca D. Williams is a writer in Oak Ridge, Tenn.

Chapter 10

Middle Ear Fluid in Young Children

About the Ear and Hearing

The ear has three parts—the outer ear, the middle ear, and the inner ear. The outer ear includes the part outside the head and the ear canal. The eardrum is a small circle of tissue about the size of a fingertip at the end of the ear canal. The middle ear is the space, usually filled with air, behind the eardrum. When a child has middle ear fluid, this is where it is found. A small tube—the eustachian tube—connects the middle ear to the back of the nose. Three tiny bones (the malleus, incus, and stapes) connect the eardrum through the middle ear to the inner ear. The inner ear is further inside the head and is important for hearing and balance.

In a healthy ear, sound waves travel through the ear canal and make the eardrum move back and forth. This makes the three bones in the middle ear move. The movement of these bones sends sound waves across the middle ear to the inner ear. The inner ear sends the sound messages to the brain. But if the middle ear has fluid in it, then the eardrum and the bones cannot move well. This could cause your child to have trouble hearing.

Purpose of This Chapter

This chapter is about middle ear fluid in children ages 1 through 3 who have no other health problems. After reading this chapter you should know more about:

Agency for Health Care Policy and Research, AHCPR Pub. No. 94-0624, July 1994.

85

- Causes of middle ear fluid.

- Tests for middle ear fluid and hearing.

- Treatments for middle ear fluid and hearing loss caused by middle ear fluid.

- How to work with your child's health care provider to find the best treatment for your child's middle ear fluid.

Another name for middle ear fluid is otitis media with effusion. Some people also call it "glue ear." Otitis media means middle ear inflammation, and effusion means fluid.

What Is Middle Ear Fluid?

If your child has middle ear fluid, it means that a watery or mucous-like fluid has collected behind the eardrum. Many children get middle ear fluid during their early years. But middle ear fluid is not the same as an ear infection.

- An **Ear Infection** usually happens in only one ear at a time. With a middle ear infection your child may have fever and sharp ear pain. When your health care provider looks into your child's ear, they might see a bulging red eardrum and some fluid in the middle ear.

- **Middle Ear Fluid** is usually found in both ears at once. Most children do not have fever or pain with middle ear fluid. A special test is needed to look for this fluid (see below).

What Causes Middle Ear Fluid?

Here are some things that may cause middle ear fluid to happen in your child:

- Past ear infection. It is common for children to have middle ear infections. And some children with middle ear infection later have middle ear fluid.

- Blockage of the eustachian tube (see Figure 10.1).

- Cold or flu.

There is no one cause for middle ear fluid. Often, your child's health care provider will not know what caused the middle ear fluid.

You may want to keep track of when your child has ear problems and medical treatments.

Why Should I Be Worried about Middle Ear Fluid?

Most health care providers and parents worry that a child who has middle ear fluid in one or both ears can have trouble hearing. Experts do not know how much middle ear fluid affects hearing. Experts are not sure if hearing loss from middle ear fluid can cause delays in learning to talk, and sometimes later on, problems with school work. They do not know for sure what the long-term effects of middle ear fluid are.

How Can Middle Ear Fluid Be Prevented?

Recent studies show that children who live with smokers and who spend time in group child care have more ear infections.

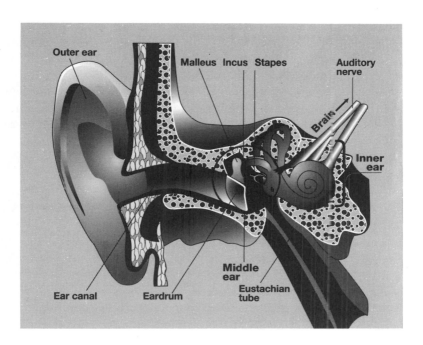

Figure 10.1. *Cross-section of the ear.*

Because some children who have middle ear infections later get middle ear fluid, you might help prevent middle ear fluid by:

- Keeping your child away from cigarette smoke.
- Trying to keep your child away from playmates who are sick.

How Do I Know If My Child Is Affected by Middle Ear Fluid?

Sometimes a child with middle ear fluid does not hear well. The most common complaint of parents whose child has middle ear fluid is that the child turns the sound up too loud or sits too close to the television set. Or sometimes the child does not seem to be paying attention.

Speak to your child's health care provider if you are concerned about your child's hearing. Often, middle ear fluid is found at a regular check-up.

Your child's health care provider may use the first two tests below to check for middle ear fluid.

- A **Pneumatic Otoscope** may be used to check for middle ear fluid (see Figure 10.2). With this tool, the health care provider looks at the eardrum. The fluid in the middle ear may be seen behind the eardrum. Even when the fluid cannot be seen, the health care provider can test for fluid with this tool by blowing a puff of air onto the eardrum to see how well the eardrum moves. The child must be still for this test to work. The child will feel the otoscope in the ear, but the test does not hurt. This test does **NOT** measure the child's hearing level. Many health care providers feel that the pneumatic otoscope is the best test for middle ear fluid.

- **Tympanometry** is another test for middle ear fluid. Tympanometry helps the health care provider find out how well the eardrum moves. For tympanometry, a soft plug that is about the size of a person's little fingertip is placed snugly into the ear canal. The probe is connected to a machine called a tympanometer. The child hears a low noise for a short time while the machine records how the eardrum reacts. An eardrum with fluid behind it does not move as well as a normal eardrum.

  Like the first test, the child must sit still for this test and will feel the probe in the ear. The test does not hurt. Tympanometry does **NOT** measure hearing level.

- **Hearing Testing** may be done to see how well your child hears. Hearing testing does not test for middle ear fluid. In this case, it measures if the fluid is affecting your child's hearing level. The type of hearing test used depends on your child's age and listening ability.

How Can Middle Ear Fluid Be Treated?

Middle ear fluid can be treated in many ways. It is important to know that a treatment that works for one child may not work for another. If one treatment does not work, another treatment can be tried. Please discuss each of the treatments listed here with your child's health care provider. Be sure to ask about the possible advantages and disadvantages of each treatment as well. Then, decide with your child's health care provider on the treatment for middle ear fluid.

- **Observation.** Middle ear fluid often goes away without treatment. Some studies show that for most children middle ear fluid clears after 3 to 6 months without treatment.

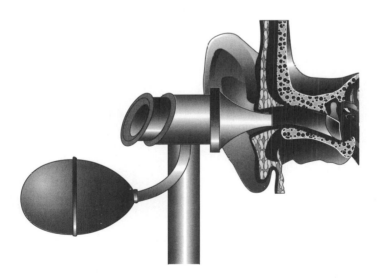

Figure 10.2. Pneumatic otoscope placed in ear.

Table 10.3. Middle Ear Fluid Treatment

Treatment: Observation

Advantages
- In about 60 percent of children, middle ear fluid goes away without treatment within 3 months; in 85 percent it goes away within 6 months.
- There is very little cost and no side effects of observation.

Disadvantages
- Middle ear fluid does not go away in about 40 percent of children in 3 months and in about 15 percent in 6 months.

Treatment: Antibiotic drug

Advantages
- May increase chance (by about 14 percent) and speed of middle ear fluid going away.
- May decrease chance of middle ear infection.

Disadvantages
- Middle ear fluid may not go away.
- Unwanted drug effects (such as diarrhea, rash).
- Development of drug-resistant strains of bacteria.
- Bother of buying and giving drug.
- Cost of drug.

Treatment: Surgery (tubes)

Advantages
- Middle ear fluid goes away right away.
- Hearing returns to normal right away.

Disadvantages
- Temporary discomfort for child.
- Risks of anesthesia.
- May need to protect ears during bathing and swimming while tubes are in place.
- Some children need another surgery to place new tubes in the ears.
- Eardrum changes possible.
- Time lost to take child for surgery.
- Most costly choice.

- **Antibiotic Drug Treatment.** Studies show that middle ear fluid cleared slightly faster in some children given antibiotic drugs than those not given antibiotics. However, antibiotics have some unwanted effects, such as diarrhea, rash, and others (see table 10.3). Also, they can be expensive and some children have trouble taking them. For these reasons, you and your child's health care provider may want to try observation first.

  Before making a decision, ask your child's health care provider about the costs and possible unwanted effects.

- **Surgery to Put "Tubes" in the Ears.** In this minor operation, a small cut is made in the child's eardrum and fluid in the middle ear is gently sucked out. Then a small metal or plastic tube is put into the slit in the eardrum. A general anesthetic is used to put the child to sleep for this operation. When the fluid is removed from the middle ear, the child's hearing returns to its normal level.

  Ask your child's health care provider about the costs and possible harms of this surgery.

  The tubes are left in place until they fall out, or until your child's health care provider feels that they are no longer needed. About one third (1 out of 3) of children with ear tubes need to have another operation to insert new tubes within 5 years after the first operation.

What Are the Advantages and Disadvantages of Middle Ear Fluid Treatments?

The advantages and disadvantages of treatment for middle ear fluid are listed in Table 10.3. Please discuss these choices further with your child's health care provider.

When Should Middle Ear Fluid Be Treated?

The treatment that your child gets for middle ear fluid depends on:

- How long your child has had middle ear fluid.
- If the fluid is causing hearing problems for your child.

Here are some examples of how your child might best be treated for middle ear fluid.

91

Remember to discuss all treatments with your child's health care provider. Be sure to ask about the advantages and disadvantages of each treatment.

If your child has had **middle ear fluid for up to 3 months,** then your child's health care provider may recommend one of these treatments:

- Observation **or** antibiotic therapy. You and your provider may choose observation because antibiotic therapy can cause some unwanted effects.

- Taking steps to prevent middle ear fluid (especially keeping your child away from cigarette smoke).

If your child has had **middle ear fluid for 3 months or more,** then your child's health care provider may recommend the following treatments:

- Observation **or** antibiotic drugs. You and your provider may choose observation because antibiotic therapy can cause some unwanted effects.

- Taking steps to prevent middle ear fluid (especially keeping your child away from cigarette smoke).

Also

- A hearing test is recommended if your child has had middle ear fluid for 3 months or more. If this shows that your child has a hearing loss in both ears, your child's health care provider may recommend surgery to put tubes in the eardrums.

- Talk to your child's health care provider about any other concerns you have about your child's development—for example, if your child does not seem to be learning to talk on schedule.

If your child has had **middle ear fluid that has lasted from 4 to 6 months with a hearing loss in both ears,** then your child's health care provider may recommend:

- Surgery to put tubes in the eardrums. Tubes in the eardrums should clear the middle ear fluid and return your child's hearing to normal. Discuss this surgery with your child's health care provider.

Also

- Find out if your child's ears should be protected from water after the surgery and when to bring your child back for a check-up.

What Treatments Are Not Recommended for My Child?

A number of medicines and surgical treatments are not recommended for young children with middle ear fluid.

The medicines not recommended are:

- Decongestants and antihistamines.
- Steroids.

Most studies show that decongestants and antihistamines used together or alone did not improve or cure middle ear fluid. There are not yet enough studies to tell whether steroids can cure or improve middle ear fluid.

The surgical treatments not recommended are:

- Adenoidectomy.
- Tonsillectomy.

There are not yet enough studies to tell if adenoidectomy (removing the adenoids—tissue at the back of the throat behind the nose) cures or improves middle ear fluid in children younger than 4 years old. But it does seem to help older children. Tonsillectomy (removing the tonsils at the back of the throat) has not been shown to cure or improve middle ear fluid in children.

If your child's health care provider suggests one of these surgeries, there may be another medical reason to do the surgery. Ask why your child needs the surgery. If you are still unsure, you may want to talk to another health care provider.

For Further Information

The information in this chapter was based on the *Clinical Practice Guideline, Otitis Media with Effusion in Young Children*. The *Guideline* was developed by a non-Federal panel of experts sponsored by the Agency for Health Care Policy and Research. Other guidelines on common health problems are available, and more are being developed.

For more information about guidelines call toll-free 800-358-9295, or write to:

Agency for Health Care Policy and Research
Publications Clearinghouse
P.O. Box 8547
Silver Spring, MD 20907

Chapter 11

Managing Otitis Media with Effusion

Purpose and Scope

Otitis media (inflammation of the middle ear) is the most frequent primary diagnosis at visits to U.S. physician offices by children younger than 15 years. Otitis media particularly affects infants and preschoolers: almost all children experience one or more episodes of otitis media before age 6.

The American Academy of Pediatrics, the American Academy of Family Physicians, and the American Academy of Otolaryngology–Head and Neck Surgery, with the review and approval of the Agency for Health Care Policy and Research of the U.S. Department of Health and Human Services, convened a panel of experts to develop a guideline on otitis media for providers and consumers of health care for young children. Providers include primary care and specialist physicians, professional nurses and nurse practitioners, physician assistants, audiologists, speech-language pathologists, and child development specialists. Because the term otitis media encompasses a range of diseases, from acute to chronic and with or without symptoms, the Otitis Media Guideline Panel narrowed the topic. Two types of otitis media often encountered by clinicians were considered:

Stool SE, Berg AO, Berman S, Carney CJ, Cooley JR, Culpepper L, Eavey RD, Feagans LV, Finitzo T, Friedman E, et al. *Managing Otitis Media with Effusion in Young Children. Quick Reference Guide for Clinicians.* AHCPR Publication No. 94-0623. Rockville, MD: Agency for Health Care Policy and Research, Public Health Service, U.S. Department of Health and Human Services. July 1994.

95

- **Acute otitis media**—fluid in the middle ear accompanied by signs or symptoms of ear infection (bulging eardrum usually accompanied by pain; or perforated eardrum, often with drainage of purulent material).

- **Otitis media with effusion**—fluid in the middle ear without signs or symptoms of ear infection.

[This text discusses only otitis media with effusion in] a very specific "target patient":

- A child age 1 through 3 years.

- With no craniofacial or neurologic abnormalities or sensory deficits.

- Who is healthy except for otitis media with effusion.

When the scientific evidence for management permitted, Guideline recommendations were broadened to include older children.

Highlights of Patient Management

Congenital or early onset hearing impairment is widely accepted as a risk factor for impaired speech and language development. In general, the earlier the hearing problem begins and the more severe it is, the worse its effects on speech and language development. Because otitis media with effusion is often associated with a mild to moderate hearing loss, most clinicians have been eager to treat the condition to restore hearing to normal and thus prevent any long-term problems.

Studies of the effects of otitis media with effusion on hearing have varied in design and have examined several aspects of hearing and communication skills. Because of these differences, the results cannot be combined to provide a clear picture of the relationship between otitis media with effusion and hearing. Also, it is uncertain whether changes in hearing due to middle ear fluid have any long-term effects on development. Evidence of dysfunctions mediated by otitis media with effusion that have persisted into later childhood, despite resolution of the middle ear fluid and a return to normal hearing, would provide a compelling argument for early, decisive intervention. There is, however, no consistent, reliable evidence that otitis media with effusion has such long-term effects on language or learning.

The following recommendations for managing otitis media with effusion are tempered by the failure to find rigorous, methodologically sound research to support the theory that untreated otitis media with effusion results in speech/language delays or deficits.

Recommendations and options were developed for the diagnosis and management of otitis media with effusion in otherwise healthy young children. The following steps parallel the management algorithm provided at the end of this chapter.

Diagnosis and Hearing Evaluation

1. Suspect otitis media with effusion in young children.

Most children have at least one episode of otitis media with effusion before entering school. Otitis media with effusion may be identified following an acute episode of otitis media, or it may be an incidental finding. Symptoms may include discomfort or behavior changes.

2. Use pneumatic otoscopy to assess middle ear status.

Pneumatic otoscopy is recommended for assessment of the middle ear because it combines visualization of the tympanic membrane (otoscopy) with a test of membrane mobility (pneumatic otoscopy). When pneumatic otoscopy is performed by an experienced examiner, the accuracy for diagnosis of otitis media with effusion may be between 70 and 79 percent.

3. Tympanometry may be performed to confirm suspected otitis media with effusion.

Tympanometry provides an indirect measure of tympanic membrane compliance and an estimate of middle ear air pressure. The positive predictive value of an abnormal (type B, flat) tympanogram is between 49 and 99 percent; that is, as few as half of ears with abnormal tympanograms may have otitis media with effusion. The negative predictive value of this test is better—the majority of middle ears with normal tympanograms will in fact be normal. Because the strengths of tympanometry (it provides a quantitative measure of tympanic membrane mobility) and pneumatic otoscopy (many abnormalities of the eardrum and ear canal that can skew the results of tympanometry are visualized) offset the weaknesses of each, using the two tests together improves the accuracy of diagnosis.

- **Acoustic reflectometry** has not been studied well enough for a recommendation to be made for or against its use to diagnose otitis media with effusion.

- **Tuning fork tests:** No recommendation is made regarding the use of tuning fork tests to screen for or diagnose otitis media with effusion, except to note that they are inappropriate in the youngest children.

4. A child who has had fluid in both middle ears for a total of 3 months should undergo hearing evaluation. Before 3 months of effusion, hearing evaluation is an option.

A change in hearing threshold is both a clinical outcome and a possible indicator of the presence of otitis media with effusion. Methods used to determine a child's hearing acuity will vary depending on the resources available and the child's willingness and ability to participate in testing. Optimally, air- and bone-conduction thresholds can be established for 500, 1,000, 2,000, and 4,000 Hz, and an air-conduction pure tone average can be calculated. This result should be verified by obtaining a measure of speech sensitivity. Determinations of speech reception threshold or speech awareness threshold alone may be used if the child cannot cooperate for pure tone testing. If none of the test techniques is available or tolerated by the child, the examiner should use his/her best judgment as to adequacy of hearing. In these cases, the health care provider should be aware of whether the child is achieving the appropriate developmental milestones for verbal communication.

Although hearing evaluation may be difficult to perform in young children, evaluation is recommended after otitis media with effusion has been present bilaterally for 3 months, because of the strong belief that surgery is not indicated unless otitis media with effusion is causing hearing impairment (defined as equal to or worse than 20 decibels hearing threshold level in the better-hearing ear).

Natural History

Longitudinal studies of otitis media with effusion show spontaneous resolution of the condition in more than half of children within 3 months from development of the effusion. After 3 months the rate of spontaneous resolution remains constant, so that only a small percentage of children experience otitis media with effusion lasting a year or longer. In most children, episodes of otitis media with effusion do not persist beyond early childhood. The likelihood that middle ear fluid will resolve by itself underlies the recommendations made for management of otitis media with effusion.

Environmental Risk Factors

Scientific evidence showed that the following environmental factors may increase potential risks of getting acute otitis media or otitis media with effusion:

- Bottle-feeding rather than breast-feeding infants.
- Passive smoking.
- Group child-care facility attendance.

Because the target child for Guideline recommendations is beyond the age when the choice of breast-feeding versus bottle-feeding is an issue, this risk factor was not considered at length.

Passive smoking (exposure to another's cigarette smoke) is associated with higher risk of otitis media with effusion. Although there is no proof that stopping passive smoking will help prevent middle ear fluid, there are many health reasons for not exposing persons of any age to tobacco smoke. Therefore, clinicians should advise parents of the benefits of decreasing children's exposure to tobacco smoke.

Studies of otitis media with effusion in children cared for at home compared to those in group child-care facilities found that children in group child-care facilities have a slightly higher relative risk (less than 2.0) of getting otitis media with effusion. Research did not show whether removing the child from the group child-care facility helped prevent otitis media with effusion.

Therapeutic Interventions

5. Observation OR antibiotic therapy are treatment options for children with effusion that has been present less than 4 to 6 months and at any time in children without a 20-decibel hearing threshold level or worse in the better-hearing ear.

Most cases of otitis media with effusion resolve spontaneously. Meta-analysis of controlled studies showed a 14 percent increase in the resolution rate when antibiotics were given. Length of treatment in these studies was typically 10 days.

The most common adverse effects of antibiotic therapy are gastrointestinal. Dermatologic reactions may occur in 3 to 5 percent of cases; severe anaphylactic reactions are much rarer; severe hematologic, cardiovascular, central nervous system, endocrine, renal, hepatic, and respiratory adverse effects are rarer still. The potential for the development of microbial resistance is always present with antibiotics.

6. For the child who has had bilateral effusion for a total of 3 months and who has a bilateral hearing deficiency (defined as a 20-decibel hearing threshold level or worse in the better-hearing ear), bilateral myringotomy with tube insertion becomes an additional treatment option. Placement of tympanostomy tubes is recommended after a total of 4 to 6 months of bilateral effusion with a bilateral hearing deficit.

The principal benefits of myringotomy with insertion of tympanostomy tubes are the restoration of hearing to the pre-effusion threshold and clearance of the fluid and possible feeling of pressure. While patent and in place, tubes may prevent further accumulation of fluid in the middle ear. Although there is insufficient evidence to prove that there are long-term deleterious effects of otitis media with effusion, concern about the possibility of such effects led the panel to recommend surgery, based on their expert opinion. Tubes are available in a myriad of designs, most constructed from plastic and/or metal. Data comparing outcomes with tubes of various designs are sparse, and so there were assumed to be no notable differences between available tympanostomy tubes.

Insertion of tympanostomy tubes is performed under general anesthesia in young children. Calculation of the risks for two specific complications of myringotomy with tympanostomy tube insertion showed that tympanosclerosis might occur after this procedure in 51 percent, and postoperative otorrhea in 13 percent, of children.

Treatment Options that Are Not Recommended

A number of treatments are not recommended for treatment of otitis media with effusion in the otherwise healthy child age 1 through 3 years.

- Steroid medications are not recommended to treat otitis media with effusion in a child of any age because of limited scientific evidence that this treatment is effective and the opinion of many experts that the possible adverse effects (agitation, behavior change, and more serious problems such as disseminated vari-cella in children exposed to this virus within the month before therapy) outweighed possible benefits.

- Antihistamine/decongestant therapy is not recommended for treatment of otitis media with effusion in a child of any age, be-cause review of the literature showed that these agents are not effective for this condition, either separately or together.

- Adenoidectomy is not an appropriate treatment for uncompli-cated middle ear effusion in the child younger than age 4 years when adenoid pathology is not present (based on the lack of sci-entific evidence). Potential harms for children of all ages in-clude the risks of general anesthesia and the possibility of excessive postoperative bleeding.

- Tonsillectomy, either alone or with adenoidectomy, has not been found effective for treatment of otitis media with effusion.

- The association between allergy and otitis media with effusion was not clear from available evidence. Thus, although close anatomic relationships between the nasopharynx, eustachian tube, and middle ear have led many experts to suggest a role for allergy management in treating otitis media with effusion, no recommendation was made for or against such treatment.

- Evidence regarding other therapies for the treatment of otitis media with effusion was sought, but no reports of chiropractic, holistic, naturopathic, traditional/indigenous, homeopathic, or other treatments contained information obtained in randomized controlled studies. Therefore, no recommendation was made re-garding such other therapies for the treatment of otitis media with effusion in children.

Treatment Outcomes

Table 11.1, presented on the following page, summarizes the ben-efits and harms identified for management interventions in the tar-get child with otitis media with effusion.

Table 11.1. Outcomes of Treating Otitis Media with Effusion[1]

Intervention	Benefits[2]	Harms[2]
Observation	Base Case	Base case
Antibiotics	Improved clearance of effusion at 1 month or less, 14.0% (95% CI [3.6%, 24.2%]).	Possible reduction in future infections. Nausea, vomiting, diarrhea (2%-32% depending on dose and antibiotic). Cutaneous reactions (less than or equal to 5%). Numerous rare organ system effects, including very rare fatalities. Cost. Possible development of resistant strains of bacteria.
Antibiotics plus steroids	Possible improved clearance at 1 month, 25.1% (95% CI [-1.3%, 49.9%]).[3] Possible reduction in future infections.	See antibiotics and steroids separately.
Steroids alone	Possible improved clearance at 1 month, 4.5% (95% CI [-11.7%, 20.6%]).[3]	Possible exacerbation of varicella. Long-term complications not established for low doses. Cost.
Antihistamine/ decongestant	Same as base case.	Drowsiness and/or excitability.[4] Cost.
Myringotomy with tubes	Immediate clearance of effusion in all children. Improved hearing.	Invasive procedure. Anesthesia risk. Cost. Tympanosclerosis. Otorrhea. Possible restrictions on swimming.
Adenoidectomy	Benefits for young children have not been established. Invasive procedure.[4]	Anesthesia risk. Cost.
Tonsillectomy	Same as base case.	Invasive procedure.[4] Anesthesia risk. Cost.

Notes to Table 11.1:

[1]*The target patient is an otherwise healthy child age 1 through 3 years with no craniofacial or neurologic abnormalities or sensory deficits.*

[2]*Outcomes are reported as differences from observation, which is treated as the base case. When possible, meta-analysis was performed to provide a mean and associated confidence interval (CI).*

[3]*Difference from base case not statistically significant.*

[4]*Risks were not examined in detail because no benefits were identified.*

Algorithm

The notes below are an integral part of the algorithm that follows.

Notes to Algorithm

A   Otitis media with effusion (OME) is defined as fluid in the middle ear without signs or symptoms of infection; OME is not to be confused with acute otitis media (inflammation of the middle ear with signs of infection). The Guideline and this algorithm apply only to the child with otitis media with effusion. This algorithm assumes followup intervals of 6 weeks.

B   The algorithm applies only to a child age 1 through 3 years with no craniofacial or neurologic abnormalities or sensory deficits (except as noted) who is healthy except for otitis media with effusion. The Guideline recommendations and algorithm do not apply if the child has any craniofacial or neurologic abnormality (for example, cleft palate or mental retardation) or sensory deficit (for example, decreased visual acuity or pre-existing hearing deficit).

C   The Panel found some evidence that pneumatic otoscopy is more accurate than otoscopy performed without the pneumatic test of eardrum mobility.

D   Tympanometry may be used as confirmation of pneumatic otoscopy in the diagnosis of otitis media with effusion (OME). Hearing evaluation is recommended for the otherwise healthy child who has had bilateral OME for 3 months; before 3 months, hearing evaluation is a clinical option.

103

E   In most cases, otitis media with effusion (OME) resolves spontaneously within 3 months.

F   The antibiotic drugs studied for treatment of otitis media with effusion (OME) were amoxicillin, amoxicillin-clavulanate potassium, cefaclor, erythromycin, erythromycin-sulfisoxazole, sulfisoxazole, and trimethoprim-sulfamethoxazole.

G   Exposure to cigarette smoke (passive smoking) has been shown to increase the risk of otitis media with effusion (OME). For bottle-feeding versus breast-feeding and for child-care facility placement, associations were found with OME, but evidence available to the Panel did not show decreased incidence of OME with breast-feeding or with removal from child-care facilities.

H   The recommendation against tonsillectomy is based on the lack of added benefit from tonsillectomy when combined with adenoidectomy to treat otitis media with effusion in older children. Tonsillectomy and adenoidectomy may be appropriate for reasons other than otitis media with effusion.

I   The Panel found evidence that decongestants and/or antihistamines are ineffective treatments for otitis media with effusion.

J   Meta-analysis failed to show a significant benefit for steroid medications without antibiotic medications in treating otitis media with effusion in children.

Algorithm for managing otitis media with effusion in an otherwise healthy child age 1 through 3 years

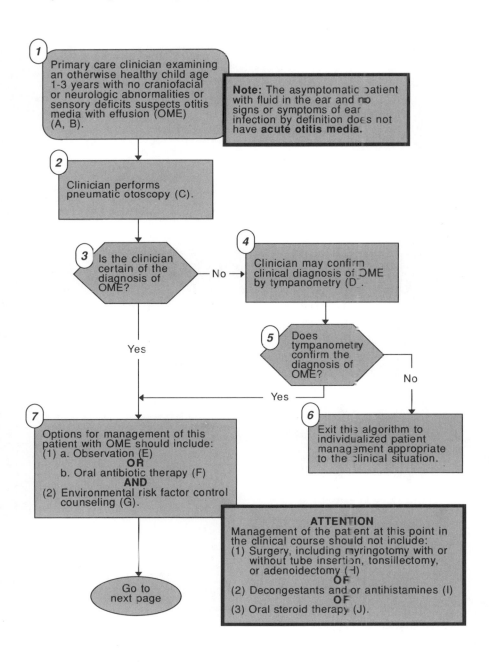

1. Primary care clinician examining an otherwise healthy child age 1-3 years with no craniofacial or neurologic abnormalities or sensory deficits suspects otitis media with effusion (OME) (A, B).

Note: The asymptomatic patient with fluid in the ear and no signs or symptoms of ear infection by definition does not have **acute otitis media.**

2. Clinician performs pneumatic otoscopy (C).

3. Is the clinician certain of the diagnosis of OME?

No →

4. Clinician may confirm clinical diagnosis of OME by tympanometry (D).

5. Does tympanometry confirm the diagnosis of OME?

No

Yes

6. Exit this algorithm to individualized patient management appropriate to the clinical situation.

Yes

7. Options for management of this patient with OME should include:
(1) a. Observation (E)
OR
b. Oral antibiotic therapy (F)
AND
(2) Environmental risk factor control counseling (G).

ATTENTION
Management of the patient at this point in the clinical course should not include:
(1) Surgery, including myringotomy with or without tube insertion, tonsillectomy, or adenoidectomy (H)
OR
(2) Decongestants and/or antihistamines (I)
OR
(3) Oral steroid therapy (J).

Go to next page

105

Algorithm (continued)

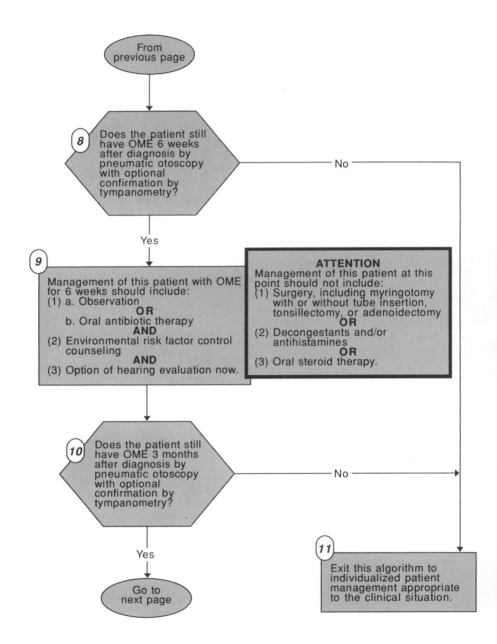

Algorithm (continued)

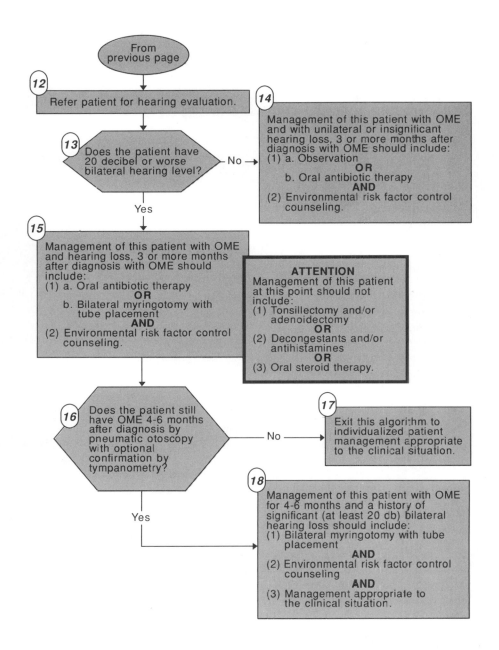

From previous page

12 Refer patient for hearing evaluation.

13 Does the patient have 20 decibel or worse bilateral hearing level? —No→

14 Management of this patient with OME and with unilateral or insignificant hearing loss, 3 or more months after diagnosis with OME should include:
(1) a. Observation
OR
b. Oral antibiotic therapy
AND
(2) Environmental risk factor control counseling.

Yes

15 Management of this patient with OME and hearing loss, 3 or more months after diagnosis with OME should include:
(1) a. Oral antibiotic therapy
OR
b. Bilateral myringotomy with tube placement
AND
(2) Environmental risk factor control counseling.

ATTENTION
Management of this patient at this point should not include:
(1) Tonsillectomy and/or adenoidectomy
OR
(2) Decongestants and/or antihistamines
OR
(3) Oral steroid therapy.

16 Does the patient still have OME 4-6 months after diagnosis by pneumatic otoscopy with optional confirmation by tympanometry? —No→

17 Exit this algorithm to individualized patient management appropriate to the clinical situation.

Yes

18 Management of this patient with OME for 4-6 months and a history of significant (at least 20 cb) bilateral hearing loss should include:
(1) Bilateral myringotomy with tube placement
AND
(2) Environmental risk factor control counseling
AND
(3) Management appropriate to the clinical situation.

107

Selected Bibliography

Black N. The aetiology of glue ear—a case-control study. *Int J Pediatr Otorhinolaryngol* 1985;9(2):121-33.

Cantekin EI, Mandel EM, Bluestone CD, Rockette HE, Paradise JL, Stool SE, Fria TJ, Rogers KD. Lack of efficacy of a decongestant-antihistamine combination for otitis media with effusion ("secretory" otitis media) in children: results of a double-blind, randomized trial. *N Engl J Med* 1983;308(6):297-301.

Casselbrant ML, Brostoff LM, Cantekin EI, Flaherty MR, Doyle WJ, Bluestone CD, Fria TJ. Otitis media with effusion in preschool children. *Laryngoscope* 1985 Apr;95:428-36.

Etzel RA, Pattishall EN, Haley NJ, Fletcher RH, Henderson FW. Passive smoking and middle ear effusion among children in day care. *Pediatrics* 1992 Aug;90(2):228-32.

Friel-Patti S, Finitzo T. Language learning in a prospective study of otitis media with effusion in the first two years of life. *J Speech Hear Res* 1990;33:188-94.

Maw AR. Development of tympanosclerosis in children with otitis media with effusion and ventilation tubes. *J Laryngol Otol* 1991;105(8):614-7.

Rosenfeld RM, Mandel EM, Bluestone CD. Systemic steroids for otitis media with effusion in children. *Arch Otolaryngol Head Neck Surg* 1991 Sept;117:984-9.

Rosenfeld RM, Post JC. Meta-analysis of antibiotics for the treatment of otitis media with effusion. *Otolaryngol Head Neck Surg* 1992;106:378-86.

Teele DW, Klein JO, Rosner B; the Greater Boston Otitis Media Study Group. Middle ear disease and the practice of pediatrics. Burden during the first five years of life. *JAMA* 1983 Feb 25;249(8):1026-9.

Teele DW, Klein JO, Rosner B; the Greater Boston Otitis Media Study Group. Otitis media with effusion during the first three years of life and development of speech and language. *Pediatrics* 1984;74(2):282-7.

Toner JG, Mains B. Pneumatic otoscopy and tympanometry in the detection of middle ear effusion. *Clin Otolaryngol* 1990;15(2):121-3.

Williams RL, Chalmers TC, Stange KC, Chalmers FT, Bowlin SJ. Use of antibiotics in preventing recurrent acute otitis media and in treating otitis media with effusion: a meta-analytic attempt to resolve the brouhaha. *JAMA* 1993 Sep 15;270(11):1344-51.

Zielhuis GA, Straatman H, Rach GH, van den Broek P. Analysis and presentation of data on the natural course of otitis media with effusion in children. *Int J Epidemiol* 1990 Dec; 19(4):1037-44.

Chapter 12

Chronic Ear Infections

Chronic Ear Infection

The diagnosis of chronic otitis media (infection of the middle ear) has been established as the cause of your ear problem. Symptoms depend upon whether the condition is active or inactive, whether or not there is involvement of the mastoid bone and whether or not there is a hole in the eardrum. There may be discharge, hearing impairment, tinnitus (head noise), dizziness, pain or, rarely, weakness of the face.

Function of the Normal Ear

The ear is divided into three parts: the external ear, the middle ear, and the inner ear. Each part performs an important function in the process of hearing.

Sound waves pass through the canal of the external ear and vibrate the eardrum which separates the external from the middle ear. The three small bones in the middle ear (hammer or malleus, anvil or incus, and stirrup or stapes) act as a transformer to transmit energy of the sound vibrations to the fluids of the inner ear. Vibrations in this fluid stimulate the delicate nerve fibers. The hearing nerve then transmits impulses to the brain where they are interpreted as understandable sound.

© 1993 House Ear Institute, 2100 West Third Street, 5th Floor, Los Angeles, CA 90057, (213) 483-4431 voice, (213) 484-2642 TDD; reprinted with permission.

Types of Hearing Impairment

The external ear and the middle ear conduct sound; the inner ear receives it. If there is some difficulty in the external or middle ear, a *conductive* hearing loss occurs. If the trouble lies in the inner ear, a *sensorineural* or nerve hearing loss is the result. When there is difficulty in both the middle and inner ear, a combination of conductive and sensorineural impairment exists.

The Diseased Middle Ear

Any disease affecting the eardrum or the three small ear bones may cause a conductive hearing loss by interfering with the transmission of sound to the inner ear. Such a hearing impairment may be due to a perforation (hole) in the eardrum, partial or total destruction of one or all of the three little ear bones, or scar tissue.

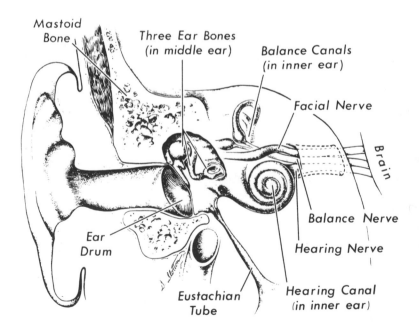

Figure 12.1. *The components of the ear.*

When an acute infection develops in the middle ear (an abscessed ear), the eardrum may rupture, resulting in a *perforation*. This perforation usually heals. If it fails to do so a hearing loss occurs, often associated with head noise (tinnitus) and intermittent or constant ear drainage.

Care of the Ear

If a perforation is present, you should not allow water to get into your ear canal. This may be avoided when showering or washing the hair by placing cotton or lambs wool in the external ear canal and covering it with a layer of vaseline. Swimming is permissible if you use a small ear plug. Your otologist can advise you in regard to this.

You should avoid blowing your nose in order to prevent any infection in your nose from spreading to the ear through the eustachian tube. Any nasal secretion preferably should be drawn backward and expectorated. If it is absolutely necessary to blow your nose, do not occlude or compress one nostril while blowing the other.

In the event of ear drainage, the ear canal should be kept clean by means of a small cotton tipped applicator. Medication, as prescribed, should be used if discharge occurs. Cotton is placed in the outer ear to catch any discharge but should not be allowed to block the ear canal.

Medical Treatment

Medical treatment frequently will stop ear drainage. Treatment consists of careful cleaning of the ear and, at times, the application of antibiotic powder or ear drops. Antibiotics by mouth may be helpful in certain cases.

Surgical Treatment

For many years surgical treatment was instituted in chronic otitis media primarily to control infection and prevent serious complications. Changes in surgical techniques now have made it possible to reconstruct the diseased hearing mechanism in most cases.

Various tissue grafts may be used to replace or repair the eardrum. These include covering of muscle from above the ear (fascia) and covering of ear cartilage (perichomdrium).

A diseased ear bone may be replaced by a plastic prosthesis (TORP or PORP), or cartilage, or may be repositioned (relocated).

113

A thin piece of plastic frequently is used behind the eardrum to prevent scar tissue from forming and to promote normal function of the middle ear and motion of the eardrum. When the ear is filled with scar tissue, or when all ear bones have been destroyed, it may be necessary to perform the operation in two stages. At the first stage a piece of stiff plastic is inserted to allow more normal healing without scar tissue. At the second operation this plastic is removed and we attempt to restore hearing. A decision in regard to staging the operation is made at the time of the first surgery.

Myringoplasty

Most ear infections subside and the structures of the middle ear heal completely. In some cases, however, the eardrum may not heal and a permanent perforation (hole) in the eardrum results.

Myringoplasty is the operation performed for the purpose of repairing a perforation in the eardrum when there is no middle ear infection or disease of the ear bones. This procedure seals the middle ear and may improve the hearing.

Surgery is usually performed under local anesthesia through the ear canal. Ear tissue is used to repair the defect in the eardrum. The patient is hospitalized for one night and may return to work in a week. Healing is complete in most cases in six weeks, at which time any hearing improvement is usually noticeable.

Tympanoplasty

An ear infection may cause a perforation of the eardrum, damage the mucosa and damage the three ear bones that transmit sound from the eardrum to the inner ear and hearing nerve. Tympanoplasty is the operation performed to eliminate any infection and repair both the sound transmitting mechanism and any perforation of the eardrum. This procedure seals the middle ear and improves the hearing in many cases.

In cases not requiring repair of the eardrum, the operation is usually performed under local anesthesia through the ear canal.

Most tympanoplasties are performed through an incision behind the ear, under a local or a general anesthesia. The perforation is repaired with ear tissue. Sound transmission to the inner ear is accomplished by repositioning or replacing diseased ear bones.

In some cases it is not possible to repair the sound transmitting mechanism and the eardrum at the same time. In these cases the eardrum is repaired first, and six months or more later, the sound transmitting mechanism is reconstructed. (See Planned Second Stage.)

The patient is usually hospitalized for one night and may return to work in a week to ten days. Healing is usually complete in eight weeks. A hearing improvement may not be noted for a few months.

Types of Mastoid Surgery

There are two techniques of mastoid surgery: canal wall up and canal wall down. The decision on which technique is usually made at the time of surgery.

Canal wall up mastoidectomy is preferred by members of the House Ear Clinic because little, if any, precautions are necessary after the ear has healed (3 to 4 months).

Canal wall down surgery is necessary 30% of the time because of the extent of the disease or the development of the mastoid bone. Healing may be prolonged. Canal wall down surgery results in a larger ear opening (meatus) but little difference in the appearance of the ear. Periodic cleaning of the mastoid (ear) cavity is necessary indefinitely and it may be necessary to avoid water in the ear.

Tympanoplasty with Mastoidectomy

Active infection may in some cases stimulate skin of the ear canal to grow through a perforated eardrum into the middle ear and mastoid. When this occurs a skin-lined cyst known as *cholesteatoma* is formed. This cyst may continue to expand over a period of years and destroy the surrounding bone. If a cholesteatoma is present the drainage tends to be more constant and frequently has a foul odor. In many cases the persistent drainage is due only to chronic infection in the bone surrounding the ear structures.

Once a cholesteatoma has developed or the bone has become infected it is rarely possible to eliminate the infection by medical treatment. Antibiotics placed in the ear and used by mouth only result in a temporary improvement in most cases. Recurrence after treatment has stopped is frequent.

A cholesteatoma or chronic ear infection may persist for many years without difficulty except for the annoying drainage and hearing loss. It may, however, by local expansion and pressure involve important surrounding structures. If this occurs the patient will often notice a fullness or a low-grade aching discomfort in the ear region. Dizziness or weakness of the face may develop. If any of these symptoms occur it is imperative that one seek immediate medical care. Surgery may be necessary to eradicate the infection and prevent serious complications.

When the destruction by cholesteatoma or infection is widespread in the mastoid the surgical elimination of this may be difficult. Surgery is performed through an incision behind the ear. The primary objective is to eliminate infection, to obtain a dry, safe ear.

In most patients with cholesteatoma it is not possible to eliminate infection and restore hearing in one operation. The infection is eliminated and the eardrum rebuilt in the first operation. This requires a general anesthetic with hospitalization for two to three nights. The patient may usually return to work in one to two weeks.

When a second operation is necessary it will be performed six to twelve months later, to restore the hearing mechanism and to reinspect the ear spaces for any residual (remaining) disease.

On rare occasions a radical mastoid operation may be necessary to control infection in a case thought originally to be suitable for tympanoplasty.

Tympanoplasty: Planned Second Stage

The purpose of this operation is to reinspect the ear spaces for disease and to improve the hearing.

Surgery may be performed through the ear canal under local anesthesia as an outpatient at the hospital.

More often than not surgery is performed from behind the ear under general anesthesia. The ear is inspected for any residual (remaining) disease. Sound transmission to the inner ear is accomplished by replacing missing ear bones.

The patient is hospitalized for one night following surgery and may return to work in four to seven days. Healing is usually complete in six weeks. Hearing improvement is frequently noted at that time.

Tympanoplasty with Revision Mastoidectomy

The purpose of this operation is to eliminate discharge from a previously created mastoid cavity defect and to improve the hearing.

The operation is performed under general anesthesia through an incision behind the ear. The mastoid cavity may be obliterated with fat from behind the ear or with bone. At times, the ear canal is rebuilt with cartilage or bone. The eardrum is repaired and, if possible, the hearing mechanism is restored. In most cases, however, a second operation is necessary to obtain hearing improvement. (See Tympanoplasty: Planned Second Stage.)

The patient is usually hospitalized for one night following surgery and may return to work after one to two weeks. Complete healing of the inside of the ear may take four months.

Modified Radical Mastoidectomy

The purpose of this operation is to eradicate the infection without consideration of hearing improvement. It is usually performed in those patients who may have very resistant infections or have infection in any only hearing ear. Occasionally it may be necessary to perform a radical mastoid operation in some case that originally appeared suitable for a tympanoplasty. This decision is made at the time of surgery. A fat or bone graft from the ear is necessary at times to help the ear heal properly.

The radical mastoid operation is performed under general anesthesia and requires one night of hospitalization following surgery. The patient may usually return to work in one to two weeks. Complete healing may require up to four months.

Mastoid Obliteration Operation

The purpose of this operation is to eradicate any mastoid infection and to obliterate (fill-in) a previously created mastoid cavity. Hearing improvement is not considered.

The operation is performed under general anesthesia through an incision behind the ear. The patient is usually hospitalized for one night following surgery and may return to work in one to two weeks. Complete healing may require up to three months.

Your Outlook with Surgery

Drainage: Eardrum grafting is successful in over 90% of patients, resulting in a healed, dry ear.

Hearing: Hearing improvement following surgery depends upon many factors, among which are the extent of the ear bone damage and the ability of the ear to heal properly.

What to Expect Following Surgery

There are some symptoms which may follow any ear operation.

Taste Disturbance and Mouth Dryness

Taste disturbance and mouth dryness are not uncommon for a few weeks following surgery. In some patients this disturbance is prolonged.

Tinnitus

Tinnitus (head noise), frequently present before surgery, is almost always present temporarily after surgery. It may persist for one to two months and then decrease in proportion to the hearing improvement. Should the hearing be unimproved or worse, the tinnitus may persist or be worse.

Numbness of Ear

Temporary loss of skin sensation in and about the ear is common following surgery. This numbness may involve the entire outer ear and may last for six months or more.

Jaw Symptoms

The jaw joint is in intimate contact with the ear canal. Some soreness or stiffness in jaw movement is very common after ear surgery. It usually subsides within one to two months.

Drainage Behind the Ear

At times the surgeon may insert a drain tube behind the ear. The necessity for this is usually not apparent before surgery. Should a drain tube be necessary, it will protrude through the skin behind the ear about ¼ of an inch and may be left in place for a week or more.

Risks and Complications of Surgery

Fortunately complications are uncommon following surgery for correction of chronic ear infection.

Ear Infection

Ear infection, with drainage, swelling and pain, may persist following surgery or, on rare occasions, may develop following surgery due to poor healing of the ear tissue. Were this to be the case, additional surgery might be necessary to control the infection.

Loss of Hearing

In 3% of the ears operated the hearing is further impaired permanently due to the extent of the disease present or due to complications in the healing process; nothing further can be done in these instances. On occasions there is a total loss of hearing in the operated ear.

In some cases a two stage operation is necessary to obtain satisfactory hearing and to eliminate the disease. The hearing is usually worse after the first operation in these instances.

Dizziness

Dizziness may occur immediately following surgery due to swelling in the ear and irritation of the inner ear structures. Some unsteadiness may persist for a week postoperatively. On rare occasions dizziness is prolonged.

Ten percent of the patients with chronic ear infection due to cholesteatoma have a labyrinthine fistula (abnormal opening into the balance canal). When this problem is encountered dizziness may last for six months or more.

Facial Paralysis

The facial nerve travels through the ear bone in close association with middle ear bones, eardrum and the mastoid. A rare postoperative complication of ear surgery is temporary paralysis of one side of the face. This may occur as a result of an abnormality or a swelling of the nerve and usually subsides spontaneously.

On very rare occasions the nerve may be injured at the time of surgery or it may be necessary to excise it in order to eradicate disease. When this happens a skin sensation nerve is removed from the upper part of the neck to replace the facial nerve. Paralysis of the face under these circumstances might last six months to a year and there would be a permanent residual weakness. Eye complications, requiring treatment by a specialist, could develop.

Hematoma

A hematoma (collection of blood under the skin) develops in a small percentage of cases, prolonging hospitalization and healing. Reoperation to remove the clot may be necessary if this complication occurs.

Complications Related to Mastoidectomy

A *cerebral spinal fluid leak* (leak of fluid surrounding the brain) is a very rare complication. Reoperation may be necessary to stop the leak.

Intracranial (brain) complications such as meningitis or brain abscess, even paralysis, were common in cases of chronic otitis media prior to the antibiotic era. Fortunately these now are extremely rare complications.

Travel Restrictions Following Surgery

You should have someone drive you from the hospital. Air travel is permissible 48 hours after surgery and is preferred to automobile or train travel for trips of over 200 miles.

General Comments

If you do not have surgery performed at this time, it is advisable to have annual examinations, especially if the ear is draining. Should you develop dull pain in or about the ear, increased discharge, dizziness or twitching, or weakness of the face, you should immediately consult your physician.

The House Ear Institute

The House Ear Institute, founded in 1946 as a private, non-profit organization, is dedicated to clinically-applied research and professional education in the diagnosis, prevention, and treatment of disorders of the ear.

The Institute is a major international center. Its associated physicians, surgeons, audiologists, and other specialists led the way in conquering the problems of the middle ear. And the House Ear Institute is setting new directions in the understanding of the inner ear and its delicate structures that are the source of "nerve" hearing impairment and many balance and facial nerve problems.

The Institute has been affiliated with the University of Southern California School of Medicine (USC) since 1960. It communicates research results and trains professionals through special courses and workshops, videotaped seminars, publications, and lectures.

Activities of the House Ear Institute are supported by grants and gifts from the private sector and the National Institutes of Health. Contributions are tax deductible.

Chapter 13

Allergy and the Ears

A Discussion of Allergies

Allergy is an over-reaction of the body to a substance that is normally harmless to most people. This substance is called an **allergen**, and one can be exposed to it in several ways. It may be *breathed* into the respiratory system, *eaten*, or *touched* by the skin to cause symptoms. Some people inherit a tendency to develop allergies.

Symptoms of Allergy

A stuffy nose, runny nose, polyps (growths) in the nose, itching and puffy eyes, frequent sore throats, asthma, skin rashes, and behavioral problems such as hyperactivity in children may be symptoms of allergy. Symptoms may occur in almost all systems of the body, including ears.

Allergy and the Ears

Outer Ear. Chronic itching or frequent infections of the ear canal may be due to allergy.

Middle Ear. Repeated ear infections and long-standing fluid behind the eardrum are often due to allergy. Both of these are more common in children.

© 1993. House Ear Institute, 2100 West Third Street, 5th Floor, Los Angeles, CA 90057, (213) 483-4431 voice, (213) 484-2642 TDD; reprinted with permission.

121

Inner Ear. Dizziness, ear fullness and pressure, tinnitus or head noise, and sensorineural (nerve) hearing loss may be due to allergy—especially food allergy. **Meniere's disease** in one or both ears may sometimes be caused by allergies.

Types of Allergy

Symptoms of allergy may be produced by inhalant (airborne), food, and contact allergens. Reactions of the immune system (autoimmune disease) may also cause symptoms.

Inhalant Allergy

Symptoms of inhalant allergy are caused by reactions to allergens that enter the body via the respiratory tract. They may develop with recurrent or prolonged exposure to the allergen. These can be pollens, dust, molds, animal dander, or other substances breathed in through the nose.

Symptoms of inhalant allergy may be year-round or seasonal. Hay fever is a form of inhalant allergy due to grass pollen.

When the nose or lungs come in repeated contact with allergens, the immune system of allergic patients makes a high level of a blood protein, or **antibody**, called **immunoglobulin E (IgE)**. The IgE attaches to special allergic cells called **mast cells**, found throughout the body. When the allergen enters the respiratory tract, a change occurs in the mast cell's outer membrane causing the cell to release substances called **mediators** which produce allergic symptoms. One of these mediators is called **histamine**; it causes congestion and swelling of tissue. That is why an **antihistamine** is frequently prescribed for allergy symptoms.

Food Allergies

Often, common foods that are eaten frequently are the ones that cause symptoms of food allergy. Allergens taken into the digestive tract such as wheat, fruit, shellfish and dairy products can cause allergic symptoms such as nasal congestion, hives, or ear infections.

Non-food substances that are ingested may cause similar symptoms. These would include medicines such as Penicillin or Sulfa, or chemicals such as food preservatives.

Contact Dermatitis (Skin Rash)

Contact dermatitis is a rash or swelling caused by direct contact of an allergen with the skin. Poison ivy, nickel earrings, wool shirts or certain ear drops may stimulate a cell called the **T-lymphocyte** to release allergic mediators which affect the skin. The rash may last many weeks or months after exposure.

Autoimmune Hearing Loss

Autoimmune hearing loss is believed to be caused by the body's immune system attacking the inner ear and damaging the hearing nerve. Autoimmune disease occurs when the body produces an immunological or allergic reaction to itself, instead of reacting to an external substance. No one knows why this occurs. Many patients have signs of other diseases caused by an overly-active immune system—arthritis, skin rash, allergy, etc.

Symptoms of inner ear involvement may include fluctuating (changing) hearing, often with dizziness and ear fullness, or a sudden loss of hearing.

Antihistamines and Non-Specific Treatment

Mild allergic symptoms require no specific test for diagnosis, and can be well controlled with some combination of antihistamines, nasal sprays, and avoidance of known allergens.

Side effects of antihistamines include dry mouth and drowsiness.

More severe or chronic allergic symptoms and those not controlled by medication—especially those involving the inner ear—may require tests to identify the specific allergens.

Diagnosis of Specific Allergies

Specific allergens may be diagnosed by skin testing, blood test, or a challenge test. Blood tests are also used in the diagnosis of autoimmune hearing loss.

Skin Testing for Inhalant Allergies

To identify inhalant allergies, small amounts of allergens are injected in rows on your arm.

Little bumps called **wheals** will form on the skin at the injection sites. After 10 minutes, these wheals are inspected. Certain larger wheals indicate an allergy to the substance that was injected at that area. The wheal size helps your doctor determine how sensitive you are and what strength your allergy injections should be.

RAST Test (Blood Test)

The Radioallergosorbent test (RAST) is a blood test sometimes used to diagnose food and inhalant allergies. It measures antibodies (such as IgE) to specific allergens, and may be used to determine your sensitivity to inhalants and some forms of food allergy.

Challenge Test for Food Allergies

Skin testing rarely helps to diagnose food allergies. Many patients crave foods to which they are allergic, and your doctor may take a food history from you to identify some of these. A RAST test may be ordered, or a challenge test may be necessary to determine what foods may cause symptoms after they have been eaten.

Foods to be tested may be either eaten or injected in a purified form. When the food has been absorbed, the allergic patient may develop common symptoms of allergy such as nasal stuffiness, a change in hearing, or ringing in the ears.

Blood Test for Autoimmune Hearing Loss

Autoimmune hearing loss is diagnosed by special blood tests to show whether the immune system is overly active. The doctor may sometimes detect evidence of involvement in other areas of the body such as the kidney or skin.

Treatment of Allergy

The type of treatment for an allergy depends on the underlying cause. It may involve desensitization (allergy shots), avoidance, or medications. At times the underlying cause can be controlled but it is necessary to do something surgical to eliminate the problem that has resulted from the allergy.

Inhalant Allergy

If your doctor suggests desensitization therapy for inhalant allergies, you will be given injections once or twice a week. These injections contain the allergens to which you are sensitive. They stimulate the production of a protective substance called **blocking antibody** to help prevent allergic symptoms. You will sometimes need to have these skin tests rechecked to adjust the allergy dose.

Food Allergies

You will be asked to eliminate, temporarily, the foods to which you are allergic. This will allow your body to lose its sensitivity to these foods. You will also be asked to rotate (vary) the other foods in your diet to prevent new food allergies from developing.

Contact Dermatitis

Your doctor will try to determine what substances may be causing your symptoms and have you avoid the allergens. An anti-inflammatory medicine called a **steroid** may also be prescribed in a pill, cream, or drop form to help decrease the inflammation.

Autoimmune Hearing Loss

Your doctor may want to prescribe a steroid to suppress or slow down an overly-active immune system. It may be necessary to prescribe other medicines to help regulate the immune system, or it may be recommended that you be tested for allergies. Affected patients may have improved hearing and balance after treatment.

Surgery

Ear symptoms due to allergy—such as fluid in the middle ear space—can be treated by the surgical placement of a ventilation tube in the eardrum. Surgery to control dizziness is necessary at times, even though the underlying problem started as a result of an allergy. Following surgery, it may be necessary to treat the underlying allergic problem itself to prevent the symptoms from recurring.

Summary

Allergies cause a number of different symptoms, many of which are found in the ear, nose, and throat. They are rarely life-threatening, but can cause discomfort and interfere with the quality of life.

Most of these symptoms can be controlled by avoiding known allergens, treating with medicine, and specific desensitization therapy.

The Future

Great progress has been made through research in the prevention and treatment of hearing and balance disorders; much still remains to be done—So All May Hear.

You can help in achieving this goal by willing your ear bones after death to the House Ear Institute, a non-profit research and education foundation. Your bones will be studied by scientists in various laboratories and compared with your symptoms and findings during life (the House Ear Institute is affiliated with the University of Southern California School of Medicine.).

When you pledge your ear bones to the Institute you will be joining many others in this research effort. As such, you will receive regular mailings from the Institute detailing progress in ear research.

Your doctor will be pleased to provide you with further information regarding this vital contribution to ear research.

The Board of Trustees of the Institute would also greatly appreciate your consideration of a bequest in your will to help support the Institute's vital research—So All May Hear.

This text was first published and copyrighted in 1978 by the doctors of the House Ear Clinic, Inc. of Los Angeles. They volunteer both time and financial support to the House Ear Institute. Much of the information herein was derived from research work at the Institute. This is a current version of the information.

Chapter 14

Perforated Eardrum

A perforated eardrum is a hole or rupture in the eardrum, a thin membrane which separates the ear canal and the middle ear. The medical term for eardrum is *tympanic membrane*. The middle ear is connected to the nose by the eustachian tube, which equalizes pressure in the middle ear.

A perforated eardrum is often accompanied by decreased hearing and occasional discharge. Pain is usually not persistent.

Causes of Eardrum Perforation

The causes of perforated eardrum are usually from trauma or infection. A perforated eardrum can occur

- if the ear is struck squarely with an open hand;
- with a skull fracture;
- after a sudden explosion;
- if an object (such as a bobby pin, Q-tip, or stick) is pushed too far into the ear canal; or
- as a result of hot slag (from welding) or acid entering the ear canal.

Middle ear infections may cause pain, hearing loss and spontaneous rupture (tear) of the eardrum resulting in a perforation. In this circumstance, there may be infected or bloody drainage from the ear. In medical terms, this is called *otitis media with perforation.*

On rare occasions a small hole may remain in the eardrum after a previously placed PE tube (pressure equalizing) either falls out or is removed by the physician.

Most eardrum perforations heal spontaneously within weeks after rupture, although some may take up to several months. During the healing process the ear must be protected from water and trauma. Those eardrum perforations which do not heal on their own may require surgery.

Effects on Hearing from Perforated Eardrum

Usually, the larger the perforation, the greater the loss of hearing. The location of the hole (perforation) in the eardrum also effects the degree of hearing loss. If severe trauma (e.g. skull fracture) disrupts the bones in the middle ear which transmit sound or causes injury to the inner ear structures, the loss of hearing may be quite severe.

If the perforated eardrum is due to a sudden traumatic or explosive event, the loss of hearing can be great and ringing in the ear (tinnitus) may be severe. In this case the hearing usually returns partially, and the ringing diminishes in a few days. Chronic infection as a result of the perforation can cause major hearing loss.

Treatment of the Perforated Eardrum

Before attempting any correction of the perforation, a hearing test should be performed. The benefits of closing a perforation include prevention of water entering the ear while showering, bathing or swimming (which could cause ear infection), improved hearing, and diminished tinnitus. It also may prevent the development of cholesteatoma (skin cyst in the middle ear), which can cause chronic infection and destruction of ear structures.

If the perforation is very small, otolaryngologists may choose to observe the perforation over time to see if it will close spontaneously. They also might try to patch a cooperative patient's eardrum in the office. Working with a microscope, your doctor may touch the edges of the eardrum with a chemical to stimulate growth and then place a thin paper patch on the eardrum. Usually with closure of the tympanic membrane improvement in hearing is noted. Several applications of a patch (up to three or four) may be required before the perforation closes completely. If your physician feels that a paper patch will not provide prompt or adequate closure of the hole in the eardrum, or attempts with paper patching do not promote healing, surgery is considered.

There are a variety of surgical techniques, but all basically place tissue across the perforation allowing healing. The name of this procedure is called *tympanoplasty*. Surgery is typically quite successful in closing the perforation permanently, and improving hearing. It is usually done on an outpatient basis.

Your doctor will advise you regarding the proper management of a perforated eardrum.

Chapter 15

Eustachian Tube Problems

The House Ear Institute

The House Ear Institute, founded in 1946 as a private, non-profit corporation, is dedicated to clinically applied research and professional education in the diagnosis, prevention, and treatment of disorders of the ear.

The Institute is now a major international center. Its associated physicians, surgeons audiologists, and other specialists led the way in conquering the problems of the middle ear. It is setting new directions in the understanding of the inner ear and the delicate structures that are the source of "nerve" hearing impairment and many balance and facial nerve problems.

The Institute is located near St. Vincent Medical Center and affiliated with the University of Southern California School of Medicine. It communicates the results of research and trains other professionals in clinical application through courses and workshops, videotaped seminars, lectures, and publications.

Loss of hearing is America's most prevalent, yet least recognized, physical ailment. More people suffer from it than from heart disease, cancer, blindness, tuberculosis, multiple sclerosis, venereal disease, and kidney disease combined.

One of every ten persons in this country is affected to some degree. Nearly one out of one hundred have extreme difficulty understanding speech. Yet we pay less attention to hearing loss than to any other major affliction.

Despite the magnitude, hearing studies attract less than one percent of the dollars spent on medical research in America today. Perhaps this is because hearing loss is invisible and usually painless. It is a hurt that does not show; therefore, it seems less important than other disabilities. But for those who are profoundly hard of hearing or deaf, and who live in a world of silence, the emotional pain is often devastating.

The House Ear Institute is supported by grants and gifts from the private sector. Contributions are tax-deductible.

Mechanism of Hearing

The ear is divided into three parts: an external ear, a middle ear and an inner ear. Each part performs an important function in the process of hearing.

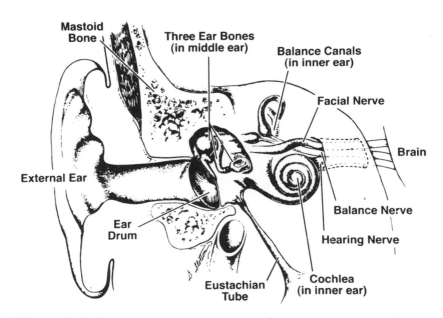

Figure 15.1. *Components of the ear.*

The external ear consists of an auricle and ear canal. These structures gather the sound and direct it towards the eardrum membrane.

The middle ear chamber lies between the external and inner ear. This chamber is connected to the back of the throat by the eustachian tube which serves as a pressure equalizing valve. The middle ear consists of an eardrum membrane and three small ear bones (ossicles): malleus (hammer), incus (anvil) and stapes (stirrup). These structures transmit sound vibrations to the inner ear. In so doing they act as a transformer, converting sound vibrations in the external ear canal into fluid waves in the inner ear. A disturbance of the eustachian tube, eardrum membrane or the bones may result in a *conductive hearing impairment*. This type of impairment is usually correctable medically or surgically.

The inner ear chamber contains the microscopic hearing nerve endings bathed in fluid. Inner ear fluid waves stimulate the delicate nerve endings which in turn transmit sound energy to the brain where it is interpreted. A disturbance in the inner ear fluids or nerve endings may result in a *sensorineural* (nerve) *hearing impairment*. This type of impairment is not correctable.

Function of the Eustachian Tube

The eustachian tube is a narrow, one and a half inch long channel connecting the middle ear with the nasopharynx, the upper throat area just above the palate, in back of the nose.

The eustachian tube functions as a pressure equalizing valve for the middle ear which is normally filled with air. When functioning properly the eustachian tube opens for a fraction of a second periodically (about once every three minutes) in response to swallowing or yawning. In so doing it allows air into the middle ear to replace air that has been absorbed by the middle ear lining (mucous membrane) or to equalize pressure changes occurring on altitude changes. Anything that interferes with this periodic opening and closing of the eustachian tube may result in hearing impairment or other ear symptoms.

Obstruction or blockage of the eustachian tube results in a negative middle ear pressure, with retraction (sucking in) of the eardrum membrane. In the adult this is usually accompanied by some ear discomfort, a fullness or pressure feeling and may result in a mild hearing impairment and head noise (tinnitus). There may be no symptoms in children. If the obstruction is prolonged, fluid may be drawn from the mucous membrane of the middle ear creating a condition we call *serous otitis media* (fluid in the middle ear). This occurs frequently in children in connection with an upper respiratory infection and accounts for the hearing impairment associated with this condition.

Occasionally pain or middle ear fluid develops when landing in an aircraft. This is due to failure of the eustachian tube to properly equalize the middle ear air pressure and the condition is called *aerotitis*. It is temporary and often can be avoided by taking precautions.

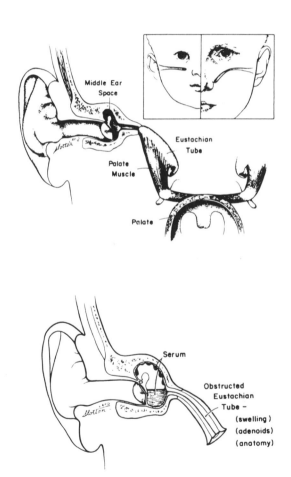

Figure 15.2. The eustachian tube.

On occasions just the opposite from blockage occurs: the tube remains open for prolonged periods. This is called *abnormal patency of the eustachian tube*. This condition is less common than serous otitis media and occurs primarily in adults. Because the tube is constantly open the patient may hear himself breathe and hears his voice reverberate. Fullness and a blocked feeling are not uncommon. Abnormal patency of the eustachian tube is annoying but does not produce hearing impairment.

Eustachian Tube Problems Related to Flying

Individuals with a eustachian tube problem may experience difficulty equalizing middle ear pressure when flying.

When an aircraft ascends, atmospheric pressure decreases, resulting in a relative increase in the middle ear pressure. When the aircraft descends, just the opposite occurs: atmospheric pressure increases and there is a relative decrease in middle ear pressure. Either situation may result in discomfort in the ear due to abnormal middle ear pressure if the eustachian tube is not functioning properly. Usually this discomfort is experienced upon aircraft descent.

To avoid middle ear problems associated with flying you should not fly if you have an acute upper respiratory problem such as a common cold, allergy attack, or sinus infection. Should you have such a problem and must fly, or should you have a chronic eustachian tube problem, you may help avoid ear difficulty by observing the following recommendations:

1. Obtain from your druggist (a prescription is not necessary) the following items: Sudafed tablets; plastic squeeze bottle of ¼ percent Neo-Synephrine nasal spray.

2. Following the container directions, begin taking Sudafed tablets the day before your air flight. Continue the medication for 24 hours after the flight if you have experienced any ear difficulty.

3. Following the container directions, use the nasal spray shortly before boarding the aircraft. Should your ears "plug up" upon ascent, hold your nose and swallow. This will help suck excess air pressure out of the middle ear.

4. 45 minutes before the aircraft is due to land again use the nasal spray every five minutes for 15 minutes. Chew gum to stimulate swallowing. Should your ears "plug up" despite this, hold your nose and blow forcibly to try to blow air up the eustachian tube into the middle ear (Valsalva maneuver).

135

5. Remember that it is unwise to fly if you have an acute upper respiratory infection. Should flying be necessary under these circumstances do not perform the Valsalva maneuver mentioned above.

None of these recommendations or precautions need be followed if you have a middle ear ventilation tube in your eardrum membrane.

The Eustachian Tube and Its Role in Serous Otitis Media

Serous Otitis media is the term we use to describe a collection of fluid in the middle ear. This may be acute or chronic.

Acute serous otitis media is usually the result of blockage of the eustachian tube from an upper respiratory infection or an attack of nasal allergy. In the presence of bacteria this fluid may become infected leading to an acute suppurative otitis media (infected or abscessed middle ear). When infection does not develop the fluid remains until the eustachian tube again begins to function normally, at which time the fluid is absorbed or drains down the tube into the throat.

Chronic serous otitis media may result from long-standing eustachian tube blockage, or from thickening of the fluids so that it cannot be absorbed or drained down the tube. This chronic condition is usually associated with hearing impairment. There may be recurrent ear pain, especially when the individual catches a cold. Fortunately serous otitis media may persist for many years without producing any permanent damage to the middle ear mechanism. The presence of fluid in the middle ear, however, makes it very susceptible to recurrent acute infections. These recurrent infections may result in middle ear damage.

Causes of Serous Otitis Media

Serous otitis media may result from any condition that interferes with the periodic opening and closing of the eustachian tube. The causes may be congenital (present at birth), may be due to infection or allergy, or may be due to blockage of the tube by adenoids.

The Immature Eustachian Tube

The size and shape of the eustachian tube is different in children that in adults. This accounts for the fact that serous otitis media is more common in very young children. Some children inherit small eustachian tubes from their parents; this accounts in part for the familial tendency to middle ear infection. As the child matures, the eustachian tube usually assumes a more adult shape.

Cleft Palate

Serous otitis media is more common in the child with cleft palate. This is due to the fact that the muscles that move the palate also open the eustachian tube. These muscles are deficient or abnormal in the cleft palate child.

Infection

The lining membrane (mucous membrane) of the middle ear and eustachian tube is connected with, and is the same as, the membrane of the nose, sinuses, and throat. Infection of these areas results in mucous membrane swelling which in turn may result in eustachian tube obstruction.

Allergy

Allergic reactions in the nose and throat result in mucous membrane swelling, and this swelling may also affect the eustachian tube. This reaction may be acute, as in a hay fever type reaction, or may be chronic, as in many varieties of "chronic sinusitis."

Adenoids

The adenoids are located in the nasopharynx, in the area around and between the eustachian tube openings. When enlarged, the adenoids may block the eustachian tube opening.

Acute Serous Otitis Media

Treatment of acute serous otitis media is medical, and is directed towards treatment of the upper respiratory infection or allergy attacks. This may include antibiotics, antihistaminics (anti-allergy drugs), decongestants (drugs to decrease mucous membrane swelling) and nasal sprays.

Acute Suppurative Otitis Media

In the presence of an upper respiratory infection, such as a cold, tonsillitis, or sinusitis, fluid in the middle ear may become infected.

This results in what is commonly called an abscessed ear or an infected ear.

This infected fluid (pus) in the middle ear may cause severe pain. If examination reveals that there is considerable ear pressure, a myringotomy (incision of the eardrum membrane) may be necessary to relieve the abscess and the pain. In many cases, antibiotic treatment will suffice.

Should myringotomy be necessary, the ear may drain pus and blood for up to a week. The drum membrane then heals and the hearing usually returns to normal within three to four weeks.

Antibiotic treatment, with or without myringotomy, usually results in normal middle ear function within three to four weeks. During this healing period there are varying degrees of ear pressure, popping, clicking, and fluctuation of hearing, occasionally with shooting pains in the ear.

Resolution of the acute infection occasionally leaves the patient with uninfected fluid in the middle ear. This is called chronic serous otitis media.

Chronic Serous Otitis Media

Treatment of chronic serous otitis media may be either medical or surgical.

Medical Treatment

As the acute upper respiratory infection subsides, it may leave the patient with a chronic sinus infection. Pus from the sinuses and nose drains over the eustachian tube opening in the nasopharynx resulting in persistent eustachian tube blockage. Antibiotic treatment may be indicated.

General health factors are particularly important in regard to the child's resistance to infection. A deficiency in some of the blood proteins may predispose to recurrent infections and prolonged colds. Periodic injections of gamma globulin may be indicated.

Allergy is often a major factor in the development or persistence of serous otitis media. Mild cases can be treated with antihistaminic drugs. More persistent cases may require allergic evaluation and treatment, including injection treatment.

In connection with medical treatment we may recommend eustachian tube inflation, the blowing of air through the nose into the obstructed eustachian tube and middle ear to help relieve the congestion and reestablish middle ear ventilation. This is done by the Valsalva maneuver or by politzerization.

Valsalva maneuver. The Valsalva maneuver is accomplished by forcibly blowing air into the middle ear while holding the nose, often called "popping the ear." This should not be done, however, if there is a cold and nasal discharge.

Politzerization. Politzerization is accomplished by blowing air with a special syringe (middle ear inflator) into one nostril while blocking the other, and at the same time swallowing. This forces air into the eustachian tube and middle ear. This likewise should not be performed when a cold is present.

Surgical Treatment

The primary objective of surgical treatment of chronic serous otitis media is to reestablish ventilation of the middle ear, keeping the hearing at a normal level and preventing recurrent infection that might damage the eardrum membrane and middle ear bones. This involves myringotomy with insertion of a ventilation tube, and at times, adenoidectomy.

Myringotomy. Myringotomy (an incision in the ear membrane) is performed to remove middle ear fluid. A hollow plastic tube (ventilation tube) is inserted to prevent the incision from healing and to insure middle ear ventilation. The ventilation tube temporarily takes the place of the eustachian tube in equalizing middle ear pressure. This plastic tube usually remains in place for three to nine months during which time the eustachian tube blockage should subside. When the tube dislodges, the eardrum heals; the eustachian tube then resumes its normal pressure equalizing function.

In rare cases the drum membrane does not heal following dislodgment of the tube. The perforation may be repaired at a later date if this occurs.

In adults myringotomy and insertion of a ventilation tube is usually performed in the office under local anesthesia. In children general anesthesia is required. The adenoids can be removed if enlarged.

More often that not, when the ventilation tube dislodges there is no further middle ear ventilation problem. Should serous otitis media recur, reinsertion of a tube may be necessary. In some difficult cases it is necessary to insert a more permanent type of tube, the "mesh" ventilation tube. This tube is more difficult to insert but frequently will remain in place until removed. In children, removal may require an anesthetic. At times a permanent drum membrane perforation (hole in the eardrum) develops when the tube is dislodged or removed. If this perforation persists it can be repaired at a later date when the eustachian tube blockage has subsided.

When a ventilation tube is in place the patient may carry on normal activities, with the exception that he must not allow water to enter the ear canal. Your doctor will recommend an ear plug for use when showering, washing the hair, or swimming.

Chronic Serous Mastoiditis and Idiopathic Hemotympanum

Chronic serous mastoiditis and idiopathic hemotympanum are uncommon conditions which have the same symptoms as chronic serous otitis media. They differ in that the middle ear fluid continues to form, either draining out the ventilation tube or blocking it completely so that the tube dislodges shortly after surgery. This persistent fluid formation is due to changes in the mucous membrane of the middle ear and mastoid.

In both of the above conditions, mastoid surgery may be necessary to control the problem and reestablish a normal middle ear mechanism.

The Abnormally Patent Eustachian Tube

Abnormal patency of the eustachian tube is a condition occurring primarily in adults, in which the eustachian tube remains "open" for prolonged periods. This abnormality may produce many distressing symptoms: ear fullness and blockage, a hollow feeling, hearing one's own breathing, and voice reverberation. It does not produce hearing impairment.

The exact cause of an abnormal patent eustachian tube is often difficult to determine. At times it develops following a loss in weight. It may develop during pregnancy, or while taking oral contraceptives or other hormones.

Treatment of this harmless condition is often difficult. A number of different medications are at times successful in alleviating the symptoms. Myringotomy and insertion of a ventilation tube (as described under the surgical treatment of serous otitis media) is often effective.

Palatal Myoclonus

Palatal myoclonus is a rare condition in which muscles of the palate (back of the mouth) twitch rhythmically many times a minute. The cause of this harmless muscle spasm is unknown.

The patient may experience a rhythmic clicking or snapping sound in the ear as the eustachian tube opens and closes. Sedatives or tranquilizers are often effective in controlling the symptoms. No treatment is needed in many cases.

In an occasional case the snapping sound in the ear is caused by simultaneous spasm of the two muscles attached to the middle ear bones. Cutting one or both of these muscles usually relieves the symptoms.

The operation is performed under local anesthesia through the ear canal. Hospitalization is necessary for one night following surgery and the patient may return to his usual activities in a few days.

The Future

Great progress has been made through research in the prevention and treatment of hearing and balance disorders; much still remains to be done—so all may hear.

You can help in achieving this goal by willing your ear bones after death to the House Ear Institute, a non-profit research and education foundation. Your bones will be studied by scientists in various laboratories and compared with your symptoms and findings during life. (The House Ear Institute is affiliated with the University of Southern California School of Medicine.)

When you pledge your ear bones to the Institute you will be joining many others in this research effort. As such you will receive regular mailings from the Institute detailing progress in ear research.

Your doctor (who is associated with the Institute) will be pleased to provide you with further information regarding this vital contribution to ear research.

The Board of Trustees of the Institute would also greatly appreciate your consideration of a bequest in your will to help support the Institute's vital research—so all may hear.

House Ear Institute
2100 West Third Street
Los Angeles, California 90057
(213) 483-4431

Chapter 16

Cholesteatoma:
A Serious Ear Condition

What Is a Cholesteatoma?

A cholesteatoma is a skin growth that occurs in an abnormal location, the middle ear behind the eardrum. It is usually due to repeated infection which causes an ingrowth of the skin of the eardrum. Cholesteatomas often take the form of a cyst or pouch which sheds layers of old skin that builds up inside the ear. Over time, the cholesteatoma can increase in size and destroy the surrounding delicate bones of the middle ear. Hearing loss, dizziness, and facial muscle paralysis are rare but can result from continued cholesteatoma growth.

How Does it Occur?

A cholesteatoma usually occurs because of poor eustachian tube function as well as infection in the middle ear. The eustachian tube conveys air from the back of the nose into the middle ear to equalize ear pressure ("clear the ears"). When the eustachian tubes work poorly, perhaps due to allergy, a cold or sinusitis, the air in the middle ear is absorbed by the body, and a partial vacuum results in the ear. The vacuum pressure sucks in a pouch or sac by stretching the eardrum, especially areas weakened by previous infections. This sac often becomes a cholesteatoma. A rare congenital form of cholesteatoma (one present at birth) can occur in the middle ear and elsewhere, such as in the nearby skull bones. However, the type of cholesteatoma associated with ear infections is most common.

What Are the Symptoms?

Initially, the ear may drain, sometimes with a foul odor. As the cholesteatoma pouch or sac enlarges, it can cause a *full feeling or pressure* in the ear, along with *hearing loss*. (An ache *behind or in* the ear, especially at night, may cause significant discomfort.) Dizziness, or muscle weakness on one side of the face (the side of the infected ear) can also occur. Any, or all, of these symptoms are good reasons to seek medical evaluation.

Is it Dangerous?

Ear cholesteatomas can be dangerous and should never be ignored. Bone erosion can cause the infection to spread into the surrounding areas, including the inner ear and brain. If untreated, deafness, brain abscess, meningitis, and rarely death can occur.

What Treatment Can Be Provided?

An examination by an otolaryngologist–head and neck surgeon can confirm the presence of a cholesteatoma. Initial treatment may consist of a careful cleaning of the ear, antibiotics, and ear drops. Therapy aims to stop drainage in the ear by controlling the infection. The extent or growth characteristics of a cholesteatoma must also be evaluated.

Large or complicated cholesteatomas usually require surgical treatment to protect the patient from serious complications. Hearing and balance tests, x-rays of the mastoid (the skull bone next to the ear), and CAT scans (3-D x-rays) of the mastoid may be necessary. These tests are performed to determine the hearing level remaining in the ear and the extent of destruction the cholesteatoma has caused.

Surgery is performed under general anesthesia in most cases. The primary purpose of the surgery is to remove the cholesteatoma and infection and achieve an infection-free, dry ear. Hearing preservation or restoration is the second goal of surgery. In cases of severe ear destruction, reconstruction may not be possible. Facial nerve repair or procedures to control dizziness are rarely required. Reconstruction of the middle ear is not always possible in one operation; and therefore, a second operation maybe performed six to twelve months later. The second operation will attempt to restore hearing and, at the same time, inspect the middle ear space and mastoid for residual cholesteatoma.

Admission to the hospital is usually done the morning of surgery, and if the surgery is performed early in the morning, discharge may be the same day. For some patients, an overnight stay is necessary. In rare cases of serious infection, prolonged hospitalization for antibiotic treatment may be necessary. Time off from work is typically one to two weeks.

Follow-up office visits after surgical treatment are necessary and important, because cholesteatoma sometimes recurs. In cases where an open mastoidectomy cavity has been created, office visits every few months are needed in order to clean out the mastoid cavity and prevent new infections. In some patients, there must be lifelong periodic ear examinations.

Summary

Cholesteatoma is a serious but treatable ear condition which can only be diagnosed by medical examination. Persisting earache, ear drainage, ear pressure, hearing loss, dizziness, or facial muscle weakness signals the need for evaluation by an otolaryngologist–head and neck surgeon.

Chapter 17

Otosclerosis

Otosclerosis

Your hearing impairment is caused by otosclerosis, a disease of the inner ear bone.

Otosclerosis is a common cause of hearing impairment and is hereditary. Someone in earlier generations of your family had the condition and passed it down to you. Similarly, your descendants may inherit this tendency from you, although the hearing impairment may not manifest itself for a generation or two. Being hereditary, diseases such as scarlet fever, ear infection, and influenza have no relationship to the development of otosclerosis.

Function of the Normal Ear

The ear is divided into three parts: the external ear, the middle ear and the inner ear. The external ear collects sound, the middle ear mechanism transforms the sound and the inner ear receives and transmits the sound.

Sound vibrations enter the ear canal and cause the ear drum membrane to vibrate. Movements of the membrane are transmitted across the middle ear to the inner ear fluids by three small ear bones. These middle ear bones (hammer or malleus, anvil or incus and stirrup or stapes) act as a transformer, changing sound vibrations in air into fluid waves in the inner ear. The fluid waves stimulate delicate nerve endings in the hearing canals. Electrical impulses are transmitted on the nerve to the brain where they are interpreted as understandable sound.

Types of Hearing Impairment

The external ear and the middle ear conduct sound; the inner ear receives it. If there is some difficulty in the external or middle ear, a *conductive* hearing impairment occurs. If the trouble lies in the inner ear, a *sensorineural* or nerve hearing impairment is the result. When there is difficulty in both the middle and the inner ear a *mixed* or combined impairment exists. Mixed impairments are common in otosclerosis.

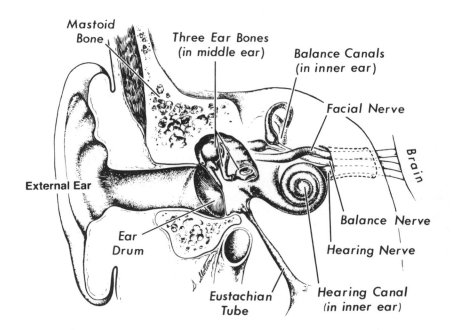

Figure 17.1. *The normal ear.*

Hearing Impairment from Otosclerosis

Had we been able to examine your inner ear bone under a microscope before a hearing impairment developed, we would have seen minute areas of both softening and hardening of the bone. This process may spread to the stapes, the inner ear, or to both these areas.

Cochlear Otosclerosis

When otosclerosis spreads to the inner ear a sensori-neural hearing impairment may result due to interference with the nerve function. This nerve impairment is called *cochlear otosclerosis* and once it develops it is permanent. In selected cases medication may be prescribed in an attempt to prevent further nerve impairment.

On occasion the otosclerosis may spread to the balance canals and may cause episodes of unsteadiness.

Stapedial Otosclerosis

Usually otosclerosis spreads to the stapes or stirrup bone, the final link in the middle ear transformer chain. This stapes rests in a small groove, the oval window, in intimate contact with the inner ear fluids. Anything that interferes with its motion results in a conductive hearing impairment. This type of impairment is called *stapedial otosclerosis* and is usually correctable by surgery.

The amount of hearing loss due to involvement of the stapes and the degree of nerve impairment present can be determined only by careful hearing tests.

Treatment of Otosclerosis

Medical

There is no local treatment to the ear itself or any medication that will improve the hearing in persons with otosclerosis.

In some cases medication may be helpful in preventing further loss of hearing.

Surgical

The stapes operation (stapedectomy) is recommended for patients with otosclerosis who are candidates for surgery. This operation is performed under local anesthesia and requires a short period of

149

hospitalization and convalescence. Over 90 percent of these operations are successful in restoring the hearing permanently.

Your Hearing

Hearing is measured in decibels (dB). A hearing level of 0 to 25 dB is considered normal hearing for conversational purposes.

Table 17.2. Conversion to Degree of Handicap

Hearing	Handicap	Degree
25dB	—	0%
30dB	mild	8%
35dB	mild	15%
45dB	moderate	30%
55dB	moderate	45%
65dB	severe	60%
75dB	severe	75%
85dB	severe	90%

Surgery Recommendations

- You have a minor degree of stapedial otosclerosis. As such we do not advise surgery at this time.

- You have *unilateral* (one ear) otosclerosis. If the stapes operation is successful you will have improved hearing from the involved side, will have less difficulty in determining the direction of sound, and should hear better in difficult listening situations.

- You have good hearing nerve function and are a very suitable candidate for the stapes operation.

- Your hearing nerve has deteriorated slightly. If the stapes operation is successful, serviceable hearing will be restored to you.

- Your hearing nerve has deteriorated to some extent. If the stapes operation is successful, you should be able to hear in many situations without an aid, but may need an aid for distant hearing.

- Your hearing nerve has deteriorated considerably. If the stapes operation is successful, you will gain more benefit from the use of a hearing aid.

- Your hearing nerve has deteriorated severely. For this reason the chances of surgery improving your hearing are reduced. If surgery should prove successful, your hearing should be improved to the extent that you may be able to use a hearing aid.

- Your hearing loss is due to inner ear and nerve involvement. As such, surgery would not be of benefit to you at this time. Many of the operations performed today were not available a few years ago. Through ear research we hope to be able to help sensori-neural (nerve) hearing impairment.

The Stapes Operation (Stapedectomy)

Stapedectomy is performed through the ear canal under local anesthesia. At times an incision may be made above the ear to remove muscle tissue for use in the operation.

Under high power magnification the eardrum membrane is turned forward and the fixed stapes partially or completely removed. The stapes may be removed with instruments, a drill, or in some cases, a laser. A prosthesis is inserted to replace it. The eardrum membrane is then replaced in its normal position.

The stapes prosthesis allows sound vibrations to again pass from the eardrum membrane to the inner ear fluids. The hearing improvement obtained is usually permanent.

The patient may return to work in seven to ten days depending upon occupational requirements. Patients residing outside the Southern California area should plan to remain in Los Angeles for a total of three days including the day of surgery.

One should not plan to drive a car home from the hospital. Air travel is permissible 48 hours following surgery.

Hearing Improvement Following Stapes Surgery

Hearing improvement may or may not be noticeable at surgery. If the hearing improves at the time of surgery, it usually regresses in a few hours due to swelling in the ear. Improvement in hearing may be apparent within 3 weeks of surgery. Maximum hearing, however, is obtained in approximately four months.

151

The degree of hearing improvement depends on how the ear heals. In the majority of patients the ear heals perfectly and hearing improvement is as anticipated. In some the hearing improvement is only partial or temporary. In these cases the ear usually may be reoperated upon with a good chance of success.

In 2 percent of the cases the hearing may be further impaired due to the development of scar tissue, infection, blood vessel spasm, irritation of the inner ear or a leak of inner ear fluid (fistula).

In less than 1 percent, complications in the healing process may be so great that there is severe loss of hearing in the operated ear, to the extent that one may not be able to benefit from a hearing aid in that ear. For this reason the poorer hearing ear is usually selected for surgery.

When further loss of hearing occurs in the operated ear, head noise may be more pronounced. Unsteadiness may persist for some time.

Tinnitus

Most patients with otosclerosis notice tinnitus (head noise) to some degree. The amount of tinnitus is not necessarily related to the degree or type of hearing impairment.

Tinnitus develops due to irritation of the delicate nerve endings in the inner ear. Since the nerve carries sound, this irritation is manifested as ringing, roaring or buzzing. It is usually worse when the patient is fatigued, nervous or in a quiet environment.

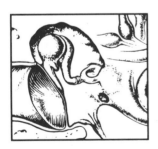 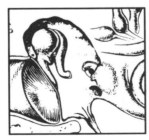 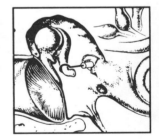

Step 1:
Stapes Otosclerosis

Step 2:
Stapes removed

Step 3:
Prosthesis replacing stapes

Figure 17.3. The Stapes Operation

Following the successful stapedectomy, tinnitus is often decreased in proportion to the hearing improvement.

Risks and Complications of Stapedectomy

Dizziness. Dizziness is normal for a few hours following stapedectomy and may result in nausea and vomiting. Some unsteadiness is common during the first few postoperative days; dizziness on sudden head motion may persist for several weeks. On rare occasions dizziness is prolonged.

Taste Disturbance and Mouth Dryness. Taste disturbance and mouth dryness is not uncommon for a few weeks following surgery. In 5 percent of the patients this disturbance may be prolonged.

Loss of Hearing. Further hearing loss develops in 2 percent of the patients due to some complications in the healing process. In less than 1 percent this hearing loss is severe and may prevent the use of an aid in the operated ear.

Tinnitus. Should the hearing be worse following stapedectomy, tinnitus (head noises) likewise may be more pronounced.

Eardrum Perforation. A perforation (hole) in the eardrum membrane is an unusual complication. It develops in less than 1 percent and usually is due to an infection. Fortunately, should this complication occur, the membrane may heal spontaneously. If healing does not occur, surgical repair (myringoplasty) may be required.

Weakness of the Face. A very rare complication of stapedectomy is temporary weakness of the face. This may occur as the result of an abnormality or swelling of the facial nerve.

Hearing Aids

If you are a suitable candidate for surgery, you are also suitable to benefit from a properly fitted hearing aid. If you have otosclerosis and are not suitable for stapes surgery, you still may benefit from a properly fitted aid.

Fortunately, patients with otosclerosis very seldom go "totally deaf," but will be able to hear with an electronic aid. The older the patient, the less the tendency for further hearing loss due to the otosclerotic process.

Hearing Aid Donation

If you regain hearing through surgery and there is no longer a need for you to wear hearing aids, it would be greatly appreciated if you would donate your hearing aids to the House Ear Clinic, Inc. Donated hearing aids are used as "loaners" for the occasional patient who requires a hearing aid for only a brief time, or who cannot afford to purchase a hearing aid.

Similarly, if one passes away and the Estate no longer has a need for the hearing aids, it would be appreciated if these instruments could be donated to us.

General Comments

If you are a suitable candidate for surgery and do not elect to have the stapes operation at this time, it is advisable to have careful hearing tests repeated at least once a year.

The Future

Great progress has been made through research in the prevention and treatment of hearing and balance disorders; much still remains to be done—so all may hear.

You can help in achieving this goal by willing your ear bones after death to the House Ear Institute, a non-profit research and educational foundation. Your bones will be studied by scientists in various laboratories and compared with your symptoms and findings during life. (The House Ear Institute is affiliated with the University of Southern California School of Medicine.)

When you pledge your ear bones to the Institute you will be joining many others in this research effort. As such you will receive regular mailings from the Institute detailing progress in ear research.

Your doctor (who is associated with the Institute) will be pleased to provide you with further information regarding this vital contribution to ear research.

The Board of Trustees of the Institute would also greatly appreciate your consideration of a bequest in your will to help support the Institute's vital research—so all may hear.

House Ear Institute
2100 West Third Street
Los Angeles, CA 90057
Telephone: (213) 483-443; TDD: (213) 484-2642

154

Chapter 18

Acoustic Neuromas

Acoustic Tumor

The diagnosis of a cerebellopontine angle tumor has been made. Most likely this is an acoustic tumor and is the probable cause of your symptoms.

General Comments

Acoustic tumors are non-malignant fibrous growths, originating from the balance or hearing nerve, that do not spread (metastasize) to other parts of the body. They constitute six to ten percent of all brain tumors.

These growths are located deep inside the skull and are adjacent to vital brain centers. The first signs or symptoms one notices usually are related to ear function and include ear noise and disturbances in hearing and balance. As the tumors enlarge, they involve other surrounding nerves having to do with more vital functions. Headache may develop as a result of increased pressure on the brain. If allowed to continue over a long period of time, this pressure on the brain is ultimately fatal.

In most cases these tumors grow slowly over a period of years. In others, the rate of growth is more rapid. In some, the symptoms are mild, and in others, severe, multiple symptoms develop rather rapidly.

Great care is exerted before, during and after surgery in these cases in order to preserve life. The preservation of life is the most important objective of surgery in these most difficult cases. A secondary objective of surgery is to preserve for future life as many vital structures as possible. For many, a completely normal life results following surgery. Some patients experience minimum physical handicap and for a few patients even maximum degrees of physical handicap may persist.

To accomplish the preservation of life with a minimum of future physical disturbance, this surgery with pre and post operative care is performed and assisted by a team. This team includes an internist, an anesthesiologist, a specially trained surgical nurse, a neurosurgeon and an otologist (ear specialist). The neurosurgeon is co-surgeon with the otologist.

Size of Tumor

Risks and complications of acoustic tumor surgery vary with the size of the tumor: The larger the tumor, the more serious the complications, and the more likelihood of complications.

The removal of an acoustic tumor, whether large or small, is a major surgical procedure, with possibilities of serious complications, including death. The risk involved in the removal of these tumors must never be minimized.

Small Tumor

A small acoustic tumor is still confined within the bony canal that extends from the inner ear to the brain. Through this canal pass the hearing, balance and facial nerves and the blood vessels which supply the inner ear.

Medium Tumor

A medium sized acoustic tumor is one which has extended from the bony canal into the brain cavity but has not yet produced pressure on the brain itself.

Large Tumor

A large acoustic tumor is one which has extended out of the bony canal into the brain cavity and is sufficiently large to produce pressure on the brain.

156

Surgical Approaches

The choice of surgical approach depends upon the size of the tumor and level of residual hearing. It is possible to save hearing in only a minority of cases; if hearing preservation is successful, the preserved hearing is not better than the preoperative level and may be worse. The larger the tumor, the lower the chances for hearing preservation. In some cases with poor preoperative hearing or large tumor, it is better to sacrifice the hearing in order to remove the tumor. All procedures are performed under general anesthesia.

Translabyrinthine approach. This involves an incision behind the ear. The mastoid and inner ear structures are removed to expose the tumor. The tumor is totally removed. Rarely, only partial removal is accomplished. The mastoid defect is closed with fat taken from the abdomen.

The translabyrinthine approach sacrifices the hearing and balance mechanism of the inner ear. Consequently the ear is made permanently deaf. Although the balance mechanism has been removed on the operated ear, the balance mechanism in the opposite ear usually provides stabilization for the patient in one to four months.

Middle fossa approach. An incision is made above the ear, and the brain is elevated to expose the tumor. The tumor is totally removed in most cases. Every effort is made to preserve the hearing and still remove the tumor. In some cases it is necessary to sacrifice the hearing to achieve tumor removal. In about 50% of cases, the tumor involves the hearing nerve or the artery leading to the inner ear and total loss of hearing results in the operated ear.

Retrosigmoid approach. An incision is made behind the ear and the brain is elevated to expose the tumor. The tumor is totally removed in most cases. Every effort is made to preserve the hearing and still remove the tumor. In some cases it is necessary to sacrifice the hearing to achieve tumor removal. In about 50% of cases, the tumor involves the hearing nerve or the artery leading to the inner ear and total loss of hearing results in the operated ear.

Following this approach, some patients may experience persistent headaches.

Partial vs. Total Removal of an Acoustic Tumor

Total removal of an acoustic tumor, without complications, is the goal of the management of these tumors.

Partial removal of the tumor, regardless of its size, may be necessary if the patient's responses during surgery indicate disturbance of the vital brain centers that control respiration, blood pressure, or heart function. If signs of vital brain center disturbance develop during surgery, it is sometimes necessary to terminate the operation before the tumor can be totally removed. This will often allow these vital brain center functions to be restored. Once they are disturbed, however, they sometimes do not recover.

If premature termination of the operation is necessary in the judgment of the operating surgeons, the remaining portion of the tumor may gradually enlarge to again produce symptoms. In this event, a subsequent operation might be necessary. This subsequent operation can often be then accomplished without significant changes in vital signs.

In the event your tumor is partially removed, you will be so informed. Usually the first operation reduces the size of the tumor sufficiently so that it has a chance to separate away from the vital brain centers and it can, therefore, be successfully removed at a later date. In most cases we wait four to six months and then electively operate again for tumor removal.

In other cases, a course of continued observation is resorted to. In this instance the tumor will be evaluated from time to time for possible regrowth and accordingly a decision made regarding its removal.

Radiation Therapy

Since acoustic tumors are benign growths, we do not routinely advise radiation treatment. Radiation therapy is not risk-free and does not result in disappearance of the tumor. Hearing loss, facial paralysis, and serious complications have also occurred after radiation therapy. After this treatment, some patients have experienced continued tumor growth and have required surgical removal, which is much more difficult due to the effects of the radiation.

Hearing Impairment Following Surgery

Following acoustic tumor surgery the patient is sometimes deaf in the operated ear. When the hearing has deteriorated prior to surgery, the patient has already become aware of problems: the location or direction of sound; hearing a person on the deaf side; and, the major problem, understanding speech in difficult listening situations.

The patient must learn to watch a speaker carefully in difficult listening situations, using their eyes to help the brain understand words which may sound very much the same, but appear different on the lips. (Example: pope, coke, soap, dope, cope.) Considerable help also may be obtained with a contralateral routing of sound (CROS) aid.

The CROS aid is an instrument that receives sound on the deaf side, amplifies it, then routes it to the good hearing ear. A small aid is worn on each ear. Although not everyone will find this type of amplification system helpful, with sufficient need and motivation, the patient will usually realize improved hearing performance with a CROS aid.

Risks and Complications of Acoustic Tumor Surgery

It is not possible to list every complication that might occur before, during or following a surgical procedure. The following discussion is included to indicate some of the risks and complications peculiar to acoustic tumor surgery.

In general, the smaller the tumor at the time of surgery, the less chance of complications. As the tumor enlarges the incidence of complication becomes increasingly greater.

Hearing Loss

In small tumors it is sometimes possible to save the hearing by removing the tumor. Most tumors are larger, however, and the hearing is lost in the involved ear as a result of the surgical procedure. Following surgery, therefore, the patient hears only with the remaining good ear.

Tinnitus

Tinnitus (ear noise) remains the same as before surgery in most cases. In 10% of the patients the tinnitus may be more noticeable.

Taste Disturbance and Mouth Dryness

Taste disturbance and mouth dryness is not uncommon for a few weeks following surgery. In 5 % of patients this disturbance is prolonged.

Dizziness and Balance Disturbance

In acoustic tumor surgery it is necessary to remove part or all of the balance nerve and, in most cases to remove the inner ear balance mechanism. Because the tumor usually damages the balance system, tumor removal frequently results in improvement in any preoperative unsteadiness. Dizziness is common following surgery and may be severe for a few days. Imbalance or unsteadiness on head motion is prolonged until the normal balance mechanism in the opposite ear compensates for the loss in the operated ear, usually in one to four months. A few patients may notice unsteadiness for several years, especially when they are fatigued.

Occasionally the blood supply to the portion of the brain responsible for coordination (cerebellum) is decreased by the tumor or the removal of the tumor. Difficulty in coordination in arm and leg movements (ataxia) may result. This complication is extremely rare.

Facial Paralysis

Acoustic tumors are in intimate contact with the facial nerve which closes the eye as well as controlling the muscles of the facial expression. Temporary paralysis of the facial nerve is common following removal of an acoustic tumor. Weakness may persist for six to twelve months. A few patients experience permanent residual weakness.

Facial paralysis may result from nerve swelling or nerve damage. Swelling of the facial nerve is common due to the fact that the nerve is usually compressed and distorted by the tumor in the internal auditory canal. Careful tumor removal, with the help of an operating microscope and facial nerve monitoring, usually results in preservation of the nerve. However, nerve stretching may result in swelling of the nerve with subsequent temporary paralysis. In these instances facial function is observed for a period of months following surgery. If it becomes certain that facial nerve function will not recover (approximately 5% of cases), a second operation may be performed to connect the facial tissue to a nerve in the neck (facial-hypoglossal anastomosis).

In 5 % of cases the facial nerve passes through the interior of the acoustic tumor. On occasion the tumor may even originate from the facial nerve (facial nerve neuroma). In either instance it is necessary to remove all or a portion of the nerve to accomplish tumor removal. When this is necessary it may be possible to immediately reconnect the facial nerve or to remove a skin sensation nerve from the upper part of the neck to replace the missing portion of the facial nerve.

When it is not possible to reconnect or replace the facial nerve, a second operation may be performed, at a later time, to reanimate the face. One option is a facial-hypoglossal anastomosis, connecting the nerve in the neck to the facial nerve. Another option is called the facial reanimation operation. The temporalis muscle (one of the chewing muscles) is attached to the muscles of the face to help move them.

Eye Complications

Should facial paralysis develop the eye may become dry and unprotected. Care by an eye specialist may be indicated. It may be necessary to apply artificial tears, to tape the eye shut, even to sew the eyelid closed. When prolonged facial nerve paralysis is expected an eye specialist may insert a spring eyelid closing device. This keeps the eye moistened as well as providing comfort and improved appearance.

Other Nerve Weaknesses

In the rare case, acoustic tumors may contact the nerves which supply the eye muscles, the face, the mouth and throat. These areas may be injured with resultant double vision, numbness of the throat, face and tongue, weakness of the shoulder, weakness of the voice and difficulty swallowing. These problems may be permanent.

Postoperative Headache

Headache following acoustic tumor removal is common in the early postoperative period. In some cases, headache may be prolonged.

Brain Complications and Death

Acoustic tumors are located adjacent to vital brain centers which control breathing, blood pressure and heart function. As the tumor enlarges it may become attached to these brain centers and usually becomes intertwined with the blood vessels supplying these areas of the brain.

Careful tumor dissection, with the help of an operating microscope, usually avoids complications. If the blood supply to vital brain centers is disturbed serious complications may result: loss of muscle control, paralysis, even death. In our experience death occurs rarely as the result of acoustic tumor removal.

Postoperative Spinal Fluid Leak

Acoustic tumor surgery results in a temporary leak of cerebral spinal fluid (fluid surrounding the brain). This leak is closed prior to the completion of surgery with fat removed from the abdomen. Occasionally this leak reopens and further surgery may be necessary to close it.

Postoperative Bleeding and Brain Swelling

Bleeding and brain swelling may develop after acoustic tumor surgery. If this occurs a subsequent operation may be necessary to reopen the wound to arrest bleeding and allow the brain to expand. This complication can result in paralysis or death.

Postoperative Infection

Infection occurs in less than 10% of the patients following surgery. This infection is usually in the form of meningitis, an infection of the fluid and tissue surrounding the brain.

When this complication occurs, hospitalization is prolonged. Treatment with high doses of antibiotics is often indicated. Complications from antibiotic treatment are rare.

Transfusion Reaction

It may be necessary to administer blood transfusions during acoustic tumor surgery. Immediate adverse reactions to transfusion are uncommon. A late complication of transfusion is viral infections. In most cases, a unit of the patient's own blood can be stored before surgery for later use.

Concluding Remarks

The standard treatment for acoustic tumors is surgical removal. The earlier they are diagnosed and removed, the less likely the possibility of serious complications.

Many patients have unilateral hearing loss, head noise, and balance difficulties. Rarely are these symptoms due to an acoustic tumor. Unfortunately, a very careful check of all patients with these symptoms does not always result in an early diagnosis of acoustic tumors. In some cases the tumor becomes relatively large before a definite diagnosis can be established. The problem must be faced as it exists at the time of diagnosis and acceptance made of whatever risks are necessary to remove these tumors. The risks of surgery are less than the risk of leaving the tumor untreated.

The statements made in this chapter are based on our personal experiences in managing a large series of acoustic tumor cases. If you have any questions about yourself and a possible acoustic tumor, please discuss them with your otologist. We can provide a list of Institute colleagues in your area upon request.

Feel free to consult a second otologist or neurotologist regarding your situation. If you are a patient of the House Ear Clinic your records can be sent to any consultant you desire.

Acoustic Neuroma Association

To provide support and information for patients who have acoustic neuromas and to offer therapeutic support to patients with tumor-related disabilities. These are the purposes of the Acoustic Neuroma Association, Inc., P.O. Box 398, Carlisle, Pennsylvania 17103.

In Canada write to P.O. Box 369, Edmonton, Alberta, Canada T5J 2V6.

Chapter 19

Information about Tinnitus

Common Questions and Facts about Tinnitus

What Is It?

Tinnitus is a subjective experience where one hears a sound when no external physical sound is present. Some call it "head noises," "ear-ringing," or use similar terms to describe it.

What Does the Word Tinnitus Mean?

The word is of Latin origin and it means "to tinkle or to ring like a bell." It has two pronunciations, both correct: "ti-night-us" or "tin-ni-tus."

What Causes It?

There are many causes; indeed almost everything that can go wrong with the ear has tinnitus associated with it as a symptom.

The chapter contains excerpts from the following publications of the American Tinnitus Association (ATA): "Information about Tinnitus" (© ATA 1994), "Tinnitus Family Information" (© ATA 1994), "If You Have Tinnitus The First Steps to Take" (© ATA 1996), "Coping with the Stress of Tinnitus" (© ATA 1994) and "Noise: Its Effects on Hearing and Tinnitus" (© ATA 1996); reprinted with permission of the American Tinnitus Association, P.O. Box 5, Portland, OR 97207-0005, (503) 248-9985. This chapter also contains information about additional resources on tinnitus from the Deafness and Other Communication Disorders subfile of the Combined Health Information Database (CHID).

Problems ranging in severity from overproduction of wax, to ear infections, to acoustic tumors can produce tinnitus. One of the most common causes of tinnitus is exposure to excessively loud sounds either on the job (musicians, carpenters, pilots) or recreationally (shooting, chain saws, loud music). Sometimes problems not associated with the ear can cause tinnitus such as disorders of the cervical vertebrae (neck) or the temporomandibular (jaw) joint. Tinnitus can also be caused by cardiovascular disease, allergies, an underactive thyroid, or degeneration of the bones in the middle ear. It's important to note that more than 200 prescription and non-prescription drugs list tinnitus as a potential side effect.

Do Many People Suffer from Tinnitus?

Yes. It is currently estimated that 50 million American adults have tinnitus to some degree. Of that number, 12 million have it severely enough to seek medical help. During an average year, patients with severe tinnitus may spend more money seeking help and treatment for their tinnitus than they do for all of their other health conditions. Some patients, however, seek no treatment in the mistaken belief that nothing can be done to help them.

What Is It Like to Have Tinnitus?

Fortunately, for most people their tinnitus is no more than a nuisance. In its severe form, however, tinnitus can be a chronic condition causing loss of concentration, sleep problems, and psychological distress. It can also make a deteriorating hearing condition or balance disorder appear worse. Tinnitus can fluctuate from day to day, and even from hour to hour.

Do We Know What Tinnitus Is?

The actual mechanism responsible for tinnitus is not yet known. We do know that it is a real—not imagined—symptom of something that has gone wrong in the auditory or neural system. There is reason to be hopeful; current research efforts using a physiological model may soon provide the necessary information for identifying its cause(s).

Is It Associated with Hearing Loss?

In most cases, tinnitus is associated with some hearing loss. For example, those who have been exposed to excessively loud sounds may have a high frequency hearing loss. Usually their tinnitus will be identified as a high pitched tone in the region of the hearing loss. Tinnitus can be perceived as being in the ears or in or around the head, and can have one or a variety of different sounds such as ringing, hissing, or roaring. In some cases tinnitus is present where there is no loss of hearing.

Does Tinnitus Mean That One Is Going Deaf?

No, tinnitus is an indication that there has been some kind of damage to the hearing mechanism, but it does not mean the patient will become deaf. Tinnitus does not cause hearing loss, and hearing loss does not cause tinnitus, although the two often exist together.

What Is Super-Sensitivity to Sound?

A small percentage of tinnitus patients also experience an acute sensitivity to sound. This tolerance problem is exhibited both in individuals who have hearing loss (recruitment) and patients who have normal or near-normal hearing (hyperacusis). Although this problem is difficult to manage, some relief can occur through the reasonable use of ear protection and/or by carefully presenting a broad band noise at a very low level and slowly increasing the level of noise thus making the ears less sensitive to environmental sounds. The Hyperacusis Support Network can provide practical information about this disorder. [The American Tinnitus Association can provide you with information about the Hyperacusis Support Network. You may also wish to consult Chapter 23 in this volume.]

What Makes Tinnitus Worse?

1. **Loud Noise.** Tinnitus patients should avoid loud sounds and protect their ears at all costs! Power tools, guns, motorcycles, noisy vacuum cleaners, etc. should be used only with ear protection—ear plugs and/or ear muffs.

2. Excessive use of **alcohol** or so-called recreational **drugs** has been found to exacerbate tinnitus in some individuals.

3. **Caffeine**, found in coffee, tea, chocolate, and cola drinks, can also increase tinnitus.

4. **Nicotine.** The vascular effects of nicotine are associated with an increase in tinnitus.

5. **Aspirin, Quinine,** some antibiotics, and hundreds of other drugs are causative tinnitus agents and can make existing tinnitus worse. If you are prescribed medication, always inform your physician of your tinnitus and discuss the drug options. A substitute medication or dosage may be available that won't affect your tinnitus. ATA can provide you and your physician with information regarding drugs that affect tinnitus.

6. **Stress.** Many people notice a reduction in the volume of their tinnitus when they are able to control their stress levels.

What Should a Tinnitus Patient Do?

Initially each tinnitus sufferer should be examined by an otologist or an otolaryngologist. The purpose of the examination is to determine if there is a medical condition causing tinnitus for which treatment could be prescribed. If that is not the case, patients might then consider nonmedical treatments such as masking or relaxation therapies for relief.

It is important to remember that a natural remission can occur, perhaps coinciding with the start of a new treatment or spontaneously with no treatment at all.

What Treatments Are Available for Tinnitus?

Several forms of treatment are currently available and several other experimental approaches hold promise for the future. These include:

1. **Amplification.** The use of hearing aids can reduce or even eliminate some forms of tinnitus. If a patient has a hearing loss and the tinnitus is in the medium or low pitches, often a hearing aid will help. The hearing aid renders the patient capable of hearing ambient environmental noises instead of the tinnitus.

2. **Masking.** Since 1977 tinnitus maskers have been used to relieve tinnitus. These units, resembling hearing aids, present a selected band of noise to the patient's ear. This external masking sound is perceived as a more pleasant sound than the internal tinnitus sound. A "tinnitus instrument" is a combination unit that includes both a hearing aid and a masker. Sometimes effective masking can be produced by the use of bedside maskers, commercial and custom-made audio tapes and even FM radio static. Masking will work for some patients, but it is

impossible to predict in advance of testing and trial which patients can be helped with this treatment. Masking does not seem to damage hearing when used over long periods of time. Residual inhibition is a term that refers to a continued masking effect after the masking noise is removed. The period of residual inhibition is usually very short, often less than a minute.

3. **Biofeedback.** Biofeedback is a relaxation process that has been very successful in the control of tension headaches. It is also effective in teaching one how to handle or cope with stress. Since stress seems to worsen tinnitus, being able to control stress and tension can be very helpful in coping with tinnitus.

4. **Drug Therapy.** Many drugs have been investigated as possible relief agents for tinnitus. These drugs have included anticonvulsant drugs, tranquilizers, antianxiety drugs, and antihistamines. For some patients, these drugs are partially effective in helping them cope with the tinnitus. It is also well established that Lidocaine will offer complete or partial relief for a large number of patients. However, because this drug must be administered intravenously and its effect is not long lasting, it is not a drug of choice for treating this symptom. Research continues in an attempt to identify a drug that can be administered orally and have a comparable effect to Lidocaine without serious side effects.

5. **Auditory Habituation.** Auditory habituation is a new technique designed to retrain the auditory system to ignore the tinnitus sounds. Therapeutic noise devices that emit stable "broad band noise"—quieter than a patient's tinnitus—are used in this treatment. The recommended course of treatment can be more than a year.

6. **Dental Treatment.** Dental treatments for temporomandibular jaw joint (TMJ) problems associated with tinnitus have been effective for some who suffer from this dual problem. Symptoms of damage to this joint, which is located just below the ear, include tinnitus, jaw clicking, and ear pain.

7. **Counseling.** Counseling, behavioral modeling, cognitive therapy, patient education, and support groups have all been shown to be useful for many patients who are having trouble coping with tinnitus.

8. **Cochlear Implants.** Currently these implants are meant for people with no usable hearing. Some of these patients report improvement in their tinnitus. Research is ongoing to determine whether a type of implanted stimulus can be devised that will be safe and effective for people with normal hearing and tinnitus.

9. **Electrical Stimulation.** Electrical stimulation is an experimental therapy involving electrical energy transmitted to the cochlea via electrodes placed near the ears. While a degree of success has been noted, some patients have reported a worsening of their tinnitus with this therapy.

10. **Other.** Additionally, some patients have found help through hypnosis, acupuncture, myotherapy, chiropractic care, naturopathic treatments, and control of allergies.

Is There an Operation for Tinnitus?

Patients sometimes report that following successful surgical treatment for ear pathologies their tinnitus will also disappear. Consequently, many patients inquire about the possibility of having the hearing nerve severed to eliminate tinnitus. This surgical procedure has not proven successful. In fact, destruction of the hearing mechanism most often leaves tinnitus still present.

Tinnitus Information for Family Members

Is Tinnitus a Common Problem?

Millions of people have tinnitus: Approximately 20% of the population experiences tinnitus at some time in their lives. Tinnitus is the perception of sound when there is none present. Although its occurrence is common, it is uncommon for most people to know the condition by name, and it is even more uncommon for people to understand how it affects those who have it. For some it is just a nuisance; for others it is a stressful, life-altering condition.

What Is It Like to Have Tinnitus?

Tinnitus, often described as "ringing in the ears," varies tremendously from person to person. Some people hear hissing, buzzing, or the sound of steam escaping from a radiator. Some hear one tone; others hear several tones. Those who do not have tinnitus can imagine what it's like by thinking of an emergency broadcast signal, the high-pitched 60-second tone often heard on the radio or television. People with tinnitus hear noises similar to that tone 24 hours every day!

How Does a Person with Tinnitus Feel?

At the onset of tinnitus, many people are worried and perhaps frightened, especially if they've never heard of tinnitus or known anyone who's mentioned it. Imagine having to explain that you're hearing something that no one else hears! It's natural to worry that others might think you're imagining things. Many people with tinnitus ask themselves: Do other people have this? How will I explain this to my family and friends? Will anyone understand? Will it go away? What if it gets worse? Will I lose my hearing? How can I sleep with all this noise? How can I work? Do other people feel this way? How do they deal with this?

These thoughts can be especially troublesome when the tinnitus is quite new. It usually helps tremendously for the person experiencing these fears to get a factual explanation from a qualified hearing professional. Questions that deal with inner thoughts and fears, on the other hand, might be better answered by someone with tinnitus, who has experienced the same type of feelings and has learned to deal with them.

Do Certain Things Make Tinnitus Worse?

Yes! The way the ear and tinnitus react to different situations varies greatly from person to person, but everyone should be aware of the following:

1. **Over-exposure to noise** can cause and worsen tinnitus and hearing loss. It is very important, especially if one already has tinnitus, to avoid or reduce further exposure. When around noise or anticipating a noisy event, always carry and use proper ear protection (ear plugs or muffs). Remember the potential danger of noise from common sources such as lawnmowers, stereos, hair dryers, chain saws, motorcycles, concerts, movies, and noise on the job.

2. **Certain medications.** Many drugs are ototoxic—damaging to the ear—and can make tinnitus worse. Consequently, tinnitus patients should tell all of their physicians (not just their ENTs) about their condition and about any prescription or OTC medications they are taking.

171

3. **Alcohol/Nicotine/Caffeine** can exacerbate tinnitus. Some tinnitus patients also I find that their tinnitus is made worse by consuming certain foods. (Cheese, salt, and red wine have been mentioned.) To determine if a particular food or substance causes an allergic reaction, it is suggested that the food or substance in question be avoided for one month then slowly reintroduced into the diet or daily routine. Any worsening of the tinnitus would be noticeable after reintroduction and could be noted in a journal for future reference.

4. **Stress.** Tinnitus causes stress; stress causes tinnitus: it can be a vicious cycle. Anything you can do to reduce stress will help break the cycle. Relaxation therapies such as yoga, meditation, and exercise can be useful.

How Can the Family Help?

- Try to empathize, not by offering sympathy but by being understanding. Tinnitus can be very distracting and irritating, and may affect a person's mood and ability to concentrate or sleep.

- Acknowledge the tinnitus as a valid condition—invisible to you but real to the people who have it.

- Remember that it is often hard to hear over the tinnitus, and parts of conversations may be lost or misunderstood. Be patient.

- Learn as much as possible about tinnitus. Not only will it help you understand the condition, but it will show the person with tinnitus that you care and are interested in helping.

- Explain tinnitus to other family members, friends, and coworkers, so that they can also understand and help.

- Learn to recognize and avoid those things that aggravate your affected family member's tinnitus. Respect that people with tinnitus must avoid exposure to loud noise, and be understanding when invitations to events are refused.

- Work in your community to reduce involuntary exposure to loud noise. Blasting speakers from open automobiles or "boom boxes" carried in public can and should be outlawed. (Young people are losing their hearing in epidemic proportions due to these and other excessive noise exposure choices.)

- Minimize needless noise in your home.

- Foster involvement in a self-help group for your affected family member and yourself. A tinnitus support group is a safe haven to air concerns and learn coping skills that can benefit everyone. Tinnitus patients and their families offer the kind of understanding that only this shared experience can inspire. Support groups, telephone contacts, and pen pals comprise ATA's nationwide network of available and helpful volunteers. ATA offers materials and on-going assistance to all of its support network participants. For information on joining the network, write to ATA for a Self-Help Packet.

- Finally, it might be helpful to hear sounds like those your family member hears. ATA has a short cassette tape available that presents some "sounds of tinnitus." An audiologist might also be able to produce the sounds for you.

What Is Being Done to Fight Tinnitus?

ATA provides information about tinnitus to patients, health professionals, and the general public through its magazine, *Tinnitus Today* and various brochures, announcements, and professional seminars. ATA has a nationwide network of hearing health professionals who take a special interest in treating tinnitus patients. Most importantly, ATA sponsors tinnitus research for better treatments and ultimately a cure. Additional research projects are sponsored by the National Institute on Deafness and other Communication Disorders (NIDCD), and various private foundations.

How Can You Fight Tinnitus?

You can become a member of ATA! Your annual contribution will help support tinnitus research and education. It will also bring you the quarterly magazine *Tinnitus Today*, which contains the latest information on research projects and technologies for tinnitus relief. Write to ATA for membership details and additional benefits.

Noise and Its Effects on Hearing and Tinnitus

What Is Noise?

Noise is, by definition, unwanted sound. It varies in its composition in terms of frequency, intensity and duration. Sounds that are pleasing to some people may be unpleasant to others. For example, loud rock music is enjoyable to some, but others find it offensive. Thus, for a sound to be categorized as noise, it must be judged as such by the listener.

Protect Your Ears from Noise!

Many of the sounds in our environment that we classify as noise are annoying but not loud enough to cause damage to our hearing. Other sounds, however, are of such high intensity that they are dangerous to the ear and may cause permanent hearing loss and/or tinnitus. Noise is everywhere and we cannot always escape being exposed to it. When noise exposure can't be avoided, protective measures can be taken to limit or possibly prevent ear damage.

Noise-Induced Hearing Loss

Continuous exposure to high levels of noise can cause hearing impairment in some individuals. There is considerable variation from person to person regarding susceptibility to noise. However, standards have been established that indicate how much sound an average person can tolerate without experiencing damage to their hearing. Although this level remains somewhat controversial, it has been established that most people will not experience a hearing loss if the noise levels do not exceed 85 to 90dBA. Therefore, the Occupational

Table 19.1. Permissible Noise Exposures

Duration per Day (hours)	Noise level (dBA)
8	90
6	92
4	95
3	97
2	100
1½	102
1	105
3/4	107
½	110
¼ or less	115

Safety and Health Act (OSHA) established criteria based upon an 8-hour duration of exposure to a 90dBA level of continuous noise. It was felt that this criteria would protect approximately 90% of the people exposed to 90dBA levels for a significant part of their lifetime. For shorter durations of exposure, higher noise levels are permissible under this regulation. There are no published noise levels that are known to specifically induce tinnitus.

Danger! Noise Can Hurt You

Many sounds in our environment exceed the OSHA standards and continuous exposure to these sounds could cause loss of hearing. The difference in decibel levels is greater than might be expected: one

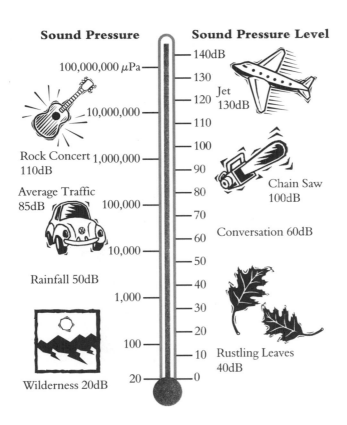

Figure 19.2. Common noise sources.

hundred times more sound energy enters the ear in a 95dB environment than in a 75dB environment. A sample of common noise sources is shown in Figure 19.2 along with their approximate sound pressure levels.

The typical hearing loss observed with patients who have a long history of on-the-job noise exposure is characterized by a loss of hearing in the frequency range between 3000 and 6000 Hz (see Figure 19.3). In the early stages of exposure, a temporary loss will be observed at the end of a working period but will disappear after several hours. Continuous exposure to the noise will result in a permanent hearing loss that will be progressive in nature and become subjectively noticeable to the employee over time. These changes in hearing thresholds can be monitored through audiometric testing and will alert clinicians that preventive measures should be initiated. In its advanced stages, a loss of hearing in the high frequencies will seriously affect the person's ability to understand normal speech. In general, patients with hearing losses limited to the high frequencies will not experience difficulty detecting speech, but will have trouble understanding it.

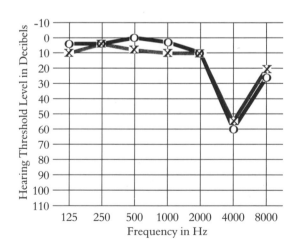

Figure 19.3. *Typical audiogram of a patient with noise-induced hearing loss. (Note: Hz = Hertz, a unit of frequency equal to one cycle per second.)*

176

Noise-Induced Tinnitus

Tinnitus, a ringing or other noise in the ears or head, is most often a subjective experience. It can be intermittent or constant; mildly annoying or, for some, very distressing. Although the exact cause of tinnitus is unknown, many patients who have a history of noise exposure have tinnitus. Noise is by far the most probable cause of tinnitus, and it may or may not occur simultaneously with hearing loss. Most patients who have tinnitus also have hearing problems, but a small percentage (fewer than 10%) have hearing within normal limits. Many patients have hearing losses without tinnitus. (It is reasonable to assume that any symptom associated with ear pathologies—hearing loss, tinnitus, sound sensitivity, dizziness, pain, or a feeling of fullness in the ear—could occur individually or without other symptoms.)

Tinnitus, as a result of noise exposure, can occur suddenly or very gradually. When it occurs suddenly, it is often perceived at a fairly loud volume and may persist at that level permanently. However, for some, the tinnitus is temporary and does not return.

More commonly, the onset of noise-induced tinnitus is gradual and intermittent in its early stages. Patients report hearing a mild form of tinnitus for a short period of time following a lengthy exposure to loud sounds. Once the patient is removed from the noise source, the tinnitus soon disappears and is inaudible until the next exposure. This intermittent pattern often continues for months or years with the periods of tinnitus becoming longer and longer. Eventually the tinnitus is constant. If exposure to the offending noise continues, the tinnitus often increases in volume.

Most patients who have a long history of noise exposure complain of tinnitus that is tonal in quality and high-pitched. Of 153 clinic patients with noise-induced tinnitus, 141 or 92.2% matched their tinnitus to external tones above 3000 Hz.

Hearing Conservation Program—What You Can Do

1. Avoid noise whenever possible.
2. Use personal hearing protection (ear plugs, ear muffs) when the noise is unavoidable.
3. Reduce the amount of time you are exposed to the noise.
4. Reduce the noise at its source.

OSHA has mandated that Hearing Conservation Programs be initiated if noise levels exceed 85dBA. Many companies have developed programs within those guidelines but others have not. Furthermore, due to differences in susceptibility to noise, some people may develop hearing loss and/or tinnitus from noise levels below 85dBA. It is important for people who observe a mild loss of hearing or the presence of tinnitus to take the initiative to implement a hearing conservation program for themselves. Personal hearing protective devices are available from safety equipment suppliers and also from hearing product distributors. These devices come in many different forms and are reasonably priced. If used properly, they can help safeguard the ears against further damage.

How Tinnitus Affects You

It is common for tinnitus patients to observe an exacerbation of their tinnitus whenever they are exposed to noise. Because of this, many people with tinnitus report they can no longer attend functions known to be noisy, such as concerts (all kinds), dances, parties, and sporting events. They sometimes need to avoid the use of motorcycles, speedboats, airplanes, trucks, buses, and sports cars. They may not be able to use lawn mowers, chain saws, vacuum cleaners, food processors, electrical tools, and firearms. Some tinnitus sufferers have even had to quit or change jobs because of work-related noise. Shortly after being removed from the noise, tinnitus patients usually notice that their tinnitus has returned to its original level.

Other Health Consequences of Noise Exposure

Noise is known to have harmful effects on more than just hearing. It can stress our circulatory, respiratory, and digestive systems as well. Continued exposure to noise may cause headaches, fatigue, and elevated blood pressure. Noise has also been shown to interfere with children's learning and even to affect an unborn child.

Whenever you contribute to the reduction of noise in your environment, every part of you and everyone around you will benefit.

If You Have Tinnitus: The First Steps to Take

An estimated 12 million Americans have severe tinnitus, a chronic ringing or other distressing noise in the ears or head. Although there is no cure, there are treatments that can help. Many people with tinnitus are unaware that useful treatments exist.

If you are interested in a treatment program but are uncertain how to access appropriate care, the following steps can help you through the process.

Step #1: Take Note of the Details Surrounding the Onset of Your Tinnitus

Were you using a new medication when it first began? Were you injured or exposed to excessive noise right before it started? Is the tinnitus in one ear, both ears, or perceived to be somewhere in the head? Does it fluctuate or is it constant in tone? Do you have a hearing loss?

These are valuable pieces of information that can potentially lead your health care provider to a solution and you to relief.

Step #2: Visit a Medical Doctor

There are several physiological causes of tinnitus—such as high blood pressure, an underactive thyroid, excessive ear wax, and in rare cases a tumor on the auditory nerve. Control of these medical problems can bring tinnitus relief.

Many people choose to see an ear, nose, and throat specialist, also referred to as an ENT or otolaryngologist. An otologist is an ears-only specialist. ENTs or otologists can perform medical tests; screen for allergies, Meniere's syndrome, or any pathology (disease or malformation); perform surgery; and prescribe drugs. In certain situations, doctors might order neurological tests (i.e. MRI or CAT scans). When a pathological cause of tinnitus is ruled out, some medical doctors refer patients to audiologists for additional tinnitus evaluation and treatment.

Step #3: Have Your Hearing Checked

An audiologist is a hearing specialist with advanced degrees—always a Master's, often a doctorate, and usually a CCC–A (Clinical Certificate of Competency–Audiology). Audiologists can perform all audiological tests and hearing evaluations. They can also, if licensed, dispense hearing aids (that can amplify everyday sounds to cover or "mask" the tinnitus), tinnitus "maskers" (hearing aid-like devices that produce a more pleasant sound than the patient's tinnitus), and tinnitus instruments (combination units that include both maskers and hearing aids). Some audiologists offer counseling, relaxation strategies, biofeedback, and a tinnitus perception retraining therapy called "auditory habituation" which uses ear-level noise generators to help in this process.

Both medical doctors and audiologists can perform diagnostic tests—such as auditory brainstem response (ABR), electrocochleography

(ECoG), electronystagmography (ENG), and a test for otoacoustic emissions (OAK)—to better determine middle ear and inner ear function.

Hearing aid specialists with a BC-HIS received certification from the National Board of Certification in Hearing Instrument Sciences. They are trained and licensed to fit hearing aids, to perform audiometric (hearing) tests and hearing aid evaluations, and to offer post-fitting follow-up care. They can also fit maskers and tinnitus instruments, and offer assistive devices such as bedside maskers or audio tapes for masking. Many offer hearing aids and tinnitus devices on a trial basis.

Be aware that not every doctor, audiologist, or hearing aid specialist is able to provide all of the services listed. There are also many health professionals who are not yet familiar with the treatments and testing protocols for tinnitus.

ATA's Professional Referral Network includes the names, addresses, phone numbers, services, and credentials of health professionals who take a special interest in treating tinnitus patients. The network list is offered to ATA members as a resource only—never as a recommendation of one provider over another. Tinnitus patients are strongly encouraged to ask questions of potential health care providers, then decide for themselves if there is a match of needs and services.

Step #4: Talk with Your Health Care Provider

It can help you understand your options and give you the assurances you need. The following questions for health care providers can be asked before or during a visit. (Remember to write down the answers and repeat them back for accuracy.)

- What tinnitus treatments do you use in your practice?
- What is your exact diagnosis?
- What is your treatment plan for me?
- Can we rule out a tumor so I can stop worrying?
- What tests do you require or suggest?
- What is the test designed to reveal?
- Will the test be uncomfortable, and if so, for how long?
- How much will each test cost?
- If I've had the test elsewhere, do I need to repeat it?

- What are the exact instructions for taking this medication? (foods, other drugs to avoid)

- What are the risks/side effects of the treatments or drugs?

- What expectations can I have for relief or an improvement in my hearing?

- Could the tinnitus be caused by a TMJ disorder or a drug I'm taking?

- Will getting a hearing aid (or getting my hearing aid refitted) affect my tinnitus?

- What else can I do on my own to help? (Diet, exercise, environmental changes.)

- How many visits do you think I will need?

- How much of this treatment will be covered by my insurance?

- Do you have written patient information about tinnitus for me to read?

- If I have to learn to tolerate this noise, how do I learn to do it?

- Can you refer me to a counselor?

- If you can't help me, do you know someone who can?

- Is there a tinnitus self-help group available in this city?

- Are you a member of the American Tinnitus Association?

- Include your own questions too.

In addition to a list of questions, it is suggested that you bring the following with you when you visit your health care provider:

- A complete, written list of your symptoms.

- Copies of all of your previous test results and audiograms.

- A written list of ALL medications (over-the-counter and prescription) you are currently taking or have just recently taken.

Step #5: Try Something!

- Hearing aids and/or maskers, drug therapy, and auditory habituation have all been used with some success.

- Counseling can help. Depression and/or anxiety occasionally accompany tinnitus in its early stages.

181

- Cognitive therapy is used to alter the way patients react to their tinnitus through the identification and elimination of negative thought and behavior patterns.

- Biofeedback therapy enables patients to consciously control their breathing, heart rate, blood pressure, and muscle tension through electronic monitoring, This treatment is usually coupled with counseling and other stress reduction techniques.

- Some cases of tinnitus appear to be of TMJ (temporomandibular jaw joint) origin. A dentist specializing in TMJ can perform this evaluation. Therapy may include orthodontia or a removable in-the-mouth appliance.

Try a treatment again. Something that did not work the first time around might work on its second try. For some patients, a combination of therapies is more effective than a single therapy.

Step #6: Take Care of Yourself

- Use hearing protection (earplugs or ear muffs) in noisy surroundings. A worsening of tinnitus can be prevented by avoiding excessive noise exposure.

- Learn how you relax best. Exercise, yoga, meditation, and environmental audio tapes (rainfall, ocean waves, etc.) are stress reduction tools that can promote relaxation and reduce fatigue. You may find that the tinnitus is better tolerated when you are relaxed.

- Get sleep. Many people are able to fall asleep by listening to FM radio static, an electric fan, or a bedside masker. Caffeine, alcohol, cigarettes, and some drugs can interfere with falling and/or staying asleep.

- Keep a diary. You might recognize a correlation between the tinnitus and your physical activities, consumption of certain foods, or drug usage.

- Be patient with the therapy you are trying. Many therapies require an investment of time to be effective. Remember that the goal is for tinnitus control, not a cure.

Step #7: Participate in a Social Network

Those who successfully adapt to their tinnitus are often those who keep busy with hobbies and work, who regularly use a social network to give and receive support, and who learn as much about tinnitus as they can.

ATA's worldwide Self-Help Network offers a variety of ways for members to exchange practical information and find emotional support with others who experience tinnitus.

If you are interested in volunteering your time as a telephone helper, pen pal, or support group leader, write to ATA for a Self-Help Packet of information.

Step #8: Join the American Tinnitus Association

ATA is a non-profit donation-supported organization dedicated to helping tinnitus patients and supporting critical tinnitus research. Your annual contribution entitles you to our quarterly journal *Tinnitus Today*, discounts on books, and referrals to professional and self-help contacts in your area. Write to ATA for a complete list of services, resource materials, and membership benefits.

Coping with the Stress of Tinnitus

Living with Tinnitus

Most tinnitus patients rate themselves as healthy and upon examination, are usually informed by their physician that there is no serious medical problem causing their tinnitus. For some people this knowledge alone is enough to allow them to adapt to the sounds they hear. For others, however, the persistent sounds of tinnitus can be disruptive and stressful. Some patients may need help learning how to cope with the sounds.

Stress and Tinnitus

With tinnitus, the body may react as if it is being constantly threatened. When this situation exceeds a person's capacity to cope, stress can result. People differ greatly in their response to stress. Therefore, if an individual is unable to cope effectively, his or her ability to lead a normal life may be hindered.

Tinnitus Severity Scale

Think for a moment about your tinnitus and rate its severity along the following scale. Rating tinnitus is not an easy task but these verbal descriptions of what each number represents might be helpful.

5.   Tinnitus is more than irritating, causing an overwhelming problem much or all of the time.

4.   Tinnitus is always present at an irritating level and often causes considerable distress.

3.   Tinnitus is difficult to ignore even with effort.

2.   Tinnitus is often irritating but can be ignored much the time.

1.   Tinnitus is there if attended to but it is not very irritating and can usually be ignored.

0.   Tinnitus not present.

If you rated your tinnitus as three or greater, you may be helped by improving your coping skills and reducing the stress in your life. You may wish to try some of the following suggestions.

Therapies in Current Use for Control of Tinnitus

Tinnitus is a medical symptom. Each patient should be seen by an otolaryngologist or an otologist to rule out any serious medical problem that could be associated with the tinnitus.

A hearing evaluation should be performed to determine whether you are correctly processing speech and other sounds. These tests can also reveal whether you perceive loudness levels in the usual way and whether your ears are functioning as they should. Other specialized tests can be performed to determine the pitch, loudness, and maskability of your tinnitus.

Based on this information the hearing professional may recommend that you be fitted with hearing aids to improve your ability to hear, or with maskers to substitute a more pleasant sound for the one you are hearing, or with "tinnitus instruments," a combination hearing-aid-masker that has proven helpful to a large group of tinnitus sufferers who need assistance with both applications.

Not all tinnitus can be relieved by the above methods. For these patients, other therapies may be useful.

Auditory Habituation is a new technique designed to retrain the auditory system to ignore the tinnitus sounds. Therapeutic noise devices that emit stable "broad band noise" quieter than a patient's tinnitus—are used in this treatment. The recommended course of treatment can be more than a year.

Biofeedback has become a popular treatment for tinnitus. It is a powerful learning tool to help people become aware of their bodily functions and learn to control them. Biofeedback therapy usually goes hand in hand with counseling and stress reduction, enabling the patient to understand stress and relaxation and to consciously exert control over the body's reactions.

Cognitive therapy is based on treating the patient's reaction to tinnitus rather than the tinnitus itself. To accomplish the desired perceptual changes, negative behaviors and thought patterns must be identified and then systematically altered via a program specifically designed for the individual.

Hypnosis therapy can help the patient enter a rapid learning state for taking suggestions into the subconscious to alter behavior. It is important to keep the patient in control of his/her reactions to tinnitus by making positive suggestions that can be set in motion for self help.

Acupuncture therapy operates on the principle that health depends on the free flow of "life energy" through the body. If the flow is disturbed, illness will result. This procedure has brought some relief for a few tinnitus patients, but usually on a temporary basis.

Temporomandibular joint specialists report tinnitus relief for numerous patients suffering from both TMJ and tinnitus. If you can alter the sound of your tinnitus by moving your jaw or pressing on it, or if you grind your teeth, experience jaw joint pain, have trouble opening your mouth wide, or have similar symptoms, it is probably worthwhile to seek out a qualified TMJ expert.

Drug therapy for tinnitus may involve the use of niacin (a vasodilator), various tranquilizers, anti-depressants, anticonvulsants, or anti-vertigo drugs. None of these are cures for tinnitus but may provide relief in some cases. Some of these same drugs have been said to cause tinnitus and therefore should be used cautiously. Future research plans of the National Institute on Deafness and Other Communications Disorders include the study of drugs to relieve tinnitus. We can be hopeful of a medical breakthrough as a result of this research.

The key to living with tinnitus is being able to remove it from immediate attention. If a person can construe tinnitus as an insignificant, repetitive noise then it is possible for the body to adjust or ignore it.

Self-Help Hints

The following suggestions are designed to help alleviate stress, thereby making the tinnitus more tolerable.

1. Learn to relax. Deep breathing is a natural relaxant. Get in the habit of stopping every so often and taking 3 or 4 deep slow breaths. Better yet, learn regular breathing from your abdomen. (Lead with your waistband as you breathe in.)

2. After you have practiced deep breathing exercises for awhile, start to pay attention to yourself: shallow breathing and frequent fast pulse are indicators of anxiety and stress. When you notice yourself breathing fast, sl-o-w-w down!

3. Simple exercises can help you to relax. Tense all of your muscles for five seconds, then let go. Do this several times a day and you'll soon recognize how you should feel with tension loosened. Many books have been written about relaxation; a classic is *You Must Relax*, by Edmund Jacobson.

4. Use mental imagery to help you relax when busy or at work. With eyes open, you can concentrate on a beautiful flower or other object for a few minutes. Force yourself to enjoy it and not think of anything else. With eyes closed, you might think of something pleasant and warm like lying on a sandy beach. These short rest periods can be better than a nap.

5. Exercise every day. Take a walk, jog, swim, play tennis. Do whatever kind of exercise you enjoy. Not only will exercising make you feel stronger and better able to cope with tinnitus, it's a great way to take out aggressions. (Some people have noted that exercise exacerbates their tinnitus, but usually only temporarily.)

6. Smile! Happiness is catching. Don't be afraid, however, to speak out about your tinnitus to let your family and friends know that you have a problem. They might surprise you with their consideration.

7. Try not to focus on the unpleasant or stressful aspects of your tinnitus. Don't feel you must fight it all the time. Try to think of tinnitus as just something you have, like your hair color, your height, or your disposition.

8. Learn more about tinnitus. The more you know about a problem, any problem, the more you are in control and the less helpless you will feel dealing with it.

9. Loud noise is the enemy of the tinnitus patient. Even a short exposure to noise can make the tinnitus worse and make you tense and irritable. Wear proper ear protection whenever you are in a noisy environment.

10. Talking to other people who also have tinnitus can be a big help. You might learn some new tips about how to get along better with your tinnitus. Go even further—join a tinnitus self-help group or start one in your area. ATA will help you with guidelines and startup information.

11. If sleep is a problem for you because of the tinnitus, there are several things that you might try. First of all, wind down and relax before going to bed. Sometimes reading for a time before retiring is helpful. Your sleeping place and your nightclothes should be comfortable. Some people benefit from having a light snack before going to bed. Soft music, FM static, bedside maskers, or pleasant sounds can often be utilized to help you fall asleep. Changing your routine so that you go to bed at a different hour might make a difference.

12. An extensive list of books, relaxation tapes, and ideas for stress reduction has been compiled based on suggestions from ATA's support group. This list is available upon request.

How Can I Learn More about Tinnitus and Find Help?

The American Tinnitus Association, a non-profit organization supported solely by private donations, is dedicated to helping tinnitus patients and supporting tinnitus research. Activities include production and distribution of public awareness materials, educational programs for the professional and lay communities, establishment and guidance for self-help groups and their leaders, and the promotion of community hearing protection programs. Write to ATA for general information and membership benefits (including subscription to ATA's quarterly journal, *Tinnitus Today*, and referrals to clinics and self-help groups in your area).

American Tinnitus Association
Post Office Box 5
Portland, OR 97207-0005
(503) 248-9984; (503) 248-0224 fax

Additional Tinnitus Resources

CHID Bibliographic Search on Tinnitus

The following information from the Deafness and Other Communication Disorders subfile of the Combined Health Information Database (CHID). CHID is a computerized bibliographic database developed and managed by health-related agencies of the Federal government to serve health professionals, patients, and the general public.

The NIDCD Information Clearinghouse has made every effort to provide accurate descriptions of the information in CHID. Please inform us of any errors or omissions. Inclusion of an item in CHID does not imply endorsement by the Clearinghouse or the National Institute on Deafness and Other Communication Disorders. All users are strongly advised to check any medical treatments or information with their own health care providers.

The materials in this search are available directly from the sources listed. Unless the NIDCD Information Clearinghouse is cited as the source, these materials are not available from the clearinghouse.

Each citation contains the producer, title, and a brief abstract describing the material. Depending upon the type of material described, the citation may also include information about a corporate author, format, where to obtain the item, and its price.

The following codes are used in this literature search:

TI Title
AU Author
CN Corporate Author
SO Source
AV Availability
AB Abstract/Description

Tinnitus Resources

TI American Tinnitus Association (ATA).
AV P.O. Box 5, Portland, OR 97207. Client Services Representative. (503) 248-9985.
AB The purpose of the American Tinnitus Association (ATA) is to carry on and support research and educational activities relating to the treatment of tinnitus and other defects or diseases of the ear. The organization provides information and referral to hearing professionals, supports self-help groups

nationwide, provides a bibliographic service, supports scientific research about tinnitus, and promotes public education concerning tinnitus and its prevention through hearing protection. ATA's target audience is people with tinnitus and their families, and hearing professionals. ATA publishes a quarterly journal, bibliography, fact sheet, and pamphlets. Informational videos (VHS) and a cassette tape are available.

TI Your Guide to Better Hearing.
CN Better Hearing Institute (BHI).
SO Washington, DC: Better Hearing Institute, 1992, 16 p.
AV Available from the Better Hearing Institute, P.O. Box 1840, Washington, DC 20013. (703) 642-0580; (800) EARWELL TTY; (703) 750-9302 FAX.
AB This booklet is a guide to better hearing for the general public. The publication discusses the causes and treatment of tinnitus. It informs those individuals with hearing impairments about improved medical assistance and the most recent auditory tests used to identify hearing loss. The pamphlet discusses hearing protection and stresses the importance of taking hearing tests.

TI Tinnitus Diagnosis/Treatment.
AU Shulman. A.; et al.
SO Malvern. PA: Lea and Febiger, 1991, 571 p.
AV Available from Lea and Febiger, 200 Chester Field Parkway, Malvern, PA 19355-9725. (215) 251-2230. PRICE: $95.00. ISBN 0-8121-1121-4.
AB This introductory text is written for basic scientists and for all professionals involved in the evaluation, treatment, and control of the symptom of tinnitus. Its goal is to provide professionals with a rationale for both diagnosis and selection of treatment methods based on a medical audiologic team approach. Section I is an introduction to tinnitus from an historical perspective. Section II is a review of the basic science of the auditory system and how its pathophysiology can be reflected in the symptom of tinnitus. Section III attempts to clinically establish the site of lesion and presents the clinical types of tinnitus. Section IV distinguishes between treatment and control of tinnitus. The concluding section considers directions for diagnosis and treatment of the symptom of tinnitus based on the results of clinical experience and basic science research.

TI F-12: Common Questions about Tinnitus (Head Noise).
CN Vestibular Disorders Association.
SO Portland, OR: Vestibular Disorders Association, n.d., 3 p.
AV Available from Vestibular Disorders Association, P.O. Box 4467, Portland, OR 97208. (503) 229-7708. (503) 229-8064 Fax. (800) 837-8428 Toll Free.
AB This free fact sheet presents some common questions asked about tinnitus. The questions deal with the causes and treatment of tinnitus, and an explanation of otolaryngology–head and neck surgery.

TI American Speech-Language-Hearing Association Answers Questions About Tinnitus.
CN American Speech-Language-Hearing Association.
SO Rockville, MD: American Speech-Language-Hearing Association, n.d., 4 D.
AV One free copy available from the American Speech-Language-Hearing Association, 10801 Rockville Pike, Rockville, MD 20852. (800) 638-8255 Voice/TTY.
AB This pamphlet, written for the patient, answers common questions about tinnitus. It defines tinnitus and discusses causes, diagnosis, and treatment.

TI Silence Ringing Ears.
AU Delaney, L.
SO *Prevention*, 1992, vol. 44, no. 4, pp. 50-54, 122-125.
AB This journal article, written for the general public, discusses the diagnosis and treatment of tinnitus. Tinnitus is not a disease, but a symptom that can be caused by any number of physical problems. The article discusses how individuals can learn to live with tinnitus through ear protection, avoidance of ear damaging substances, hearing aids, maskers and tinnitus devices, emotional relief techniques, and social support. In addition, a personal account of a woman who lives with tinnitus is presented.

TI "Doctor, what causes the noise in my ears?"
CN American Academy of Otolaryngology–Head and Neck Surgery, Inc., 1992, 6 p.
AV Available from American Academy of Otolaryngology Head and Neck Surgery, Inc. One Prince Street, Alexandria, VA 22314. (703) 836-4444; (703) 683-5100 Fax. PRICE: Single copy free.

AB   This leaflet presents information about tinnitus in a question and answer format. Causes and treatments are discussed, although it is noted that sometimes no cause can be identified. A list of 8 do's and don'ts to lessen the tinnitus are included, which may provide some relief when no specific cause is identified. The leaflet concludes with a reminder to seek medical attention and an explanation of otolaryngology–head and neck surgery.

Chapter 20

Management of Tinnitus

Part I—Medical Intervention

Objective Tinnitus

To understand tinnitus, it is best to recall that there are two forms of this perplexing disorder. In the first instance is the condition known as *objective tinnitus*. Objective tinnitus is best defined as an acoustic-like sensation which can be confirmed by appropriate tests and examination. For example, vascular abnormalities (bruits) can create awareness of the blood flowing through a restricted orifice of arterial or venal systems. This objective tinnitus is reported as an acoustic sensation which is pulsating in nature and coincidental with the heart beat. Also, chronic spasm of the stapedial or tensor tympani muscle creates a "clicking" sensation to which the person will react negatively. Further, spasm of the muscles of the Eustachian tube can create an objective tinnitus that can be very irritating and frustrating to the person experiencing this condition. Temporal mandibular joint (TMJ) dysfunction can produce a tinnitus that is bothersome to the patient.

Fortunately, most objective tinnitus conditions can be treated effectively with appropriate medical, surgical or therapeutic management. For these reasons, objective tinnitus does not constitute a major problem and is of less concern, relative to the frequency of occurrence. Obviously, if the hearing health professional can differentiate between

"The Management of Tinnitus—Parts I and II," *Audecibel*, January-February-March 1994, and April-May-June 1994; reprinted with permission.

193

objective and subjective tinnitus, an appropriate referral can be made and proper counseling or care given.

Subjective Tinnitus

Subjective tinnitus can best be defined as an apparent acoustic sensation for which there is no external cause. That is, the person hears the tinnitus but it can not be heard by others or objectively assessed by existing instrumentation. Subjective tinnitus has been described in many ways. To some it is a high pitched ringing. To others it is a persistent roar that permeates the very soul of the individual. For many it is a cacophony of sounds. Still others describe their experience as an exposure to music-like sounds that make their presence known twenty four hours a day. Some complain that they hear a hissing sound, while others state their tinnitus sounds more like the constant chirping of crickets.

The sensation may be bilateral or unilateral. Several patients will tell you that their tinnitus is louder in one ear than the other. For some, the presence of this subjective tinnitus is intolerable and they would go to any extreme to end themselves of its constant and irritating presence. Others acknowledge its presence but are not bothered by it and proceed in carrying out their normal daily activities of living without appreciable difficulty. Unfortunately, there are those few who have been so troubled by tinnitus that they have paid the ultimate price—suicide.

Relative to subjective tinnitus, we do know some of those conditions which cause it. For example, noise exposure, various ear pathologies, physical trauma or whiplash injury, excessive use of aspirin, temporal mandibular joint dysfunction and aminoglycocides are thought to be among the rather common causes of tinnitus. For many with tinnitus, the cause is unknown but the symptoms are present and unrelenting and offer a significant problem.

Essentially, there are two major modes of treatment that have emerged over the past several years. The first part of this two part chapter will concentrate on the medical model. The reader should be aware that this is not an exhaustive review of medical intervention but rather an attempt to emphasize some related methods of treatment.

The Medical Model

This model suggests that control of tinnitus (the apparent absence or reduction In subjective loudness) can be achieved through the administration of drugs, application of direct electrical stimulation of the cochlear substance, or surgical procedures which destroy the functional contributions of the ear by sectioning the cochlear branch of the VIII nerve. Sectioning of the VIII nerve for controlling tinnitus is not without considerable risk.

Although procedures based on medical models have had some success in ameliorating the person's response to the presence of tinnitus, none has been sufficiently compelling to gain universal acceptance by the clinician. However, let us examine in somewhat more detail treatment procedures based on medical intervention.

Drug Therapy

Intravenous Lidocaine. This is a local anesthetic that alters central nervous system function and is used frequently in treating those patients having intractable pain. The drug is administered locally and appears to be of limited benefit to the tinnitus sufferer. Its effect is short lived and it is necessary to administer the drug intravenously. Because of these two factors, Lidocaine is not used very often to treat subjective tinnitus. There was a chemical analog of Lidocaine, Tocanide, developed that could be taken orally. However, subsequent controlled studies have revealed that Tocanide provided very limited benefit to those with tinnitus.

Tegretol. This drug is a carbamazepine derivative and its primary use is for the treatment of those with epilepsy, in that it has been demonstrated to have anticonvulsant properties. It is important to remember that most pharmacologists stress that Tegretol is not a simple medication and should not be considered as a proper method of treatment for the relief of minor aches and pains. Somewhat by chance, Tegretol was found to have some positive effect on reducing the apparent loudness of subjective tinnitus. However, this drug must be administered with close medical supervision; especially the monitoring of blood levels. Some of the more dire side effects from the use of Tegretol include aplastic anemia, agranulocytosis (an acute disease characterized by leukopenia, with ulcerative lesions of the throat and other mucous membranes), thrombocytopenia, (causing aplastic anemia and hemorrhaging), and leukopenia (a reduction of the number of leukocytes in the blood).

Mysoline. Here, again, this drug is intended for the management of patients with focal epileptic seizures, grand mal, or psychomotor seizures. It does not produce the same side effects as does Tegretol,

195

but the physician and the clinician must be aware of the possibility of nausea, anorexia, vomiting, fatigue, hyperirritability, emotional disturbances, sexual impotency, diplopia, nystagmus and drowsiness. Its effect on tinnitus is similar in nature to that of Tegretol. Again, close monitoring of the patient is most important to avoid deleterious side effects.

In general, there is no significant body of evidence to demonstrate the consistent value of either Mysoline or Tegretol. Although the initial indications suggested a positive correlation between the drugs and reduction of tinnitus, later placebo controlled, double blind studies indicated that neither drug was effective for most. The assumption, of course, was that these anticonvulsant drugs had some effect on neuronal activity of the central auditory system thought to be hyperactive.

Xanax. A recently completed study (Johnson, et al. 1992) at the Oregon Hearing Research Center investigated Xanax (Alprazolam) as a possible treatment for subjective tinnitus. Xanax is an anti-anxiety that has been used successfully for those individuals suffering from depressional episodes. Xanax is a dependent drug and must be prescribed and controlled by the physician. In the Oregon study of Xanax, forty adult patients participated in a double blind experiment. Seventeen of 20 patients in the experimental group (Xanax) and 19 of 20 patients in the placebo (lactose) group completed the study. Of the 17 patients receiving Xanax, 13 (76%) had a reduction in the loudness of their tinnitus when measurements were made using both a tinnitus synthesizer and a visual analog scale. Only one of the 19 patients who received the placebo showed any improvement in the loudness of their tinnitus. No changes were observed in the audiometric data or in tinnitus masking levels for either group. Individuals differed with regard to the dosage required to achieve benefit from the alprazolam and the side effects were minimal for this 12 week study.

Furosemide. Dobie (1993) of the Department of Otolaryngology–Head and Neck Surgery, the University of Texas Health Science Center in San Antonio, Texas, reported his findings on the clinical effects of Furosemide (Lasix). Twenty subjects with subjective tinnitus were involved initially in the study. The mean duration of tinnitus among the experimental group was about 11 years. Each subject was given 80 mg. b.i.d. for the first two weeks. The dosage was increased to 40 mg. t.i.d. for the third and fourth weeks and then to 40 mg. q.i.d. for the fifth and sixth weeks. Several tinnitus scales were used in rating any change in the subjective loudness of the tinnitus during the course of the study.

Of the twenty subjects starting the study, only 12 finished the full course of Furosemide. Only 4 patients of the final 12 answered yes to a global satisfaction question: "Has the drug helped you in any way?" However, two of these mentioned benefits unrelated to tinnitus, (perceived improvement of hearing in one case and reduction of edema in another). Only two of twelve patients answered yes to a second global question, "Is your tinnitus improved?" It would appear that, although there were some positive statements regarding the benefit of Furosemide, the results did not strongly support the value of this drug in reducing or eliminating subjective tinnitus. It was interesting to note that the greatest benefit seemed to be achieved by those who had tinnitus for the shortest period of time.

Guth, et al. (1991), stated that the clinical administration of Furosemide may indicate that tinnitus is of a peripheral origin if its loudness is reduced. If, on the other hand, Furosemide does not alter the patient's perception of tinnitus, then tinnitus is of a central origin, and Xanax may be the drug of choice.

Dr. Robert Brummett of the Oregon Hearing Research Center states that, *"Because we to do not understand the mechanisms by which tinnitus is produced, it is impossible to rationally select a drug that should control tinnitus. However, because so many people are taking a wide variety of drugs for many different reasons, it has been possible to capitalize on some people's spontaneous reports that their tinnitus is relieved when they take certain drugs. These serendipitous discoveries have led to the current armamentarium of drug therapy for tinnitus. At best, though, the current state of knowledge about drug therapy for tinnitus is woefully inadequate."* (*The Hearing Journal*, November 1998, pp.34-37.)

According to tinnitus specialist Dr. Robert Johnson (personal communication) there are, nonetheless, those investigators who feel that if a more permanent relief is found for tinnitus patients, it most likely will be in the area of drug therapy. In order to achieve this treatment goal, much more research is needed, using a variety of drugs.

Although drug therapy is still used in the treatment of the tinnitus patient, many practitioners prefer other modalities that do not pose the same degree of compromise and uncertainty as do most drugs.

Direct Electrical Stimulation

The application of an electric stimulus to the ear is not of recent origin. As early as 1800, Volta made the first battery consisting of some

30 separate plates (silver and zinc). Although he did not specifically experiment with relieving tinnitus, it is recorded that attempts to apply a direct current to the ear resulted in an acoustic sensation that was "altogether disagreeable." Shortly thereafter, Grapengiesser applied a direct electrical stimulus to each ear. Although he was hoping to develop a cure or treatment for deafness, he did report the effects of direct current on tinnitus. He simply maintained that some patients responded positively to the stimulus and others did not. He reported, however, that in deaf ears where there was no tinnitus, electrical stimulation produced it. In those deaf ears where there was tinnitus, direct current would often suppress it.

The first use of an alternating current developed by Faraday was that of Duchenne de Boulogne in 1855. He claimed to have cured 8 out of 10 patients through the use of electrical stimulation. What he meant by cure is open to considerable speculation, in view of recent investigations using more sophisticated methods of stimulus control and response assessment.

Based on experiment with cochlear implant devices, it was discovered that for some people, electrical stimulation of neural tissue within the cochlea had an apparent positive effect on eliminating or reducing subjective tinnitus, as long as the stimulus was present. However, some cases of residual inhibition have been reported following electrical stimulation. For example, House (1990) reported the results of transtympanic electrical stimulation on 125 patients with severe tinnitus. A 60 Hz and 16000 Hz current stimulated the promontory. The stimulation time was 20 minutes. Some 20% of the patients stimulated reported some lessening of their tinnitus.

One should point out that success of this magnitude is not statistically significant. Chouard (1982) reported that many of his cochlear implant patients with tinnitus experienced noticeable relief when using the implant device. Again, House, et al. (1982) reported that about 50% of his implanted patients had some relief from their ongoing tinnitus. It should be noted that 8% of his implanted patients experienced a worsening of their tinnitus while using the implant.

Through the years, various forms of electrical stimulation have been investigated. As with some other forms of treatment, direct electrical stimulation is not without risk. That is, the length, magnitude, and type of electrical stimulus employed will determine the adverse affects on neural and other structures within the cochlea.

In general, studies have demonstrated that the most effective electrical stimulus for the relief of tinnitus is a positive phase direct current. Recall, however, that sinusoidal and bipolar pulses have had positive effects on the reduction of tinnitus for some people. Studies have indicated that the point of electrical stimulation, i.e., extra or intra-tympanic sites, will determine what effect, if any, it has on the elimination or reduction of ongoing, subjective tinnitus. It would appear that the closer the stimulating electrode is to the neural structures of the cochlea the more positive the effect, if indeed there is any alteration of the tinnitus sensation at all. Although there may be significant promise relative to effective management of subjective tinnitus, there is not sufficient data to warrant a great deal of clinical optimism at this time.

Summary

It has been the purpose of the first part of this chapter to inform the hearing health professional of the complexity of subjective tinnitus. It is not a simple human disorder that is amenable to an "easy fix." Neither has it been the intent of this chapter to suggest that the hearing aid specialist become involved in some type of management involving the medical model. However, it is important to realize that medical management can be a very significant contribution to the treatment of tinnitus. There is no common consensus as to the causes or cures of tinnitus. There is no single treatment modality, medical or non medical, which has proven sufficiently compelling to have been embraced by all who work with the tinnitus sufferer. In Part II, the role of the hearing health professional in the management of the patient with subjective tinnitus will be stressed.

There is no doubt that the hearing aid specialist can play a very important role in the treatment of tinnitus. However, it is equally as important for the specialist to realize that it is not a simple matter of recommending a hearing aid or a masker device. The management strategy used is of utmost importance, if the individual is to realize lasting benefit. These issues will be discussed in Part II.

References

Chouard, H. 1982. Comments Made at Symposium of Artificial Auditory Stimulation. Erlangen, September.

Dobie, R.A. 1993. Furosemide open trial for treatment of tinnitus, *Tinnitus Today*, March 18:11, pp.6–9.

Guth, P.S., Risey, J., Amedee, R., and Norris, C.H. (1991) A pharmaceutical approach to the treatment of tinnitus. 14th Midwinter Research

Meeting of the Association for Research in Otolaryngology, February 3-7, St. Petersburg Beach, Florida, p.4.

House, W.F. (1983). Effects of electrical stimulation on tinnitus. 2nd International Tinnitus Seminar, New York, June 10 & 11, Supplement No. 9, *Jour. Laryn. & Oto.* pp.139–140.

House, W.F. & Berliner, K.I. editors. 1982. Cochlear implants Progress in perspective *Annals of Oto. Rhino & Laryn.*, 94:124.

Johnson, R.M., Brummett, R. & Schleuning, A. (1993). Use of Alprazolam for relief of tinnitus. *Arch. Otolaryngol Head Neck Surg.* 119 pp.842–845.

Part II—Non-Medical Strategies

Part One of this article discussed some management strategies associated with the medical model. It was suggested that the hearing health professional be aware of various management approaches in order to provide more appropriate counseling of the tinnitus patient.

Part Two covers some of the more common non-medical management strategies which have proven effective for some tinnitus patients.

No one treatment modality, medically or non-medically based, has been effective in dealing with all patients having some form of subjective tinnitus. However, almost every patient can be helped to some degree with an effective management program.

As mentioned in Part One, tinnitus is not a simple disorder to deal with. There are many complexities involving not only neurophysiological phenomena but patient behavioral and emotional responses to subjective tinnitus.

For many who work with the tinnitus patient, it is becoming increasingly evident that the psychological state of the individual often determines the effectiveness of any therapeutic modality employed in the treatment of this disorder. One cannot emphasize too strongly the necessity of having some awareness of the psychological status of the individual.

Studies by House (1981) and Reich (1984) regarding personalities of tinnitus patients suggest there are abnormal patterns associated with a number of psychological disorders. Among them are those associated with various forms of depression and neuroses. The presence of such aberrant behavior often interferes with the patient's ability to cope with the disorder.

Following is an actual case history that took place 14 to 15 years ago. The client was a white female in her mid-fifties who was the wife a naval captain. She had complained of bilateral tinnitus for about two years prior to her visit to our clinic. Her history suggested she was having an extremely difficult time coping with her problem.

She had, on more than one occasion, considered the possibility of ending her life. Further, she stated her social and intimate relationships were affected by the constant presence of the tinnitus. She had been examined by several physicians, none of whom offered treatment or medication which provided relief.

When questioned about those kinds of activities which brought some relief to her, she responded by saying she took 10 to 12 showers a day. This statement was somewhat surprising until it was determined that the water beating down on her head was providing "masking" of her tinnitus. As long as she was in the shower, there was considerable relief.

She was a logical candidate for a masker device. Subsequent clinical testing supported that thinking and she became a very effective user of a tinnitus masker. So successful that she appeared on local radio and TV extolling the virtues of the clinic and exclaiming that her social and interpersonal life were now pleasant experiences.

The euphoria, however, only lasted a few months until the patient said the masker device was no longer effective and her tinnitus had returned to its former, irritating level. She was scheduled for a re-evaluation and it was discovered that her ongoing tinnitus could no longer be masked, regardless of the intensity of the masker signal applied. The audiometric and speech discrimination data were not changed, yet her tinnitus had returned and could not be masked.

This inability to mask her ongoing tinnitus is mentioned because it represents, somewhat, our ignorance as clinicians of the course the disorder will follow and those forces that shape it. After extensive questioning it was determined that her tinnitus became uncontrollable after she was told that she could not accompany her husband to Alaska to a new military post.

Although there is no assurance a correlation existed between her husband's transfer and the inability to mask her tinnitus, it was felt strongly that there was. It is known, for example, there is a positive correlation between stress and an increase in subjective loudness of on-going tinnitus.

This case history is presented only to underscore clinical problems associated with management of the tinnitus patient. The person's psychological or emotional status can greatly affect the success of any clinical modality used in the treatment program.

There are a number of psychologically oriented programs which have been used in treating the tinnitus patient. Space restrictions do not permit the review of each of the programs; which may range from psychiatric care to other counseling strategies. It is valuable to discuss, however, cognitive therapy as an adjunct treatment for the tinnitus sufferer.

Cognitive Therapy

The primary intent of cognitive therapy is to modify or alter maladaptive behaviors—behaviors which reduce the quality or conduct of life due to the presence of some physical, mental or emotional condition. If, in the application of cognitive therapy, one can modify these unwanted behaviors, then the individual can better cope with the stresses generated by the disorder.

If one is to employ cognitive therapy as a method of treating the tinnitus patient, it would seem logical to design a well-organized and structured set of procedures. Sweetow (1989) suggests three behavioral techniques employing cognitive therapy, which have proven useful in the treatment of the tinnitus patient. They are:

1. Direct modification of overt or covert behaviors through the application of specific behavioral techniques;

2. Manipulation of environmental antecedents or situational demands, and;

3. Manipulation of environmental consequences (Sweetow, p. 38).

What Sweetow refers to is the process by which the patient learns to understand the relationship between his or her maladaptive behaviors caused by the presence of tinnitus. In a sense, one may refer to these behaviors as a type of cognitive distortion. It is the resolution of these distortions that provides positive relief from tinnitus. Relief does not imply that the tinnitus is absent, but rather that one's behavior to it has been significantly modified. Some distortions are:

1. Mental filter—dwelling on a negative event so that all reality becomes clouded. (This kind of behavior is seen often in tinnitus patients. They often feel that the tinnitus will never go away and any comment or suggestion to the contrary is automatically denied.)

202

2. "Should" statements—e.g., creating guilt by believing you "should" have done something differently. (This is a common behavior seen in tinnitus patients. Many feel they should have done something different, or should have been more solicitous to their health or should have been kinder to others, etc. Some feel they are being punished because they should have done something else and failed to do so. This kind of behavior is seen more often in those patients for whom the tinnitus was of violent and sudden onset.)

3. Disqualifying the positive—e.g., positive experiences don't count. (There are those patients who will discredit any positive experience relating to tinnitus. For example, the tinnitus may be greatly reduced or even absent for a period of time. However, these positive experiences don't count because the patient is certain the tinnitus will return and they will be as miserable as ever.)

There are a number of other cognitive distortions of which the reader should be aware. See Sweetow (1989) for a more in-depth analysis. Suffice it to say that one of the effective management strategies for subjective tinnitus is cognitive therapy.

Biofeedback

Biofeedback is not new to the medical or applied sciences. It stemmed from the practice of Eastern religions and was adapted to other pursuits such as meditation and physiological processes involving the heart and its function as well as the physiology of other body organs (Grossman 1976).

It is well documented that through meditation one is able to alter physiological states. We know, for example, that such ailments as migraine headaches, abnormal muscle tension, and anxiety can be effectively modified through conscious effort and appropriate mental focusing.

It has been generally accepted among practitioners working with tinnitus patients, that stress can exacerbate the subjective loudness. Although the mechanism for this phenomenon is unknown, it is apparent that stress can create a number of physiological disturbances that may have negative consequences. Therefore, it seems rather straightforward to employ some treatment modality which would eliminate or reduce stress contributing to increased loudness of the tinnitus.

Biofeedback has been most instrumental in providing a means by which the patient can control his or her stress level. Apparently it makes little difference what the stressor is, or the environment in which it is generated. Biofeedback, if properly managed, can be effective in teaching the patient a means of relaxation. When in a relaxed state it becomes an easier task for the patient to visualize that part of the body to be relaxed. Relaxation through biofeedback intervention not only provides a means by which muscle relaxation is possible, but provides a means of visualizing other sensory sensations such as warmth and coolness.

Relative to tinnitus, it has been suggested by Grossman (1989, Section 9, p. 2), that...

> *"...tinnitus is measured before treatment as to tonal content and subjective loudness. The same assessment is repeated after treatment. Even though the patient may feel better and be appreciative of having been improved, when the actual measurement of tinnitus is made it is usually still there. What has been removed is that portion of the symptom caused by anxiety reinforcement. As a matter of fact, if the patient has no element of anxiety reinforcing his tinnitus, biofeedback may not be particularly beneficial."*

Biofeedback is often coupled to other methods of patient management such as counseling or other forms of psychologically-based intervention. This is not to suggest that biofeedback must be coupled to other treatment modalities, but rather that for some a multidisciplinary approach is more productive.

Biofeedback, as with all other current forms of treatment, is not a panacea. It does not promise an absolute resolution of the problem. It is, however, a method which has proven beneficial to some. To that extent it is important the hearing instrument dispenser be aware of its contribution to the treatment of tinnitus.

Tinnitus Maskers and Combination Devices

The application of a controlled noise to the offending ear(s) to reduce tinnitus loudness is well known and has an extended history. Johnson and his colleagues (1989) tell us that *"...Aristotle in the 3rd century B.C. reported that the buzzing in his ears ceased when he was in the presence of other sounds."* Since this time, others have reported the effects of a masking noise on the reduction of tinnitus loudness (Jones and Knudsen, 1928; Feldmann, H., 1987 and Vernon, 1977).

Such observations and subsequent practices are of great importance to the hearing health professional. Although commercially available masker devices do not work for all individuals, the frequency of success is such that it plays a major role in the clinical management of tinnitus.

A *masker device* produces a controlled narrow or broad band of noise. Often, these devices have a potentiometer controlling frequency shaping of the output response as well as the volume. Such devices are selected on the basis of a tinnitus evaluation to determine whether the patient can be masked by a noise band and whether there is a period of residual inhibition following the withdrawal of the noise to the offending ear.

Residual inhibition is best defined as the absence or reduction of tinnitus loudness following a specified period of exposure to a noise source. In general, residual inhibition is greater the longer the patient is exposed to the masking signal. Although many patients report some degree of residual inhibition following masker use, the neurophysiological mechanisms are not understood entirely. Parenthetically, it is interesting to note that hearing aid devices alone do not promote significant residual inhibition.

A combination device is simply a masker signal and a hearing aid in the same physical housing. The patient has independent control over the output of the hearing aid and the masking signal. Johnson and his co-researchers (1989) report that a combination device is more effective than just a masker device alone.

Success underlying the use of a masker or combination device is most probably a psychological phenomenon. Most individuals with tinnitus complain of the constant presence of an unwanted sound in their head or at their ear(s). For the majority, subjective tinnitus is present 24 hours a day. Although it may vary in intensity and frequency composition, it is ever-present. It can interfere with social interaction, concentration, sleep and emotional stability. There is no way for the individual to ignore the tinnitus. With the introduction of an external noise (via a masker or combination device) sufficient to mask the ongoing tinnitus, the noise is "external" to the head. That is, the noise is outside the head and part of the acoustic environment. It is a much easier task for one to ignore an external stimulus than an internally generated one.

All of us experience noises of our external acoustic environment and, normally, are not bothered by them. We are psychologically able to ignore environmental sounds unless they have immediate significance to us. For example, a young mother is exposed to a number of everyday sounds in the home and is oblivious to them. Yet, when the baby cries, she is immediately alerted and takes appropriate action. This ability to ignore one's acoustic environment makes it possible for the tinnitus masker to be effective as a method of treatment.

There is no doubt that the use of a masker or combination device has been beneficial to many. Unfortunately, not all who have tinnitus can benefit from masker use (Johnson et al. 1969, Johnson and Agnew, 1993). There is no general consensus among serious investigators why masker devices are effective for some and of no value to others. The etiology of subjective tinnitus is most likely multicausal. That is, the site of lesion (neurogenerating site) causing tinnitus can occur at any point along the auditory pathway; from the cochlea to the auditory cortex.

There is even some evidence to suggest that sensory systems, other than auditory, can cause subjective tinnitus. It may be that masker devices are effective for those who have the same or similar etiological factors creating tinnitus. If such is the case, then it is logical to assume that masker device effectiveness is restricted to that group having common causal factors.

Regardless of the percent of individuals helped by masker or combination devices, the hearing health professional should evaluate the person's response to the administration of a controlled masking signal. However, when so doing, it is important to realize that maximum effectiveness may be achieved after an extended period of use. The person should be counseled relative to reasonable expectations from a masker device and a structured follow up evaluation should be formulated.

The intent of this two-part chapter has been to present rather basic information about tinnitus and its management. It was not the intent to offer exhaustive commentary or extensive review of therapeutic practices, but rather to present an overview of major considerations in dealing with people with subjective tinnitus.

There is a clinical responsibility that hearing health professionals can exercise when working with those having subjective tinnitus. It is hoped that this chapter has added to the information needed to effectively deal with the tinnitus patient.

References

Feldmann, H. (1987). Historical remarks. Proceedings III International Tinnitus Seminar (Munster, Germany). Harsch Verlag, Karlsruhe. pp. 210–213.

Grossan. M. (1976). Treatment of subjective tinnitus with biofeedback. *Ear, Nose & Throat*. 55; pp. 314–318.

Grossan, M. (1989). The biofeedback program. In R. Sandlin (Ed.), *The Understanding and Treatment of Tinnitus*. Published by the American Tinnitus Association. Portland, Oregon.

House, P. (1981). Personality of the tinnitus patient. In D. Everest and G. Lawrenson (Eds.). *Tinnitus*, Ciba Foundation Symposium 85. London Pitman.

Johnson, R., Press, L., Griest, S., Storter, K. and Lentz, B. (1989). A tinnitus masking program: Efficacy and safety. *Hear. Jour.* (November), pp. 18–21.

Johnson, R. and Agnew, J. (1993). New tinnitus masking devices allow patient clinician tuning. *Hear. Instrum.* 44:1, pp.25–26.

Jones, I. and Knudsen, V. (1928). Certain aspects of tinnitus, particularly treatment. *Laryngoscope*, pp. 597–611.

Reich, G. and Johnson, R. (1984). Personality characteristics of tinitus patients. Supplement 9, *Jour. Laryng. & Oto.*, Proceedings of the II International Tinnitus Seminar (New York, New York). pp. 228–232.

Sweetow, R. (1986). Cognitive aspects of tinnitus patient management. *Ear & Hear.* 7:6 pp. 390–396.

Sweetow, R. (1989). Adjunctive approaches to the tinnitus-patient management. *Hear. Jour.* (November). pp. 38–43.

— by Dr. Robert E. Sandlin, Ph.D.

Chapter 21

Noise, Ears, and Hearing Protection

How Prevalent Is Noise-Related Hearing Loss?

One in 10 Americans has a hearing loss that affects his ability to understand normal speech. Excessive noise exposure is the most common cause of hearing loss.

Can Noise Really Hurt My Ears?

Yes—noise can be dangerous. If it is loud enough and lasts long enough, it can damage your hearing.

The damage caused by noise, called *sensorineural hearing loss* or *nerve loss*, can be caused by several factors other than noise, but noise-induced hearing loss is different in one important way—it can be reduced or prevented altogether.

Can I "Toughen Up" My Ears?

No. If you think you have grown used to a loud noise, it probably has damaged your ears, and there is no treatment—no medicine, no surgery, not even a hearing aid—that truly corrects your hearing once it is damaged by noise.

How Does the Ear Work?

The ear has three main parts: the outer, middle, and inner ear. The outer ear (the part you can see) opens into the ear canal. The eardrum separates the ear canal from the middle ear. Small bones in the middle ear help transfer sound to the inner ear. The inner ear contains the auditory (hearing) nerve, which leads to the brain.

Any source of sound sends vibrations or sound waves into the air. These funnel through the ear opening, down the ear canal, and strike your eardrum, causing it to vibrate. The vibrations are passed to the small bones of the middle ear, which transmit them to the hearing nerve in the inner ear. Here, the vibrations become nerve impulses and go directly to the brain, which interprets the impulses as sound: music, a slamming door, a voice, etc.

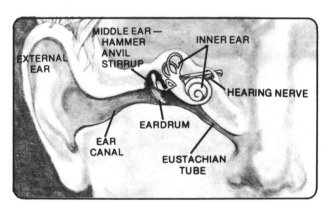

Figure 21.1. The normal ear.

When noise is too loud, it begins to kill the nerve endings in the inner ear. As the exposure time to loud noise increases, more and more nerve endings are destroyed. As the number of nerve endings decreases, so does your hearing. **There is no way to restore life to dead nerve endings: the damage is permanent.**

How Can I Tell If a Noise Is Dangerous?

People differ in their sensitivity to noise. As a general rule, noise may damage your hearing if you have to shout over background noise to make yourself heard, the noise hurts your ears, it makes your ears ring, or you are slightly deaf for several hours after exposure to the noise.

Sound can be measured scientifically in two ways. Intensity, or loudness of sound, is measured in decibels. Pitch is measured in frequency of sound vibrations per second. A low pitch such as a deep voice or a tuba makes fewer vibrations per second than a high voice or violin.

What Does Frequency Have to Do with Hearing Loss?

Frequency is measured in cycles per second, or Hertz (Hz). The higher the pitch of the sound, the higher the frequency.

Young children, who generally have the best hearing, can often distinguish sounds from about 20 Hz, such as the lowest note on a large pipe organ, to 20,000 Hz, such as the high shrill of a dog whistle that many people are unable to hear.

Human speech, which ranges from 300 to 4,000 Hz, sounds louder to most people than noises at very high or very low frequencies. When hearing impairment begins, the high frequencies are often lost first, which is why people with hearing loss often have difficulty hearing the high pitched voices of women and children.

Loss of high frequency hearing also can distort sound, so that speech is difficult to understand even though it can be heard. Hearing impaired people often have difficulty detecting differences between certain words that sound alike, especially words that contain S, F, SH, CH, H, or soft C, sounds, because the sound of these consonants is in a much higher frequency range than vowels and other consonants.

What about Decibels?

Intensity of sound is measured in decibels (dB). The scale runs from the faintest sound the human ear can detect, which is labeled O dB, to over 180 dB, the noise at a rocket pad during launch.

Decibels are measured logarithmically. This means that as decibel intensity increases by units of 10, each increase is *10 times* the lower figure. Thus, 20 decibels is 10 times the intensity of 10 decibels, and 30 decibels is 100 times as intense as 10 decibels.

How High Can the Decibels Go Without Affecting My Hearing?

Many experts agree that continual exposure to more than 85 decibels may become dangerous.

211

Does the Length of Time I Hear a Noise Have Anything to Do with the Danger to My Hearing?

It certainly does. The longer you are exposed to a loud noise, the more damaging it may be. Also, the closer you are to the source of intense noise, the more damaging it is.

Every gunshot produces a noise that could damage the ears of anyone in close hearing range. Large bore guns and artillery are the worst because they are the loudest. But even cap guns and firecrackers can damage your hearing if the explosion is close to your ear. Anyone who uses firearms without some form of ear protection risks hearing loss.

Recent studies show an alarming increase in hearing loss in youngsters. Evidence suggests that loud rock music along with increased use of portable radios with earphones may be responsible for this phenomenon.

Table 21.2. Examples of approximate decibel levels.

Approximate Decibel (dB) Level	Example
0	faintest sound heard by human ear.
30	whisper, quiet library.
60	normal conversation, sewing machine, typewriter.
90	lawnmower, shop tools, truck traffic; 8 hours per day is the maximum exposure (protects 90% of people).
100	chainsaw, pneumatic drill, snowmobile; 2 hours per day is the maximum exposure without protection.
115	sandblasting, loud rock concert, auto horn; 15 minutes per day is the maximum exposure without protection.
140	gun muzzle blast, jet engine; Noise causes pain and even brief exposure injures unprotected ears. Maximum allowed noise *with* hearing protectors.

Can Noise Affect More Than My Hearing?

A ringing in the ears, called *tinnitus*, commonly occurs after noise exposure, and it often becomes permanent. Some people react to loud noise with anxiety and irritability, an increase in pulse rate and blood pressure, or an increase in stomach acid. Very loud noise can reduce efficiency in performing difficult tasks by diverting attention from the job.

Who Should Wear Hearing Protectors?

If you must work in an excessively noisy environment, you should wear protectors. You should also wear them when you are using power tools, noisy yard equipment, or firearms.

What Are the Laws for On-the-Job Exposure?

Habitual exposure to noise above 85 dB will cause a gradual hearing loss in a significant number of individuals, and louder noises will accelerate this damage. For unprotected ears, the allowed exposure time decreases by **one-half for each 5 dB increase** in the average noise level. For instance, exposure is limited to 8 hr at 90 dB, 4 hr at 95 dB, and 2 hr at 100 dB. The highest permissible noise exposure for the **unprotected** ear is 115 dB for 15 **minutes/**day. Any noise above 140 dB **is not permitted.**

The Occupational Safety and Health Administration, in its Hearing Conservation Amendment of 1983, requires hearing conservation programs in noisy work places. This includes a yearly hearing test for the approximately five million workers exposed to an average of 85 dB or more of noise during an 8-hour work day.

Ideally, noisy machinery and work places should be engineered to be more quiet or the worker's time in the noise should be reduced; however, the cost of these actions is often prohibitive As an alternative, individual hearing protectors are required when noise averages more than 90 dB during an 8-hour day.

When noise measurements indicate that hearing protectors are needed, the employer must offer at least one type of earplug and one type of earmuff without cost to employees. If the yearly hearing tests reveal hearing loss of 10 dB or more in higher pitches in either ear, the worker must be informed and must wear hearing protectors when noise averages more than 85 dB for an 8-hour day.

Larger losses of hearing and/or the possibility of ear disease should result in referral to an ear, nose and throat physician (otolaryngologist).

What Are Hearing Protectors? How Effective Are They?

Hearing protection devices decrease the intensity of sound that reaches the eardrum. They come in two forms: earplugs and earmuffs.

Earplugs are small inserts that fit into the outer ear canal. To be effective they must totally block the ear canal with an airtight seal. They are available in a variety of shapes and sizes to fit individual ear canals and can be custom made. For people who have trouble keeping them in their ears, they can be fitted to a headband.

Earmuffs fit over the entire outer ear to form an air seal so the entire circumference of the ear canal is blocked, and they are held in place by an adjustable band. Earmuffs will not seal around eyeglasses or long hair, and the adjustable headband tension must be sufficient to hold earmuffs firmly around the ear. Earplugs must be snugly sealed so the entire circumference of the ear canal is blocked. An improperly fitted, dirty or worn-out plug may not seal and can irritate the ear canal.

Properly fitted earplugs or muffs reduce noise 15 to 30 dB. The better earplugs and muffs are approximately equal in sound reduction, although earplugs are better for low frequency noise and earmuffs for high frequency noise.

Simultaneous use of earplugs and muffs usually adds 10 to 15 dB more protection than either used alone. Combined use should be considered when noise exceeds 105 dB.

Why Can't I Just Stuff My Ears with Cotton?

Ordinary cotton balls or tissue paper wads stuffed into the ear canals are very poor protectors: they reduce noise only by approximately 7 dB.

What Are the Common Problems of Hearing Protectors?

Studies have shown that one-half of the workers wearing hearing protectors receive one-half or less of the noise reduction potential of their protectors *because these devices are not worn continuously while in noise or because they do not fit properly.*

A hearing protector that gives an average of 30 dB of noise reduction if worn continuously during an 8-hour work day becomes equivalent to only 9 dB of protection if taken off for one hour in the noise. This is because decibels are measured on a logarithmic scale, and there is a 10-fold increase in noise energy for each 10 dB increase.

During the hour with unprotected ears, the worker is exposed to 1,000 times more sound energy than if earplugs or muffs had been worn.

In addition, noise exposure is cumulative. So the noise at home or at play must be counted in the *total* exposure during any one day. A maximum allowable while on-the-job followed by exposure to a noisy lawnmower or loud music will definitely exceed the safe daily limit.

Even if earplugs and/or muffs are worn continuously while in noise, they do little good if there is an incomplete air seal between the hearing protector and the skin.

When using hearing protectors, you will hear your own voice as louder and deeper. This is a useful sign that the hearing protectors are properly positioned.

Can I Hear Other People and Machine Problems If I Wear Hearing Protectors?

Just as sunglasses help vision in very bright light, so do hearing protectors enhance speech understanding in very noisy places. Even in a quiet setting, a normal-hearing person wearing hearing protectors should be able to understand a regular conversation.

Hearing protectors do slightly reduce the ability of those with damaged hearing or poor comprehension of language to understand normal conversation. However, it is essential that persons with impaired hearing wear earplugs or muffs to prevent further inner ear damage.

It has been argued that hearing protectors might **reduce** a worker's ability to hear the noises that signify an improperly functioning machine. However, most workers readily adjust to the quieter sounds and can still detect such problems.

What If My Hearing Is Already Damaged? How Can I Tell?

Hearing loss usually develops over a period of several years. Since it is painless and gradual, you might not notice it. What you might notice is a ringing or other sound in your ear (called *tinnitus*), which could be the result of long-term exposure to noise that has damaged the hearing nerve. Or, you may have trouble understanding what people say: they may seem to be mumbling, especially when you are in a noisy place such as in a crowd or at a party. This could be the beginning of high-frequency hearing loss, a hearing test will detect it.

215

If you have any of these symptoms, you may have nothing more serious than impacted wax or an ear infection, which might be simply corrected. However, it might be hearing loss from noise. In any case, take no chances with noise—the hearing loss it causes is permanent. If you suspect a hearing loss, consult a physician with special training in ear care and hearing disorders (called an otolaryngologist or otologist). This doctor can diagnose your hearing problem and recommend the best way to manage it.

Chapter 22

Treatment of
Sensorineural Hearing Loss

Abstract

Of the 25 million people who are hearing impaired, 85% suffer from sensorineural hearing loss (SNL). In the past decade, the identification and treatment of SNL have evolved from futile efforts to active intervention. This chapter identifies nine forms of inner ear disorders causing SNL for which medical/surgical treatment is available. Physicians must realize that, with appropriate diagnosis and treatment, hearing nerve loss can have a satisfactory outcome.

Introduction

During the past decade, otologists have focused their attention on identifying and treating sensorineural hearing loss (SNL). Before this time, a loss of hearing due to decreased hearing nerve function was untreatable, except by amplification.

The conquest of middle ear deafness by replacing ossicles, restoring the tympanic membrane or removing diseased tissue using microsurgical techniques has become an accomplished fact. The success in conductive deafness treatment has overshadowed recent progress in hearing improvement in the larger population of sensorineurally deaf patients. Conductive deafness affects only 15% of the 25 million people who are hearing-impaired.

Indiana Medicine, Journal of the Indiana State Medical Association, August 1991; reprinted with permission.

217

There are nine forms of inner ear disorders causing SNL for which medical/surgical treatment is available. Although responses to treatment vary, any relief is appreciated by the afflicted patient.

This chapter will review the progress in managing sensorineural deafness and outline nine forms of SNL for which treatment should be instituted.

Meniere's Disease

Meniere's disease is a clear-cut clinical entity characterized by hearing loss, vertigo, ear fullness and tinnitus. Substantial benefit is obtained from dietary, medical and/or surgical treatments. The major spells can be stopped in more than 90% of patients, and hearing can be improved or stabilized in two-thirds of patients.

All patients are placed on a salt- and caffeine-restricted diet and advised to stop smoking. Other medications such as diuretics, vasodilators and vestibular suppressants can be used. Diazepam frequently is used and is beneficial in the latter category. Meclizine is seldom beneficial.

Surgery is offered to patients who do not improve with medical and dietary therapies. If hearing is salvageable, an endolymphatic sac-mastoid shunt is usually the first choice. The shunt is an outpatient surgical procedure offering more than an 80% chance of controlling dizziness and, especially in the early stages of the disease, about a 60% chance of stabilizing or reversing sensorineural hearing loss. If this procedure fails to control the vertigo and there is reasonably good hearing, a retro-sigmoid or suboccipital vestibular nerve section is performed to save auditory nerve function.

Intraoperative surgical monitoring is recommended to minimize risk to the facial and auditory nerves. This procedure does nothing to alter the basic disease process in the cochlea and, after a period of time, hearing can deteriorate severely. If no useable hearing is present and tinnitus is severe, total VIIIth nerve section is done to provide relief of tinnitus and vertigo. If tinnitus is not a primary complaint, labyrinthectomy usually is curative.

The goals of therapy today are not only to relieve dizzy spells but also to improve and stabilize hearing.

Perilymph Fistula

Perilymph fistula is a leakage of fluid (perilymph) from the inner ear (labyrinth) into the middle ear through the round and/or oval windows. A history of exertion, barotrauma or an audible "pop" in the ear at the time of the hearing loss suggests this entity. A fistula within the cochlea also can develop, causing a mixing of the inner ear fluids (endolymph and perilymph). This condition disrupts the delicate balance of electrolytes within the inner ear compartment. Although symptoms characteristically are fluctuating hearing loss alone (15%) or vestibular symptoms alone (12%), both symptoms commonly are present. Developmental anomalies, such as a widely patent cochlear aqueduct or cochlear modiolar defects, may predispose the involved ear to this condition.

Historical features suggesting fistula of the inner ear include compressive/decompressive episodes, heavy lifting or straining, head injury or stapedectomy. Conservative treatment consists of bed rest, stool softeners and avoiding heavy lifting, coughing or straining. Sensorineural hearing loss that continues to progress, with or without positional vertigo and ataxia while walking, indicates the need for surgery. A tympanotomy with tissue sealing of the oval and round windows will eliminate dizzy symptoms in 95% of patients and improve or stabilize hearing in 50% of patients.

Autoimmune Sensorineural Deafness

Autoimmune sensorineural deafness is a treatable form of severe hearing loss when the body's immune system attacks and progressively destroys the inner ear. Reports indicate that it may involve patients of any age. It may take the form of sudden or fluctuating hearing losses. Any patient with a bilateral or asymmetric sensorineural deafness for which the cause is not readily apparent is suspect for this disease. It is important to recognize it since there is no treatment other than immunosuppression that may salvage or restore hearing. Without treatment, all hearing is lost.

Any patient suspected of having this disease should have an immune screen (sedimentation rate, rheumoid factor, anti-nuclear antibody with and without culture cells and quantitative IgA and IgG). If any two of these are positive, treatment should be started.

Our treatment is dexamethasone, 16 mg daily in divided doses for a period of approximately three months before tapering the medication begins. Twice weekly audiograms are used to monitor the patient. In severe bilateral cases, some investigators have used cyclophosphamide infusion. We have not needed to use this medication. Patients who cannot tolerate steroid therapy are candidates for plasmaphoresis.

Identifying this cause of sensorineural deafness is of paramount importance since it can be reversed totally.

Syphilitic Deafness

Sensorineural hearing loss due to syphilis has been around for years. The benefits of steroid therapy after appropriate antibiotic treatment are well-documented. This form of deafness and vertigo may mimic Meniere's disease; thus, all patients suspected of Meniere's must have appropriate testing for tertiary syphilis. A fluorescent treponemal antibody/absorbed is suggested.

Steroid therapy eliminates vertigo and allows patients to hear for up to 10 years. Steroid therapy every other day can provide relief without significant side effects.

Cochlear Otosclerosis

Cochlear otosclerosis is characterized by a flat audiometric loss and good to excellent speech understanding and starts in the third or fourth decade of life. Although a positive family history of proven stapedial otosclerosis is usually present, this is not necessary. This type of hearing nerve loss can be arrested (85%) or even reversed (15% of the 85%) with appropriate doses of daily fluoride, Vitamin D and calcium. Since fluoride therapy can prematurely close the epiphyseal plate in developing bones, it must be used with caution in children or pregnant women.

Sudden Deafness

Sudden hearing loss is defined as a loss of at least 30 dB in three contiguous frequencies in less than 72 hours and occurs in about 10 people per 100,000 per year. Both men and women are affected, with an average age of 43 years at onset. In most cases, the etiology cannot be determined. Most commonly, the sudden loss is attributed to either viral infection or compromised circulation to the inner ear.

Our treatment for this idiopathic loss is primarily steroid therapy. The prognosis for recovery depends upon: 1) the hearing loss configuration, 2) the patient's age; 3) the degree of vestibular injury defined by the electro-nystagmogram; 4) the presence or absence of vertigo; and 5) the duration of the loss. Patients with a mild mid-frequency hearing loss often recover all of the lost hearing. Patients with a moderate sensorineural hearing loss will have a partial recovery rate, ranging from 40% to 80%. Patients with severe to profound loss have a 20% chance of recovery.

Administering intravenous iodinated contrast media is another treatment that we have used for sudden idiopathic hearing nerve deafness. Inhaling carbogen (95% O_2 and 5% CO_2), which has a strong vasodilating effect, also has been useful.

Toxic Deafness

Physicians must be aware of the potentially toxic effects of medications on the hearing and balance nerves of the inner ear. Aminoglycosides and loop diuretics are especially hazardous, especially when used in combination. Chemotherapeutic agents, such as cisplatin, are capable of producing a devastating effect on the auditory/vestibular apparatus. Preoperative audiometric and vestibular testing with close monitoring during treatment is strongly advised.(see Table 22.1).

Profound Sensorineural Deafness: Cochlear Electrode Implant

Total bilateral hearing nerve deafness is untreatable with the most powerful means of hearing aid amplification but can be treated with cochlear electrode implants. Although there are not many suitable candidates, selected centers can provide this treatment for adults and children with total deafness.

Noise-Induced Hearing Loss

Sensorineural hearing loss due to loud noise exposure can be arrested in its early stages and reversed with appropriate sound protection devices and, occasionally, with medication. The early warning signs after noise exposure include fullness in the ear, tinnitus and a temporary decrease in hearing and should be seriously addressed.

Evaluation

As with all medical disorders, a thorough history forms the basis for diagnosis and treatment. Particular attention is paid to antecedent ear disease or surgery, trauma, activity at the time of onset and symptoms of hearing fluctuation, tinnitus, vertigo and ear pressure. Physical examination should include microscopic ear examination and neurological examination. Audiologic evaluation should include measuring the air

Table 22.1. Medications that effect the hearing or balance function of the inner ear.

The medications listed below have toxic effects on the hearing or balance function of the inner ear. The prescribing physician should consult the *Physicians' Desk Reference*, a pharmacist or similar source before prescribing these medications.

This list is not exhaustive but provides guidance in using some common medications. Hearing and balance function monitoring is recommended when potentially ototoxic medications are used.

Chemical Name	Trade Name
Aminoglycoside Antibiotics	
Streptomycin	—
Neomycin	Mycifradin, Neobiotic
Kanamycin	Dantrex, Klebcil
Tobramycin	Nebcin
Paromomycin	Humatin
Gentamicin	Garamycin
Sisomycin	Sispetin
Amikacin	Amikin
Netilmicin	Netromycin
Chemotherapeutic Agents	
Cisplatin	Platinol
Salicylic Acid Derivatives	
Asprin	Various (effects reversible)
Other Antibiotics	
Vancomycin	Vancocin
Erythromycin	Various (rarely ototoxic)
Capreomycin	Capastat (rarely ototoxic)
Metal Antagonist	
Deferoxamine	Desferal (usually reversible)
Loop Diuretics	
Ethacrynic acid	Edecrin
Furosemide	Lasix
Bumetanide	Bume
Drug Combinations	
Neomycin	Aminoglycoside
Polymyxin B	Loop Diuretics
Dexamethasone	

and bone conduction with speech discrimination. Auditory brain stem responses will show the status of eighth nerve and brain stem structures if hearing is not too depressed.

Electrocochleography (ECoG) measures the electrical activity within the cochlea in response to sound stimuli. It can distinguish between nerve loss originating in the cochlea versus the eighth nerve or higher structures. Meniere's disease often gives a distinctive signature on ECoG. Vestibular evaluation consists of electronystagmography (ENG) and a fistula test with ENG-impedance testing if fistula is suspected. Posturography often is helpful in cases of confusing balance findings. Radiologic studies include magnetic resonance imaging (MRI) and computed tomography (CT). MRI is used when a tumor is suspected, and CT may be helpful if a fracture or other bony abnormality is suspected. Laboratory work consists of an FTA/ABS, complete blood count and erythrocyte sedimentation rate, unless a specific clinical entity is suspected.

Summary

Sudden or rapid progressive sensorineural hearing loss is an otologic emergency demanding expeditious evaluation and initiation of therapy if the patient's hearing is to be preserved. Nine distinct entities have been identified in which a patient's hearing can be preserved, stabilized or restored to normal. Early intervention is of great importance.

—by George W. Hicks, M.D.,
J. William Wright III, M.D.

References

1. Nagahara K, Fisch U, Dillier N: Experimental study on the perilymphatic pressure. *Am J Otolaryngol*, 3:1–8, 1981.

2. Coats AC: The summating potential and Meniere's disease. *Arch Otolaryngol*, 107:199–208, 1981.

3. Maddox HE III: Endolymphatic sac surgery. *Laryngoscope*, 88:1676–1679, 1977.

4. Gibson WPR: A study of endolymphatic sac surgery. *Otolaryngol Clin North Am*, 16(1):181–188, 1983.

5.   Anderson RG, Meyerhoff WL: Sudden sensorineural hearing loss. *Otolaryngol Clin North Am*, 16(1):189–195, 1983.

6.   Daspit CP, Churchill D, Linthicum FH: Diagnosis of perilymph fistula using ENG and impedance. *Laryngoscope*, 90:217–223, 1980.

7.   Hicks GW, Wright III JW: Delayed endolymphatic hydrops. *Laryngoscope* 98(8): 840–845, 1988.

8.   Wright Jr JW, Wright III JW, Hicks GW: Valve implants: Comparative analysis of the first year's experience with results in other sac operations. *Otolaryngol Clin North Am*, 16(1):175–179, 1983.

9.   Silverstein H, Norrell H, Rosenberg S: The resurrection of vestibular neurectomy: A 10-year experience with 115 cases. *J Neurosurg*, 72:533–539,1990.

10.   McCabe B: Autoimmune sensorineural hearing loss. *Ann Otol Rhinol Laryngol*, 88:585–589, 1979.

11.   Guzya AJ: Sudden sensorineural hearing loss. *The Hearing Journal*, 40(2):23–31, 1987.

12.   Schuknecht HF, Donovan ED: The pathology of idiopathic sudden sensorineural hearing loss. *Arch Otolaryngol*, 243:1–15, 1986.

13.   Sismanis A, Hughes GB, Butts F: Bilateral spontaneous perilymph fistula: a diagnostic and management dilemma. *Otolaryngol Head Neck Surg*, 103(3):436–438, 1990.

14.   Wilson WR, Byl FM, Laird N: The efficacy of steroids in the treatment of idiopathic sudden hearing loss: a double-blind study. *Arch Otolaryngol*, 106:772–776, 1980.

Chapter 23

Hyperacusis

What Is Hyperacusis?

Hyperacusis is defined as a collapsed tolerance to normal environmental sounds. It is a rare hearing disorder where an individual becomes highly sensitive to noise. Sometimes people think they have hyperacusis because they are bothered by loud sounds like music, heavy equipment, jet airplanes or sirens. This is not hyperacusis because these sounds are loud to normal ears. Individuals with hyperacusis have difficulty tolerating sounds which do not seem loud to others (running faucet water, riding in a car, walking on leaves, dishwasher, fan on the refrigerator, handling paper). The ears lose much of their dynamic range, and everyday noises sound unbearably or painfully loud. Even quick shifts in sound are difficult to tolerate. It is like the volume control on our ears is stuck on HIGH! Hyperacusis can affect people of all ages and is usually accompanied by tinnitus (ringing in the ears). Hyperacusis and tinnitus may affect one or both ears. Recruitment is a similar hearing disorder often confused with hyperacusis. Individuals with hyperacusis are highly sensitive to sound but have no hearing loss. Individuals with recruitment are very sensitive to sound but have hearing loss documented by a nose diving line on their audiogram. Hyperacusis, recruitment and tinnitus

From http://www.visi.com/~minuet/hearing/hyperacusis/hdef_sht.html provided by the Hyperacusis Network, 444 Edgewood Drive, Green Bay, WI 45302-4873; reprinted with permission granted in March 1998.

225

are not life threatening but, depending on their severity can be very traumatic.

What Causes Hyperacusis?

Hyperacusis is very rare therefore little is known about it. The onset is usually caused by either exposure to loud noise or head injury. Some experts speculate there has been a breakdown or dysfunction in the efferent portion of the auditory nerve. Efferent meaning fibers that originate in the brain which serve to regulate or inhibit incoming sounds. It is possible that the efferent fibers of the auditory nerve are selectively damaged even though the hair cells that allow us to hear pure tones in an audiometric evaluation remain intact. Hearing tests on hyperacusis individuals usually appear to be normal. This shows how inadequate current testing is in evaluating hyperacusis. This complicates our efforts to secure reasonable accommodations from an employer or obtaining disability. No one clearly understands how the brain interprets sound and the mechanisms in the ear which receive sound are so microscopic and deep in the inner ear they are hard to examine. Medicine has much to learn about the auditory system before hyperacusis or many other hearing problems are fully understood. Other contributing causes of hyperacusis are Temporomandibular Joint (TMJ), Meniere's Disease, Lyme's Disease, William's Syndrome, Bell's Palsy and Tay-Sachs Disease. As many as 40% of all autistic children are also very sound sensitive. Although their reaction to sound is similar to hyperacusis sufferers, their condition is called hyperacute hearing. Autistic children can currently receive Auditory Integration Therapy (AIT) to help resolve their sound sensitivities. This therapy does not work for hyperacusis and can actually worsen our condition—particularly the tinnitus because the treatment is administered at uncomfortably loud sound levels. Because many autistic children are non-verbal, parents learn much from individuals with hyperacusis on what it is like to have hypersensitive hearing.

What Can Be Done?

Currently, there are a few treatments available for hyperacusis. The most promising comes from Dr. Pawel Jastreboff of the University of Maryland. The therapy requires individuals listen to static (white noise) from a specific ear appliance (masker) called the Starkey viennetone AM/ti. By listening to a specific kind of white noise at barely audible levels for a disciplined period of time each day it is thought that the efferent system of the auditory nerve may be re-trained to once again tolerate normal environmental sounds. The treatment usually improves one's tolerance to sound for those who complete the program which may last from 12-16 months. Usually no improvement is seen during the first 6 months. The biggest obstacle for individuals considering this therapy is themselves. Those who are extremely sound sensitive seek quiet places and tend to isolate them-selves. It is only natural to feel this way because our natural instinct for survival tells us to do so. Initially abstinence from noise is essen-tial following a significant noise injury (to begin healing) however, over the long hall there is a tendency for individuals with hyperacusis to wear ear protection even when they are in relatively quiet surround-ings. Over a period of time this tends to make one's tolerance to sound collapse even further. The very idea of undergoing a therapy which involves sound (no matter how gentle) is offensive. For this reason, the University of Maryland feels counseling is every bit as important as the (masking/noise generator) therapy is.

How Rare Is Hyperacusis?

Although there may be as many as 1% of the population who are sound sensitive, hyperacusis sufferers go well beyond the definition of sound sensitive. Because hyperacusis has received little publicity (latest article—August issue of Prevention Magazine) it is hard to get a handle on how rare hyperacusis really is. At this point rough esti-mates would put it as little as one in every 100,000 people. That is extremely rare! Recruitment and hyperacute hearing are far more common and tinnitus sufferers have been estimated to be approxi-mately 50 million! Tinnitus is associated with most hearing disorders and is a common thread which affects more and more in our culture where the noise level continues to escalate.

Where Can I Turn for Help?

The most difficult thing an individual suffering from severe hyperacusis must endure is a family who does not believe. Without the support of their family, this can turn into a nightmare. It is hard enough to deal with an indifferent medical community who has no idea what is wrong with us. Furthermore they often subject our ears to tests which may involve loud sounds—deteriorating our condition even worse. A sound tolerance test must be performed by an audiologist before any further testing is performed. This would give the E.N.T. a sound level guideline to conduct any further testing which the doctor may feel is necessary. Most hyperacusis patients wear ear protection— either foam ear plugs or ear muffs when they are in areas which are not sound friendly (on their terms). When ears are initially trauma- tized, it is even difficult to sleep because the sufferers stress level is so high. Sleep is extremely important in stress management and some sedative may initially be required to help at the very beginning. The Hyperacusis Network is an international support network to help individuals and their families with a collapsed tolerance to sound. No one knows more about hyperacusis than we do. The network also edu- cates the medical community and offers a 20 page supplement which explains hyperacusis in great detail. To receive the free quarterly newsletter, a subscription form must completed and sent to:

The Hyperacusis Network
444 Edgewood Drive
Green Bay, Wisconsin 54302-4873

Chapter 24

Ears and Altitude

Have you ever wondered why your ears pop when you fly on an airplane? Or why, when they fail to pop, you get an earache? Have you ever wondered why the babies on an airplane fuss and cry so much during descent?

Ear problems are the most common medical complaint of airplane travelers, and while they are usually simple, minor annoyances, they occasionally result in temporary pain and hearing loss.

The Ear and Air Pressure

It is the middle ear that causes discomfort during air travel, because it is an air pocket inside the head that is vulnerable to changes in air pressure.

Normally, each time (or each 2nd or 3rd time) you swallow, your ears make a little click or popping sound. This occurs because a small bubble of air has entered your middle ear, up from the back of your nose. It passes through the eustachian tube, a membrane-lined tube about the size of a pencil lead that connects the back of the nose with the middle ear. The air in the middle ear is constantly being absorbed by its membranous lining and resupplied through the eustachian tube. In this manner, air pressure on both sides of the eardrum stays about equal. If, and when, the air pressure is not equal the ear feels blocked.

Blocked Ears and Eustachian Tubes

The eustachian tube can be blocked, or obstructed, for a variety of reasons. When that occurs, the middle ear pressure cannot be equalized. The air already there is absorbed and a vacuum occurs, sucking the eardrum inward and stretching it. Such an eardrum cannot vibrate naturally, so sounds are muffled or blocked, and the stretching can be painful. If the tube remains blocked, fluid (like blood serum) will seep into the area from the membranes in an attempt to overcome the vacuum. This is called "fluid in the ear," serous otitis or aero-otitis.

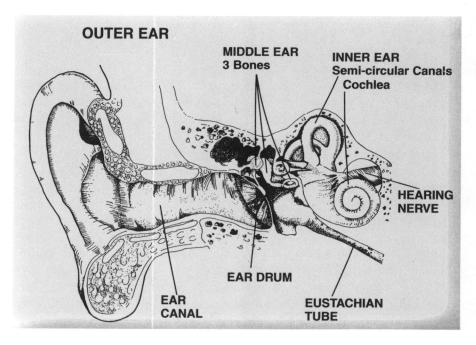

Figure 24.1. The ear is divided into three parts:

1. **The outer ear:** the part that you can see on the side of the heard plus the ear canal leading down to the eardrum.

2. **The middle ear:** the eardrum and ear bones (ossicles), plus air spaces behind the eardrum and in the mastoid cavities (vulnerable to air pressure).

3. **The inner ear:** the area that contains the nerve endings of the organs of hearing and balance (equilibrium).

The most common cause for a blocked eustachian tube is the common cold. Sinus infections and nasal allergies (hay fever, etc.) are also causes. A stuffy nose leads to stuffy ears because the swollen membranes block the opening of the eustachian tube.

Children are especially vulnerable to blockages because their eustachian tubes are narrower than in adults.

How Can Air Travel Cause Problems?

Air travel is sometimes associated with rapid changes in air pressure. To maintain comfort, the eustachian tube must open frequently and wide enough to equalize the changes in pressure. This is especially true when the airplane is landing, going from low atmospheric pressure down closer to earth where the air pressure is higher.

Actually, any situation in which rapid altitude or pressure changes occur creates the problem. You may have experienced it when riding in elevators or when diving to the bottom of a swimming pool. Deep sea divers are taught how to equalize their ear pressures; so are pilots. You can learn the tricks too.

How to Unblock Your Ears

Swallowing activates the muscle that opens the eustachian tube. You swallow more often when you chew gum or let mints melt in your mouth. These are good air travel practices, especially just before take-off and during descent. Yawning is even better. Avoid sleeping during descent, because you may not be swallowing often enough to keep up with the pressure changes. (The flight attendant will be happy to awaken you just before descent.)

If yawning and swallowing are not effective, unblock your ears as follows:

1. Pinch your nostrils shut.

2. Take a mouthful of air.

3. Using your cheek and throat muscles, force the air into the back of your nose as if you were trying to blow your thumb and fingers off your nostrils (see "Precautions").

When you hear a loud pop in your ears, you have succeeded. You may have to repeat this several times during descent.

231

Babies' Ears

Babies cannot intentionally pop their ears, but popping may occur if they are sucking on a bottle or pacifier. Feed your baby during the flight, and do not allow him or her to sleep during descent.

Precautions

- When inflating your ears, you should not use force. The proper technique involves only pressure created by your cheek and throat muscles.

- If you have a cold, a sinus infection, or an allergy attack, it is best to postpone an airplane trip.

- If you recently have undergone ear surgery, consult with your surgeon on how soon you may safely fly.

What about Decongestants and Nose Sprays?

Many experienced air travelers use a decongestant pill or nasal spray an hour or so before descent. This will shrink the membranes and help the ears pop more easily. Travelers with allergy problems should take their medication at the beginning of the flight for the same reason.

Decongestant tablets and sprays can be purchased without a prescription. However, they should be avoided by people with heart disease, high blood pressure, irregular heart rhythms, thyroid disease, or excessive nervousness. Such people should consult their physicians before using these medicines. Pregnant women should likewise consult their physicians first.

If Your Ears Will Not Unblock

Even after landing you can continue the pressure equalizing techniques, and you may find decongestants and nasal sprays to be helpful. (However, avoid making a habit of nasal sprays. After a few days, they may cause more congestion than they relieve.) If your ears fail to open, or if pain persists, you will need to seek the help of a physician who has experience in the care of ear disorders. He/she may need to release the pressure or fluid with a small incision in the ear drum.

Chapter 25

Understanding Otoplasty: Ear Surgery

Probably no other physical characteristic cries out for facial plastic surgery more than protruding ears. Children, long the victims of cruel nicknames like "Dumbo" or "Mickey Mouse," are the most likely candidates for otoplasty, but this surgery can be performed at any age after the ears have reached full size, usually around five to six years of age. Even if the ears are only mildly distorted, the condition can lead to self-consciousness and poor adaptation to school. When it comes to otoplasty, conventional wisdom is the earlier the better.

Adults may also benefit from this procedure, which improves self-esteem with relative ease. Often, adults choose this surgery in conjunction with other facial plastic surgical procedures. Not only is it possible to "pin back" ears, but ears can also be reshaped, reduced in size, or made more symmetrical.

If you are wondering how otoplasty can improve the way you look, you need to know how otoplasty is performed and what you can expect from this procedure. This chapter can address many of your concerns.

Successful facial plastic surgery is a result of good rapport between patient and surgeon. Trust, based on realistic expectations and exacting medical expertise, develops in the consulting stages before surgery. Your surgeon can answer specific questions about your specific needs.

Is Otoplasty for You?

General good health and realistic expectations are prerequisites. It is also important to understand the surgery. Otoplasty will not alter hearing ability. What is important for successful otoplasty is that the ears be in proportion to the size and shape of the face and head.

When considering otoplasty, parents must be confident that they have their child's best interests at heart. A positive attitude toward the surgery is an important factor in all facial plastic surgery, but it is especially critical when the patient is a child or adolescent.

Adult candidates for otoplasty should understand that the firmer cartilage of fully developed ears does not provide the same molding capacity as in children. A consultation with a facial plastic surgeon can help parents decide what is best for their child, not only aesthetically, but also psychologically and physically. Timing is always an important consideration. Having the procedure at a young age is highly desirable in two respects: the cartilage is extremely pliable, thereby permitting greater ease of shaping; and secondly, the child will experience psychological benefits from the cosmetic improvement.

Making the Decision for Otoplasty

Your choice of a qualified facial plastic surgeon is of paramount importance. During the consultation, the surgeon will examine the structure of the ears and discuss possibilities for correcting the problems. Even if only one ear needs "pinning back," surgery will probably be recommended on both ears to achieve the most natural, symmetrical appearance.

After the surgeon and patient decide that otoplasty is indicated, your surgeon will discuss the procedure. Following a thorough medical history, your surgeon will explain the kind of anesthesia required, surgical facility, and costs. Typically, your surgeon will suggest a general anesthesia for young patients and a local anesthetic combined with a mild sedative for older children and adults. Under normal conditions, otoplasty requires approximately two hours.

Understanding the Surgery

Surgery begins with an incision just behind the ear, in the natural fold where the ear is joined to the head. The surgeon will then remove the necessary amounts of cartilage and skin required to achieve the right effect. In some cases, the surgeon will trim the cartilage, shaping it into a more desirable form and then pin the cartilage back with permanent sutures to secure the cartilage. In other instances, the surgeon will not remove any cartilage at all, using stitches to hold the cartilage permanently in place. After sculpting the cartilage to the desired shape, the surgeon will apply sutures to anchor the ear until healing occurs to hold the ear in the desired position.

What to Expect After the Surgery

Soft dressings applied to the ears will remain for a few days. Most patients experience some mild discomfort. If you are accustomed to sleeping on your side, your sleep patterns may be disrupted for a week or so because you cannot put any pressure on the ear areas. Headbands are sometimes recommended to hold the ears in the desired position for two weeks after the surgery.

The risks are minimal. There will be a thin white scar behind the ear after healing. Because this scar is in a natural crease behind the ear, the problem of visibility is inconsequential. Anything unusual should be reported to the surgeon immediately.

Facial plastic surgery makes it possible to correct many facial flaws that can often undermine one's self-confidence. By changing how you look, cosmetic surgery can help change how you feel about yourself.

Insurance does not generally cover surgery that is purely for cosmetic reasons. Surgery to correct or improve birth defects or traumatic injuries may be reimbursable in whole or in part. It is the patient's responsibility to check with the insurance carrier for information on the degree of coverage.

Facial Plastic Surgery

American Academy of Facial Plastic and Reconstructive Surgery, Inc.
1110 Vermont Avenue, N.W., Suite 220
Washington, D.C. 20005-3522
(202) 842-4500

The American Academy of Facial Plastic and Reconstructive Surgery, Inc. (AAFPRS) is the world's largest association of facial plastic and reconstructive surgeons—those physicians performing cosmetic and reconstructive surgery of the face, head, and neck. The Academy's bylaws provide that AAFPRS fellows be board-certified surgeons with training and experience in facial plastic surgery and be fellows of the American College of Surgeons.

Part Three

Vestibular Disorders

Chapter 26

Understanding Vestibular Function

Prevalence of Balance Disorders

The vestibular sense organs, located in the inner ear, are critical for control of balance. However, their importance and function are poorly understood by the general public. Perhaps this is because the control of balance is largely an unconscious process. The importance of balance function is typically recognized only after a failure of the vestibular system results in incapacitating problems. Disorders of the vestibular system cause a variety of serious problems, including falls, imbalance, dizziness, spatial disorientation and a blurring of vision. These problems interfere with most activities of everyday life and may prevent employment and limit personal independence.

Although the precise incidence of balance disorders, disequilibrium and dizziness from vestibular disturbance is difficult to determine, it is clear that these disorders constitute a major public health problem. For example, primary disorders of balance and dizziness are often hidden by their acute and serious consequences, such as falls; motor vehicle, boat and airplane accidents; and on-the-job injuries. Falls are experienced by more than 18 percent of persons over the age of 65 and more than 25 percent of individuals over the age of 75. Among individuals who are institutionalized, the incidence of falls nearly doubles. It has been estimated that, among elderly people, up

Excerpted from *National Strategic Research Plan*, National Institute on Deafness and Other Communication Disorders, 1994-1995; NIH Pub. No. 97-3217.

to 50 percent of those who fall and 20 to 25 percent of those who are hospitalized after falling have vestibular disorders. It has been suggested that disequilibrium may be responsible for many of the fractures caused by falling, including 200,000 hip fractures, that occur annually in Americans over the age of 65. Data from the National Institute on Aging (1990) indicates that combined medical and surgical costs for care of individuals with hip fractures exceed $8 billion per year. Furthermore, within this age group, morbidity may be as high as 50 percent and mortality may exceed 35 percent. Vestibular disorders have serious economic and social costs.

Community surveys have demonstrated that, among elderly individuals living at home, over half believe that dizziness prevents them from doing things that they could otherwise do. Overall, it is estimated that 12.5 million Americans over the age of 65 have dizziness that significantly interferes with their life, thereby extracting not only a physical but also a serious psychological toll. For individuals over the age of 65, disequilibrium is one of the two most common diagnoses among short-stay hospital admissions. In fact, the National Ambulatory Medical Care Survey for 1981 found that dizziness was the most common symptom presented to primary care physicians by individuals 75 years of age and older.

Disorders of balance are also common in younger individuals and children. Up to two-thirds of children with acquired deafness have severe vestibular deficits. In most cases their parents and health professionals have not identified their vestibular-related disabilities, often attributing the deficit to motor clumsiness, disorientation or cognitive or emotional limitations. In addition, many individuals who have sustained head injuries have long-lasting balance and dizziness problems related to vestibular system damage.

Although nearly everyone knows someone who has experienced dizziness and/or balance problems, these problems take many forms. The most common type of dizziness is provoked by inclining the head into certain positions, thereby interfering with occupational safety and daily activities. Although dizziness itself can lead to balance problems, disorders of the inner ear can cause severe balance problems even without dizziness. Slow degeneration of the vestibular sensors in the inner ear with aging is associated with postural instability in the dark or on uneven surfaces. Unfortunately, many individuals are not aware that they have an inner ear problem until they sustain a serious injury from a fall.

The psychological impact of vestibular symptoms should not be underestimated. The fear of falling, with the chance of physical injury, adversely affects an individual's sense of independence and affects the quality of life. Similarly, the fear of a sudden attack of dizziness, accompanied by socially embarrassing gait instability (ataxia), nausea and vomiting, can cause individuals to become reclusive. Subconscious fear of movement may play a role in the fear of being in large, open areas (agoraphobia). Subtle dysfunction of the vestibular system may underlie difficulties in learning, writing and reading. Vestibular dysfunction adversely affects an individual's ability to perform the most routine activities, such as taking a shower, performing housekeeping duties or driving an automobile. It may also prevent individuals from holding risk-intensive jobs (for example, telephone lineman, mechanic or bus driver).

With at least half of the people living in the United States being affected by balance or vestibular system impairment sometime during their lives, tremendous health care resources are committed to the medical, surgical and rehabilitative therapy for persons with vestibular disorders. Millions of dollars are spent each year on specific and symptomatic pharmacotherapy for vestibular disorders. The costs of surgical procedures and rehabilitation add many more millions. Advances in basic research, pathology and diagnostic methods have led to more specific medical and surgical treatment. However, the remaining gaps in professional and public knowledge of vestibular disorders and their management result in quality-of-life compromises for those individuals who suffer from vestibular impairment.

In 1976, an estimated $500 million was spent on visits to physicians for dizziness or vertigo. In 1994, the costs for medical care alone are estimated to exceeded $1 billion. To this total must be added the cost of diagnostic testing and treatment. The cost of falls from poor balance, which potentially lead to fractured limbs, hospitalization, surgery, pneumonia and sometimes death, add significantly to this amount.

Balance disorders also exact a military cost. Each year, the Army, Navy and the Air Force lose an average of 30 pilots and their aircraft to accidents caused by pilot disorientation and subsequent error. This loss of material conservatively represents an estimated cost of $300 million per year. In times of armed conflict, this cost increases three to four times. Also, two-thirds of all astronauts experience motion sickness that can severely reduce their effectiveness for the first three days into orbital flight.

A better scientific understanding of balance disorders is needed to identify and treat all of these problems. New research is needed to identify how vestibular pathology causes so many different types of dizziness and balance problems. The current lack of understanding of balance disorders results in misdiagnosis and failed therapy. Individuals with balance disorders see a variety of health care professionals before an accurate diagnosis is made. Some suffering could be partly remedied by improving health provider education on the clinical presentation and management of vestibular disorders.

Although considerable progress has been made over the past decade in understanding balance disorders, research is critically needed: (1) to learn the actual incidence and social effects of balance disorders, (2) to understand how the vestibular organs sense movements, (3) to understand how development, aging, regeneration and genetics affect normal and disordered vestibular function, (4) to characterize normal and disordered balance, gaze and perception of spatial orientation, and (5) to improve the diagnosis and treatment of balance disorders. This research provides the basis for eliminating the excessive, unnecessary suffering, dependence and social and economic costs associated with balance disorders.

Signal Transduction and Transmission

To understand the fundamental basis of balance and balance disorders and to identify and treat individuals with such disorders, further investigations are needed to explain how the vestibular sense organs inform the nervous system about body position and movement.

Signal Transduction

In mammals, there are five vestibular sensors located in each inner ear, adjacent to the structures for hearing. Two of these sensors, the utricular and saccular maculae, transduce linear acceleration forces acting on the head. The other three, the cristae of the semicircular canals, transduce angular or rotational acceleration forces. The five vestibular sensors are contained within the membranous labyrinth, a series of interconnected tubes and sacs filled with a high-potassium fluid called endolymph. The outside of the membranous labyrinth is bathed in perilymph, a fluid low in potassium and high in sodium, like most other extracellular fluids. The components of the labyrinth are so arranged in the temporal bone that they collectively provide the brain with a three-dimensional reconstruction of the position and motion of the head in space.

Each vestibular end-organ contains dark and transitional cells involved in endolymph homeostasis and a sensory epithelium composed of supporting cells and sensory hair cells. Bundles of mechanosensitive stereocilia (hair bundles) protrude from the apical surfaces of hair cells. Gelatinous accessory structures, the otoconial membranes of the maculae and the cupulae of the cristae, are moved by forces associated with active or passive head movements or by certain static head positions (head tilts). Displacement of these structures deflect the hair bundles to which they attach. These mechanical links between head perturbations or displacements and hair-bundle deflection are poorly understood. Deflection of hair bundles opens mechanically sensitive ion channels that allow potassium ions to flow from endolymph into the hair cell to depolarize the cell membrane. The change in membrane voltage modulates currents through other ion channels, located in the basolateral membrane, which modify the receptor potential. Calcium ion influx through channels at presynaptic sites on the hair cell modulates the release of glutamate or possibly other (as yet unknown) chemical transmitters, initiating the neural signal.

Signal Transmission

To transmit sensory information to the central nervous system, vestibular sensory nerve terminals in the labyrinth respond to hair cell transmitters by increasing or decreasing the frequency of nerve impulses from a resting level. These afferent nerve fibers are structurally and physiologically diverse. They innervate one or more hair cells, and afferents innervating different regions of the maculae and cupulae have different response properties. The functional significance of this heterogeneity is currently unclear but is actively being investigated. Vestibular afferents transmit signals to nuclei in the brain stem and cerebellum. At all points in the pathway, resting neural activity is biased upward or downward by positive or negative deflection of the hair bundles or by efferent activity.

Hair cells and sensory afferent terminals receive synapses from cholinergic, efferent fibers that originate in the brain stem. Efferent activity modifies the afferent response and may modulate vestibular responses on a longer time scale.

The afferent vestibular nerves enter the brain stem and contact cells in the vestibular nuclei and cerebellum. Transmission at these contacts involves the release of excitatory neurotransmitter molecules. The receiving cells carry receptors that are highly specialized for the detection of these specific molecules. Excitatory amino acid and gamma amino butyric acid (GABA) receptors have been shown to be present in the vestibular nuclei. However, the molecular subtypes of

243

these receptors, as well as the subtypes of various other neurotransmitter receptors in this region, have not been analyzed in detail. Because these receptors are critical to normal synaptic transmission or activation of intercellular communication, knowledge of their distribution and association with specific vestibular pathways is important for developing specific pharmacotherapy for vestibular disorders.

Development, Aging, Regeneration and Genetics

Normal Development

During embryonic development, the inner ear arises from the otic placode, an invagination of surface and neural ectoderm that closes off to form the otic vesicle. Topological elongations and distortions of the otic vesicle produce the six organs of the inner ear: the three semicircular canals, the saccule and utricle of the vestibular system and the cochlea of the auditory system. Specialized epithelia within each organ produce the mechanosensory hair cells for balance and hearing relatively late in the developmental sequence. The transcription factors and growth factors driving morphogenesis and cellular differentiation are not well understood. Differentiation of epithelial cells into hair cells is apparently inhibited by contact with other hair cells, but the proteins that mediate this interaction are just beginning to be identified.

Aging

Parsing out the causes of balance problems has been difficult, because balance is achieved by a complex interaction of vestibular transduction, joint and touch sensation, vision, multisensory integration in the central nervous system and motor output. Nevertheless, the age-related progressive loss of vestibular hair cells and afferents has been observed in postmortem studies and is known to reach 40 percent by the age of 80. In fact, the extent of afferent loss with aging is greater in the vestibular system than reported in any other sensory system. It is not known why so many individuals lose vestibular function as they age or how to prevent the loss.

Regeneration

Damage to the sensory hair cells caused by ototoxic antibiotics or certain diuretics can cause severe vestibular defects. Although individuals can learn adaptive strategies, the fundamental defect is not curable because human hair cells generally do not regenerate. Hair cells are apparently added to the sensory epithelia of fish, birds and amphibians throughout life, and some hair cell regeneration has been observed in mammalian vestibular organs in culture following ototoxic damage. It is not yet understood how to manipulate chemical factors to promote regeneration.

Genetic Disorders

Some vestibular disorders are caused by defective genes encoding the proteins involved in vestibular transduction and processing; therefore, these disorders can be inherited in families. For example, Ushers syndrome (type I), causing episodic vertigo, is one of the most common syndromic auditory and vestibular disorders. There is a genetic predisposition for developing Meniere's disease, resulting in hearing deficits as well as devastating vertigo and balance disorders in some families, but other inherited vestibular disorders are less well characterized.

Identification of markers for the genes defective in other inherited vestibular deficits will become an important component of diagnosis and treatment. Genetic linkage markers enable prenatal diagnosis to be performed and provide a basis for genetic counseling. They also are the starting point for identification of the defective gene itself. Knowledge of the protein encoded by the defective gene can clarify pathophysiology and help to suggest treatment. Ultimately, methods for gene therapy will be available for treatment of some of these genetic disorders.

Identification of gene defects in mouse mutants, in which experimental manipulation is possible, can aid in identifying human homologues. A number of mouse strains with genetic vestibular disorders have been found, usually having problems with balance or gait. Some of these problems are degenerative disorders that may elucidate the aging process.

Vestibular Functions: Posture, Gaze and Motion Perception

Natural behavior entails a nearly continuous sequence of complex head movements that are registered by the semicircular canals (angular motion sensors) and otolithic organs (linear motion and static tilt sensors); all of these inputs are capable of driving stabilizing movements of the eyes, head and body. These functions are subserved by two classes of central pathways. Vestibular signals drive eye movements through the vestibulo-ocular reflexes and control head and body orientation and movement through the vestibulospinal reflexes. One vestibulospinal reflex is the vestibulocollic reflex, which specifically controls head stability by activating the neck muscles.

Control of Gaze

The vestibulo-ocular reflexes compensate for head movement by generating compensatory eye movements. These compensatory eye movements help maintain binocular fixation on visual targets in the environment and enable a stable image. This reflex operates in response to either passive or active, linear or angular head movements. Because the eyes are automatically driven by head movements, eye and head movements must be closely coordinated during purposeful shifts of the line of sight called gaze. The vestibulo-ocular and vestibulocollic reflexes typically are closely linked and generate complementary results. Together, vestibular influences on eye and head movements are often referred to as gaze control.

Like all vestibular reflexes, those that control gaze are mediated through the vestibular nuclei, with important links to other brainstem structures, the cerebellum, and higher brain regions. Even at the level of the vestibular nuclei, however, it is clear that vestibular pathways serve to integrate inputs from other sensory modalities (that is, vision and somatosensory), as well as motor-related signals relevant to equilibrium, spatial orientation and control of eye and head movement. Indeed, natural eye/head coordination usually occurs while a person is looking at, or shifting gaze between, objects. The vestibulo-ocular reflex typically operates in conjunction with visual influences on eye movements, part of which share brain-stem neural circuitry closely associated with the vestibular system.

Despite the superficial simplicity of vestibular control of eye motion, three important complexities exist. First, input signals from the semicircular canals and otolithic organs maintain planar and directional properties that must be matched with the pulling directions of the extraocular muscles and muscles of the head and neck if proper compensatory eye and head movements are to be achieved. Second, the effectiveness of ocular responses to head motion, especially linear motion, depends upon the line of sight relative to the direction of motion and the viewing distance. This proper adjustment requires that the vestibulo-ocular reflex be rapidly modulated by nonvestibular signals that convey the current state of the positions of the eyes in the head. Third, vestibular reflexes are under constant, though more gradual, adjustment by virtue of adaptive plastic mechanisms that serve to maintain or restore proper performance despite the physical and neural changes entailed by development, aging and disease. Adaptive modifications in the vestibulo-ocular reflex occur whenever mismatch arises between vestibular inputs and the visual feedback received during compensatory eye movements. These processes have been best characterized for rotational motion and remain largely uncharted or rudimentary for linear motion.

Control of Posture

As a sensor of gravity and head movement, the vestibular system is one of the nervous system's most important tools in controlling posture. It contributes to balance and movement as both a sensory and motor system. As a sensory system, vestibular information combines with visual and somatosensory information to construct an internal representation of the position and movement of the body relative to its environment. As a motor system, vestibular information combines with visual and somatosensory information to control static head and body postures and to coordinate postural movements. Thus, postural stability results from the integration of vestibular signals with other sensory and motor systems to control the forces that maintain equilibrium and appropriate postural alignment.

The particular role played by the vestibular system in any given postural task depends upon the nature of the task and on the environmental conditions. For example, when head stability is critical for good performance or when somatosensory and/or visual information is not available, vestibular information assumes a more dominant role for postural control. Although it was once assumed that the abnormal balance of individuals with vestibular disorders is the simple and necessary consequence of the loss of vestibular reflexes, it is now known that the role of the vestibular system in control of posture is much more complex. This complexity enables some individuals with severe vestibular loss to compensate sufficiently by using other sensory and motor systems to achieve postural stability and coordinated motor function in a certain range of environments and activities. A better understanding of the contribution of the semicircular canals and otolithic system to posture and movement will make it possible to facilitate maximal compensation in individuals with vestibular disorders, and thereby promote maximal functional independence.

247

Motion Perception

Dysfunction of the vestibular system, particularly the inner ear and its interconnections with the brain, may cause abnormal perception of body movement and position, described by such terms as dizziness, disorientation, vertigo, spinning, floating, rocking, lightheadedness, giddiness, sense of falling, imbalance and unsteadiness or difficulty in walking.

These movement illusions may be accompanied by autonomic (cardiovascular, respiratory and gastrointestinal) dysfunction, resulting in changes in blood pressure and heart rate, as well as the occurrence of nausea and vomiting.

Disorientation (wrongly perceived tilt or motion of the body relative to the environment) is one form of position and movement illusion that can arise from abnormalities in the vestibular system or result from subjecting the normal vestibular system to an artificial environment. Artificial environments include many modes of travel, from highway driving to space flight.

Motion sickness is currently regarded as the brain's response to conflicting sensory messages about the body's orientation and state of motion. The sensors involved include the vestibular part of the inner ear, the eyes and body pressure and joint-position sensors. Nausea, vomiting and associated consequences, including poor concentration, are symptoms provoked by so-called sensory mismatch.

Difficulty in Diagnosis and Treatment

Evaluation of vestibular function has improved in the last 15 years due to the development of tests based on modern anatomic and physiologic concepts and the application of technical advancements. For example, studies of individual neurons are providing data upon which models are being developed to provide a more precise understanding of the vestibular, visual and somatosensory inputs involved in gaze stabilization, balance and orientation.

Technical advancements are making it possible to use angular and linear acceleration devices in clinical testing laboratories for measures of both eye movement responses and postural stability. New video techniques are being developed to record torsional, vertical and horizontal eye movements. New brain-imaging techniques, too, are helping to identify structural lesions in both the peripheral and central aspects of the vestibular system.

In many ways, though, the diagnosis of individuals with vestibular disorders remains primitive and inadequate. Unlike the assessment of hearing or vision, there is no easy way of quantifying the functional status of the vestibular receptors. The need to use reflex motor responses to infer the functional integrity of the labyrinthine sensors complicates the interpretation of what is normal and abnormal. One's sense of the body's orientation and motion in the environment, vestibular perception, is much more difficult to describe quantitatively than are visual or auditory perceptual experiences. Other sensory inputs, especially vision and proprioception, also contribute to balance and spatial orientation, and they must be tested alone and in combination with labyrinthine stimuli.

Furthermore, the relatively crude tests of vestibular function are largely limited to testing the function of the lateral semicircular canals. Usually these are restricted to assessing the contribution to the vestibulo-ocular reflex. Measurements of torsional and vertical eye movements resulting from otolithic organs and vertical canal inputs are not yet clinically available. Quantitative tests of vestibulospinal control of the head stability and balance are not yet possible except for a few sophisticated, research-intensive testing laboratories.

The rudimentary state of vestibular testing means that many individuals with symptoms attributable to vestibular dysfunction from a variety of causes, including trauma, infection, infarction and toxins, are not being properly diagnosed and, consequently, are not being properly treated. Clearly, if knowledge about vestibular disorders, their diagnosis, epidemiology, natural history and response to treatment, is to be increased, better tests of the function of the vestibular system must be developed.

Treatment of vestibular disorders include medical, surgical and behavioral strategies. Behavioral rehabilitation programs that include training in mobility, gait, balance, eye/head coordination and vertigo habituation have demonstrated improvement in balance. This improvement prevents falls and reduces vertigo in elderly persons and others with balance disorders. Specific exercise programs have been shown to facilitate the rate and final level of recovery from vestibular deficits. The use of orthotic/prosthetic devices such as canes and walkers is also beneficial in improving balance and preventing falls. Over 50 medical centers in the United States now offer rehabilitation services to treat vestibular disorders.

Limited understanding of the underlying pathology and neurochemistry of vestibular disorders, combined with the rudimentary state of vestibular testing and the lack of standardized diagnostic criteria, has hampered the development of effective treatment. To relieve suffering from balance and vestibular disorders, better treatment methods must be developed.

Chapter 27

Dizziness

The Vestibular System

Special organs called vestibular receptors are located in the inner ear. The vestibular system is responsible for maintaining the body's orientation in space, balance, and posture. The vestibular system also regulates locomotion and other purposeful motions and helps keep objects in visual focus as the body moves.

When balance is impaired, the capability for normal movement is affected. Dizziness and impairment of balance also can affect one's motivation, concentration, and memory. The primary symptoms of vestibular disorders include a sensation of dizziness, spinning or vertigo, falling, imbalance, lightheadedness, disorientation, giddiness, or visual blurring. A person also may experience nausea and vomiting, diarrhea, faintness, changes in heart rate and blood pressure, fear, anxiety, panic attacks, drowsiness, fatigue, depression, impaired memory, and decreased concentration.

Many Americans, age 17 and older, have at some time experienced a dizziness or balance problem. Some groups, especially older people, are particularly at risk for developing balance disorders. In a study of people age 65 to 75, one-third experienced dizziness and imbalance. Other people at risk include those with diseases of the vestibular system, such as Meniere's disease, and those who suffer from motion sickness. Meniere's disease is a disorder that affects the inner ear and

This article, published in April 1993, is an update of the original NIDCD booklet on Dizziness.

causes periods of vertigo, hearing loss, and tinnitus (roaring or ring-ing in the ear). Motion sickness is a common cause of dizziness and occurs in healthy people who are exposed to unusual motion condi-tions as well as to patients with vestibular disorders.

Vestibular function results in specialized reflexes. A reflex is a spon-taneous or involuntary reaction or movement. The vestibular reflexes are the body's mechanisms for regulating the position of the eyes and body in relation to changes in head position and motion. A particular reflex called the vestibulo-ocular reflex (VOR) causes the eyes to move in reaction to head motion so it is possible to look steadily at some-thing and keep it in focus when the head moves. When the head is turned to the right, for example, fluid movement in the semicircular canals excites a vestibular receptor in the right ear but inhibits the

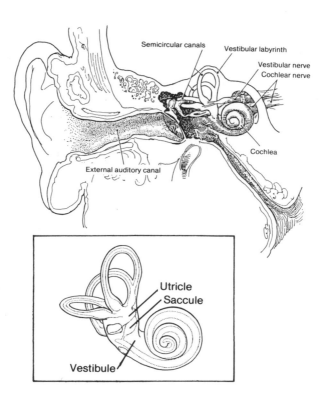

Figure 27.1. *The semicircular canals and vestibule of the inner ear con-tain a fluid called endolymph that moves in response to head movement.*

receptor in the left ear. This sets off a pattern of nerve signals resulting in the eye-stabilizing reflex that allows you to keep your eyes focused on a target while turning your head.

Orientation and Balance

Orientation is knowing the relationship of one's body to the environment. Balance is maintaining the desired body position in the environment. For orientation and balance to be maintained, information from the motion, visual and position receptors located in the ears, eyes, skin, muscles, and joints must be integrated to produce coordinated patterns of muscle activity to maintain balance.

Sometimes the information received from these sensory systems provide conflicting information to the brain. The feeling of continued motion experienced by an individual who steps off a merry-go-round is an example of a sensory conflict situation. When illusions like this are prolonged, motion sickness results.

People with balance or dizziness problems often do not know what is making them feel ill. Physicians may also have difficulty determining the exact cause of their symptoms. This is because the vestibular system is complex, and it interacts with other major systems usually at an unconscious level.

Recent Advances

Basic Mechanisms of Vestibular Function

The vestibular system has the remarkable ability to compensate and recover following injury. The system adapts its performance to maintain gaze and postural stability in response to body and environmental changes. Scientists are currently studying how these adaptations are accomplished. They have identified and mathematically modeled some of the features of the neural pathways underlying adaptive changes of the VOR. An understanding of the adaptive capabilities of the vestibular system at the cellular and molecular levels will provide much needed insight into the medical treatment of balance disorders.

Diagnosis of Vestibular Disorders

Physicians need to know which structures of the vestibular system cause different symptoms. Disorders may affect one or both ears and can develop gradually or suddenly. The inner ear, the vestibular nerve, the vestibular nuclei or other structures of the vestibular nervous system may be involved. NIDCD-supported scientists have developed new computerized techniques that are helping physicians evaluate balance disorders. Physicians can identify, measure, and localize the source of balance disorders by using the VOR and vestibulospinal reflex evaluation techniques. By precisely measuring the reflexes that stabilize the eyes and body posture under different conditions, scientists can relate these reflex responses to the underlying balance control system.

New computer-controlled rotational chairs and eye movement analysis computer software enable physicians to measure precisely both caloric and rotationally induced vestibular eye movement responses in the clinic. Powerful rotation devices allow physicians to test an expanded range of the VOR. Vestibular responses to rotation in a variety of body positions are being studied at several centers, including the Massachusetts Eye and Ear Infirmary, the Eye and Ear Institute of Pittsburgh, Johns Hopkins University, and the University of California at Los Angeles. A new recording device, called the magnetic search coil system, enables these scientists to measure vertical and "rolling" eye movements as well as horizontal eye movements. Scientists can use this new technology to separate and study eye movements driven by the different vestibular organs of the inner ear.

Other new technology includes imaging techniques, such as magnetic resonance imaging (MRI). Physicians use imaging techniques to identify lesions affecting various parts of brain, cranial nerves, and the inner ear structures. They are also able to screen for blood vessel diseases that cause balance disorders by using MRI and other imaging techniques.

Treatment of Vestibular Disorders

Scientists are developing new treatments for people with vestibular disorders. These treatments include new surgical techniques, drug therapy, and physical therapy.

Because of improved diagnostic tests, physicians can locate small tumors of the vestibular nerve. Often, surgery can be performed before tumors enlarge and compress the brain stem, sparing hearing as well as other important functions. Facial nerve and auditory brain stem response monitoring, as well as improved anesthesia techniques, make these operations safer and reduce the risk of complications. A variety of lasers are also now being used to remove tumors.

Surgeons have developed new operations that have been successful in correcting balance and preserving hearing. For example, surgeons can repair fluid leaks caused by fistulae or ruptures from the inner-ear fluid space to the middle-ear air space to treat dizziness. Surgeons are using new techniques to interrupt the nerve pathways from the inner ear vestibular organs to the brain for treatment of persistent vertigo.

NIDCD-supported scientists at the University of Oklahoma Health Sciences Center are analyzing the chemical changes in the brain that occur when the vestibular system compensates for injury. A description of these chemical changes may help clinical investigators develop drug therapy to help patients recover from vestibular injury. Scientists at Good Samaritan Hospital in Portland, Oregon, are determining the relationships between the recovery of the control of posture and the role of central nervous system compensatory mechanisms.

Scientists at the Johns Hopkins University School of Medicine are studying the effectiveness of certain exercises as a treatment for vertigo caused by degenerative fragments from the inner ear lodged in the receptor region of a posterior semicircular canal. These small fragments make the canal unusually sensitive to changes in the position of the head, causing dizziness. When the head positions of patients in the study were manipulated to dislodge the debris, their dizziness resolved. After treatment, most of the patients in the study had improved enough to return to a normal life. In another study, scientists at the University of Michigan have shown preliminary evidence that suggests that a customized physical exercise program that repeatedly exposes the patient to sensory conflict and provokes vertigo and imbalance is more effective than general exercises for recovery. Such exercises may be a safe and effective alternative to surgery.

Investigators at the Johns Hopkins University School of Medicine have demonstrated the beneficial effects of even brief periods of physical exercise in patients recovering from unilateral vestibular loss. These investigators are studying the effectiveness of patients viewing moving visual scenes and of inducing VOR adaptation with magnifying lenses in the rehabilitation from vestibular disorders. Balance disorders frequently cause falls. According to the National Institute on Aging, falls are the most common cause of fatal injury in older people. In the past, research has focused on the visual-stabilizing reflexes in balance disorders rather than on postural-stabilizing reflexes. Research at the Johns Hopkins University School of Medicine is underway on adaptive strategies of people with balance problems to stabilize posture. Scientists are studying people with and without vestibular disorders to understand these adaptive capabilities. They are comparing the adaptation of the visual reflex with that of the postural reflex. The results of this project will be used to design and assess physical therapy programs.

NIDCD continues to support research concerning the basic mechanisms of balance function, diagnostic procedures, and treatment. The vestibular system is a complex set of inner ear and central nervous system mechanisms that is capable of adapting to changes in the body and the environment. Because of the system's complexity and its interaction with other sensory and motor systems, symptoms are many and varied. As scientists learn more about the vestibular system and its adaptive capabilities, they can develop better diagnostic procedures, medical treatments, surgical techniques, and nonmedical rehabilitative procedures to help patients recover from debilitating disorders of balance.

About the NIDCD

The NIDCD conducts and supports research and research training on normal and disordered mechanisms of hearing, balance, smell, taste, voice, speech, and language. The NIDCD achieves its mission through a diverse program of research grants for scientists to conduct research at medical centers and universities around the country and through a wide range of research performed in its own laboratories.

The institute also conducts and supports research and research training related to disease prevention and health promotion; addresses special biomedical and behavioral problems associated with people who have communication impairments or disorders and supports efforts to create devices that substitute for lost and impaired sensory communication function. The NIDCD is committed to understanding how certain diseases or disorders may affect women, men, and members of underrepresented minority populations differently.

The NIDCD has established a national clearinghouse of information and resources. Additional information on dizziness may be obtained from the NIDCD Clearinghouse. Write to:

NIDCD Clearinghouse
P.O. Box 37777
Washington, DC 20013-7777

or call:
Voice (800) 241-1044
TDD/TT (800) 241-1055

Chapter 28

BPPV
(Benign Paroxysmal
Positional Vertigo)

Benign Paroxysmal Positional Vertigo (BPPV) causes dizziness due to debris which has collected within a part of the inner ear. You can think of this debris as "ear rocks." Chemically, ear rocks are small crystals of calcium carbonate. They are derived from structures in the ear called "otoliths" that have been damaged by head injury, infection, or other disorder of the inner ear, or degenerated because of advanced age.

The symptoms of BPPV include dizziness or vertigo, lightheadedness, imbalance, and nausea. Activities which bring on symptoms will vary in each person, but symptoms are almost always precipitated by a position change of the head or body. Getting out of bed or rolling over in bed are common "problem" motions. Some people will feel dizzy and unsteady when they tip their heads back to look up, and for this reason sometimes BPPV is called "top shelf" vertigo. Women with BPPV may find that use of the hair dryers in beauty parlors brings on symptoms. An intermittent pattern is the usual situation. BPPV may be present for a few weeks, then stop, then come back again.

What Causes BPPV?

The most common cause of BPPV in people under age 50 is head injury. In older people, the most common cause is degeneration of the

From http://www.teleport.com/~veda; last modified December 22, 1997. Provided by the Vestibular Disorders Association, P.O. Box 4467, Portland, OR 97208-4467, (503) 229-7705; reprinted with permission. This document is not intended as a substitute for professional health care.

vestibular system of the inner ear. However, in perhaps half of all cases, BPPV is called "idiopathic," which means it occurs for no known reason.

How Is the Diagnosis of BPPV Made?

Your physician can make the diagnosis based on your history, findings on physical examination, and the results of vestibular and auditory tests. Blood pressure will be checked lying flat and standing. Other diagnostic studies may be required. An ENG may be needed to look for the characteristic nystagmus (jumping of the eyes). An MRI scan will be performed if there is any possibility of a stroke or brain tumor. A rotatory chair test may be used for difficult diagnostic problems. It is possible to have BPPV in both ears (bilateral), which may make diagnosis and treatment more challenging.

How Is BPPV Treated?

BPPV has often been described as "self-limiting" because symptoms often subside or disappear within six months of onset. Symptoms tend to wax and wane. Motion sickness medications are sometimes helpful in controlling the nausea associated with BPPV but are otherwise rarely effective. However, various kinds of physical maneuvers and exercises have proved effective. Three varieties of conservative treatment involve exercises, and another involves surgery.

Office Treatment of BPPV (The Epley and Semont Maneuvers)

There are two treatments of BPPV that are usually performed in the doctor's office. Both are very effective, with roughly an 80% cure rate, according to a study by Herdman and others (1993).

The maneuvers are named after their inventors. They are both intended to move debris or "ear rocks" out of the sensitive back part of the ear (posterior canal) to a less sensitive location. Both maneuvers take about 15 minutes to accomplish. The Semont maneuver (also called the "liberatory" maneuver) involves a procedure whereby the patient is rapidly moved from lying on one side to the other. The Epley maneuver (also called the particle repositioning, canalith repositioning procedure, and modified liberatory maneuver) involves sequential movement of the head into four positions. The recurrence rate for BPPV after these maneuvers is about 5 percent, and in some instances a second treatment may be necessary.

After either of these maneuvers, you should be prepared to follow the instructions below, which are aimed at reducing the chance that debris might fall back into the sensitive back part of the ear.

Instructions for Patients After Office Treatments (Epley or Semont Maneuvers)

- Wait for 10 minutes after the maneuver is performed before going home. This is to avoid "quick spins," or brief bursts of vertigo as debris re-positions itself immediately after the maneuver. Don't drive home yourself; have someone else drive you.

- Sleep semi-recumbent for the next two days. This means sleep with your head halfway between being flat and upright (a 45 degree angle). This is most easily done by using a recliner chair or by using pillows arranged on a couch. During the day, try to keep your head vertical. You must not go to the hairdresser or dentist. No exercise which requires head movement. When men shave under their chins, they should bend their bodies forward in order to keep their head vertical. If eyedrops are required, try to put them in without tilting the head back. Shampoo only under the shower.

- For at least 1 week, avoid provoking head positions that might bring this on again.

  - Use two pillows when you sleep.

  - Avoid sleeping on the "bad" side.

  - Don't turn your head far up or far down.

  - Be careful to avoid head-extended positions, in which you are lying on your back, especially with your head turned towards the bad side. This means be cautious at the beauty parlor, dentist's office, and if having minor surgery done. Ask them to keep you as upright as possible. If appropriate, exercises for low-back pain should be stopped for a week. No "sit-ups" for at least one week. No "crawl" swimming. (Breast stroke is OK.)

    - Avoid far head-forward positions such as might occur in certain exercises (i.e. touching the toes).

- At one week after treatment, put yourself in the position that usually makes you dizzy. Position yourself cautiously and under conditions in which you can't fall or hurt yourself. Let your doctor know how you did.

What If the Maneuvers Don't Work?

These maneuvers don't always work (only 80% of the time), and if they don't, then your doctor may wish you to proceed with the Brandt-Daroff exercises. They are more arduous but can be done at home, with your doctor's guidance. The Brandt-Daroff exercises as well as the Semont and Epley maneuvers are compared in an article by Brandt (1994), listed in the reference section below.

Surgical Treatment of BPPV (Posterior Canal Plugging)

If exercises are ineffective in controlling symptoms and they have persisted for a year or longer, a surgical procedure called "canal plugging" may be recommended. Canal plugging completely stops the posterior canal's function without affecting the functions of the other canals or parts of the ear. This procedure poses a small risk to hearing.

How Might BPPV Affect My Life?

Certain modifications in your daily activities may be necessary to cope with your dizziness. Use two or more pillows at night. Avoid sleeping on the "bad" side. In the morning, get up slowly and sit on the edge of the bed for a minute. Avoid bending down to pick up things, and extending the head, such as to get something out of a cabinet. Be careful when at the dentist's office, beauty parlor, or in sports activities or positions where your head is flat or extended.

References

Brandt T, Daroff RB. Physical therapy for benign paroxysmal positional vertigo, *Arch Otolaryngol*, 1980, 106:484-485 (Brandt-Daroff Exercises).

Brandt T, Steddin S, Daroff RB. Therapy for benign paroxysmal positioning vertigo, revisited. *Neurology* 1994, 44:796-800.

Epley JM. The canalith repositioning procedure: For treatment of benign paroxysmal positional vertigo. *Otol Head Neck Surg* 1992: 107: 399-404 (Epley Maneuver).

Froehling DA, Silverstein MD, Mohr DN, Beatty CW, Offord KP, Ballard DJ. Benign positional vertigo: incidence and prognosis in a population-based study in Olmsted county, Minnesota. *Mayo Clinic Proc*, 66, 1991, 596-602.

Harvey S, Hain T, Adamiec L. Modified liberatory maneuver: effective treatment for benign paroxysmal positional vertigo. *Laryngoscope* 104: October 1994 (Epley Maneuver).

Herdman, S. Treatment of benign paroxysmal vertigo, *Physical Therapy* 70, 1990, 381-388 (All maneuvers).

Herdman S, Tusa R, Zee D, Proctor LR, Mattox DE. Single treatment approaches to benign paroxysmal positional vertigo. *Arch Otol Head Neck Surg* 1993, 119;450-454 (Epley and Semont maneuvers).

Parnes LS, McClure JA. Posterior semicircular canal occlusion for intractable benign paroxysmal positional vertigo. *Ann Otol Rhinol Laryngol* 1990, 99:330-334 (surgical treatment).

Parnes LS, Price-Jones RG. Particle repositioning maneuver for benign paroxysmal positional vertigo. *Ann Otol Rhinol Laryngol* 1993,102:325-331 (Epley maneuver).

Semont A, Freyss G, Vitte E. Curing the BPPV with a liberatory maneuver. *Adv Otolaryngol* 1988, 42, 290-293 (Semont Maneuver).

Welling DB, Barnes DE. Particle Repositioning maneuver for benign paroxysmal positional vertigo. *Laryngoscope* 104; 1994, 946-949 (Epley Maneuver).

— by Timothy C. Hain, MD

Chapter 29

Labyrinthitis and Neuronitis

The inner ear consists of a system of fluid-filled tubes and sacs called the *labyrinth* as well as the nerves that connect the labyrinth to the brain. The labyrinth, which rests inside the bone of the skull, contains both an organ devoted to hearing, called the *cochlea*, and other organs, called the *vestibular system*, which are devoted to the control of balance and eye movements.

The terms *labyrinthitis* and *neuronitis* refer to inflammations of the inner ear or the nerves connecting the inner ear to the brain. The inflammation can be caused by either bacterial or viral infections. If the inflammation affects the cochlea, it will produce disturbances in hearing, such as ear noises (*tinnitus*) or hearing loss. If the vestibular system is affected, the symptoms will include dizziness and difficulty with vision and/or balance.

Since the whole inner ear is about the size of a dime, many infections affect both the hearing and balance systems and produce both kinds of symptoms. The symptoms can be mild or severe, temporary or permanent, depending on the severity of the infection. Although the symptoms of bacterial and viral infections may be quite similar, the two disorders require very different treatments, and it is therefore important for your doctor to make a proper diagnosis before starting a course of treatment.

Bacterial Labyrinthitis

Bacteria may cause damage to the labyrinth in two different ways. Bacteria that infect the middle ear or the bone surrounding the inner ear can produce toxins that inflame the cochlea or the vestibular system or both. This sort of inflammation is called *serous labyrinthitis*. Alternatively, bacteria may invade the labyrinth itself, causing what is called *suppurative labyrinthitis*. Serous labyrinthitis is most frequently caused by chronic, untreated middle ear infections (*chronic otitis media*) and is the more common type of bacterial inner ear infection. The bacteria that cause suppurative labyrinthitis can enter the inner ear as a result of bacterial meningitis, which is an inflammation of the protective sheath surrounding the brain. Bacteria can also enter the labyrinth if the membranes that separate the middle ear from the inner ear are ruptured by a disease, like otitis media, or by an injury, as in the case of perilymph fistula.

The symptoms caused by serous labyrinthitis may be very mild at first. If the infection is not treated, however, symptoms can become more severe and eventually end in total loss of hearing and vestibular function. The symptoms associated with suppurative labyrinthitis are similar to those of serous labyrinthitis, but they are usually pronounced from the beginning and rapidly become very severe. Suppurative labyrinthitis often results in permanent loss of hearing and vestibular function. Regardless of the type of bacterial infection, the treatment consists of destroying the bacteria by means of antibiotics. If the labyrinthitis is caused by a break in the membranes separating the middle and inner ears, surgery may also be required to repair the membranes to prevent a recurrence of the disease.

Viral Labyrinthitis and Neuronitis

Viruses can also enter the inner ear and inflame the labyrinth or the nerves that connect the labyrinth to the brain. It is almost impossible to distinguish whether the labyrinth or the nerve is the site of the infection based on symptoms alone, and so the terms *labyrinthitis* and *neuronitis* are used almost interchangeably. Less is known about viral infections than about bacterial infections of the inner ear; it is assumed that the viruses that cause the inflammation enter the inner ear through the blood stream. This may result from a systemic infection, in which the rest of the body is also affected by the virus, or the virus may damage the inner ear without affecting other organs. Some of the more common viruses that have been associated with viral labyrinthitis include influenza, measles (rubeola), mumps, German measles (rubella), herpes, hepatitis, polio, and Epstein-Barr. Because it is impossible to take a sample of inner ear tissue to identify the viruses growing there without destroying the labyrinth, we are probably unaware of other viruses that can also cause labyrinthitis.

The symptoms of viral labyrinthitis are similar to those of bacterial infections, and they consist of trouble with hearing or with balance or with some combination of the two. Symptoms can be mild or severe, ranging from slight loss of hearing or mild dizziness to sudden total loss of hearing or violent spinning sensations (called *vertigo*). Unlike bacterial infections, however, many viral infections cause no permanent damage in adults. Almost half of the patients recover completely, and most of the rest improve substantially. This is very fortunate, because viruses are not killed by antibiotics, and there are no other treatments that have been proven scientifically to be of any help in viral labyrinthitis. If the nausea and vertigo are severe, your doctor may give you medicines that relieve these symptoms, but they do not affect the virus itself, which must simply be allowed to run its course.

Diagnosing the Disorder

If you suddenly begin having trouble with your hearing or trouble with dizziness and imbalance, seek medical help. Because the consequences of bacterial infections of the inner ear can be quite severe if left untreated, it is important for your doctor to make a correct diagnosis and begin antibiotics promptly if a bacterial infection is present. If there are signs of middle ear infection or meningitis or other infections in or around the ear, a diagnosis of bacterial labyrinthitis will often be made. If there is no sign of bacterial infection, the doctor will suspect a viral infection, particularly if you or a member of your family has had a viral disease recently. Your doctor will need to rule out some other causes for your symptoms as well.

The symptoms of an inner ear infection can sometimes be mimicked when one of the small blood vessels in the inner ear becomes blocked; if you have a history of high blood pressure or hardening of the arteries, your doctor may suspect a blockage.

A blow to the head that damages the inner ear may also mimic the symptoms of an inner ear infection, and your doctor will probably carefully question you about recent accidents. If your symptoms consist primarily of dizziness, your doctor will attempt to rule out many other problems that can cause dizziness, including side effects of prescription or nonprescription drugs (including alcohol, tobacco, caffeine, and many illegal drugs), cardiovascular disease, allergies, neurological disorders, and anxiety.

Getting Well Again

If treated promptly, many inner ear infections cause no permanent damage. In some cases, however, permanent loss of hearing, ranging from barely detectable to total, can result. Your doctor will be able to advise you about the usefulness of hearing aids in your individual case. Permanent damage to the vestibular system can also result. Fortunately, the brain can adapt to damage to the vestibular system, particularly when the damage is partial and/or confined to one side. This adaptation may take days to months, depending on how severe the damage is and how quickly the body is able to recover from the infection. Symptoms of dizziness, difficulty with vision, and imbalance may persist as long as the adaptation is incomplete. This adaptation can only occur if the patient makes an effort to keep moving around despite the symptoms of dizziness and imbalance. Sitting or lying with the head still, while more comfortable, can prolong or even prevent the adaptation process, and should be avoided if at all possible once the worst of the infection is over.

— by Charlotte L. Shupert, Ph.D.

An important source of information for this chapter was *Clinical Neurophysiology of the Vestibular System* by Robert W. Baloh, M.D., and Vincente Honrubia, M.D. (F. A. Davis Company, Philadelphia, 1990, 2nd edition).

Chapter 30

Meniere's Disease

What Is Meniere's Disease?

Meniere's disease is an abnormality of the inner ear causing a host of symptoms, including vertigo or severe dizziness, tinnitus or a roaring sound in the ears, fluctuating hearing loss, and the sensation of pressure or pain in the affected ear. The disorder usually affects only one ear and is a common cause of hearing loss. Named after French physician Prosper Meniere who first described the syndrome in 1861, Meniere's disease is now also referred to as endolymphatic hydrops.

What Causes Meniere's Disease?

The symptoms of Meniere's disease are associated with a change in fluid volume within a portion of the inner ear known as the labyrinth. The labyrinth has two ports: the bony labyrinth and the membranous labyrinth. The membranous labyrinth, which is encased by bone, is necessary for hearing and balance and is filled with a fluid called endolymph. When your head moves, endolymph moves, causing nerve receptors in the membranous labyrinth to send signals to the brain about the body's motion. An increase in endolymph, however, can cause the membranous labyrinth to balloon or dilate—a condition known as endolymphatic hydrops.

Many experts on Meniere's disease think that a rupture of the membranous labyrinth allows the endolymph to mix with perilymph,

NIH Publication No. 95-3404, November 1994.

another inner ear fluid that occupies the space between the membranous labyrinth and the bony inner ear. This mixing, scientists believe, can cause the symptoms of Meniere's disease. Scientists are investigating several possible causes of the disease, including environmental factors, such as noise pollution and viral infections, as well as biological factors.

What Are the Symptoms of Meniere's Disease?

The symptoms of Meniere's disease occur suddenly and can arise daily or as infrequently as once a year. Vertigo, often the most debilitating symptom of Meniere's disease, forces the sufferer to lie down. Vertigo attacks can lead to severe nausea, vomiting, and sweating and often come with little or no warning.

Some individuals with Meniere's disease have attacks that start with tinnitus, a loss of hearing, or a full feeling or pressure in the affected ear. It is important to remember that all of these symptoms are unpredictable. Typically, the attack is characterized by a combination of vertigo, tinnitus and hearing loss lasting several hours. But people experience these discomforts at varying frequencies, durations, and intensities. Some may feel slight vertigo a few times a year. Others may be occasionally disturbed by intense, uncontrollable tinnitus while sleeping. And other Meniere's disease sufferers may notice a hearing loss and feel unsteady all day long for prolonged periods. Other occasional symptoms of Meniere's disease include headaches, abdominal discomfort and diarrhea. A person's hearing tends to recover between attacks but over time becomes worse.

How Is Meniere's Disease Treated?

There is no cure for Meniere's disease. Medical and behavioral therapy, however, are often helpful in managing its symptoms. Although many operations have been developed to reverse the disease process, their value has been difficult to establish. And, unfortunately, all operations on the ear carry a risk of hearing loss.

The most commonly performed surgical treatment for Meniere's disease is the insertion of a shunt, a tiny silicone tube that is positioned in the inner ear to drain off excess fluid.

In another more reliable operation, a vestibular neurectomy, the vestibular nerve which serves balance is severed so that it no longer sends distorted messages to the brain. But the balance nerve is very close to the hearing and facial nerves. Thus, the risk of affecting a patient's hearing or facial muscle control increases with this type of surgical treatment. Also, older patients often have difficulty recovering from this type of surgery.

A labyrinthectomy, the removal of the membranous labyrinth, is an irreversible procedure that is often successful in eliminating the dizziness associated with Meniere's disease. This procedure, however, results in a total loss of hearing in the operated ear—an important consideration since the second ear may one day be affected. Also, labyrinthectomies themselves may result in other balance problems.

Some physicians recommend a change of diet to help control Meniere's symptoms. Eliminating caffeine, alcohol and salt may relieve the frequency and intensity of attacks in some people. Eliminating tobacco use and reducing stress levels may lessen the severity of the symptoms. And medications that either control allergies, reduce fluid retention or improve blood circulation in the inner ear may also help.

How Is Meniere's Disease Diagnosed?

Scientists estimate that there are 3 to 5 million people in the United States with Meniere's disease, with nearly 100,000 new cases diagnosed each year. Proper diagnosis of Meniere's disease entails several procedures, including a medical-history interview and a physical examination by a physician; hearing and balance tests; and medical imaging with magnetic resonance imaging (MRI). Accurate measurement and characterization of hearing loss are of critical importance in the diagnosis of Meniere's disease.

Through the use of several types of hearing tests, physicians can characterize hearing loss as being *sensory*, arising from the inner ear, or *neural* arising from the hearing nerve. An auditory brain stem response, which measures electrical activity in the hearing nerve and brain stem, is useful in differentiating between these two types of hearing loss. And under certain circumstances, electrocochleography, recording the electrical activity of the inner ear in response to sound, helps confirm the diagnosis.

To test the vestibular or balance system, physicians irrigate the ears with warm and cool water. This flooding of the ears, known as caloric testing, results in nystagmus, rapid eye movements that can help a physician analyze a balance disorder. And because tumor growth can produce symptoms similar to Meniere's disease, magnetic resonance imaging is a useful test to determine whether a tumor is causing the patient's vertigo and hearing loss.

What Research Is Being Done?

Scientists are investigating environmental and biological factors that may cause Meniere's disease or induce an attack. They are also studying how fluid composition and movement in the labyrinth affect hearing and balance. And by studying hair cells in the inner ear, which are responsible for proper hearing and balance, scientists are learning how the ear converts the mechanical energy of sound waves and motion into nerve impulses. Insights into the mechanisms of Meniere's disease will enable scientists to develop preventive strategies and more effective treatment.

Where Can I Get More Information?

The NIDCD currently supports research on Meniere's disease in medical centers and universities throughout the nation. For more information about Meniere's disease, you can contact:

American Academy of Otolaryngology–Head and Neck Surgery
One Prince Street
Alexandria, VA 22314
Telephone: (703) 836-4444; TTY: (703) 519-1585

Deafness Research Foundation
9 East 38th Street
New York, NY 10016
Telephone: (212) 684-6556
TTY: (212) 684-6559; 1-800-535-DEAF

Ear Foundation
2000 Church Street, Box 111
Nashville, TN 37236
Telephone: (615) 329-7807
TTY: (615) 329-7809; 1-800- 545-HEAR

Vestibular Disorders Association
P.O. Box 4467
Portland, OR 97208-4467
Telephone: (503) 229-7705; 1-800-837-8428

NIDCD Information Clearinghouse
1 Communication Avenue
Bethesda, MD 20892-3456
1-800-241-1044 (Voice); 1-800-241-1055 (TTY)

Chapter 31

Perilymph Fistula

A **perilymph fistula** is a tear or defect in one or both of the small, thin membranes between the middle and inner ears.

These membranes, the **oval window** and the **round window**, separate the middle ear from the fluid-filled inner ear. The changes in air pressure that occur in the middle ear (for example, when your ears "pop" in an airplane) normally do not affect your inner ear.

When a fistula is present, changes in middle ear pressure will directly affect the inner ear, stimulating the balance and/or hearing structures within and causing typical symptoms.

The **symptoms of perilymph fistula** may include dizziness, vertigo, imbalance, nausea, and vomiting. Some people experience ringing or fullness in the ears, and many notice a hearing loss. Most people with fistulas find that their symptoms get worse with changes in altitude (elevators, airplanes, travel over mountain passes) or air pressure (weather changes), as well as with exertion and activity.

Causes

Head trauma is the most common cause of fistulas, usually involving a direct blow to the head or in some cases a "whiplash" injury. Fistulas may also develop following rapid or profound changes in intracranial or atmospheric pressure, such as may occur with SCUBA diving, aerobatic maneuvers in airplanes, weight lifting, or childbirth. Fistulas may be present from birth or may result from chronic, severe ear infections. Rarely, they appear to occur spontaneously.

Fistulas may occur in one or both ears.

Diagnosis

The only positive way the diagnosis can be confirmed is by performing a tympanotomy (operation) and directly viewing the area of the suspected fistula. If a fluid (perilymph) leak is seen, a perilymph fistula is assumed to be present.

Your physician will also use information from your history and physical examination, as well as objective vestibular and audiometric test results, to assist in establishing the diagnosis of perilymph fistulas.

Treatment

In many cases, a fistula will heal itself if your activity is markedly restricted. In such cases, strict bed rest is recommended to give the fistula a chance to close.

If your symptoms are severe and have not responded to conservative treatment (bed rest), or if you have a progressive hearing loss, surgical repair of the fistulas may be required. This procedure involves placing a graft over the fistula defect in the oval and/or round window.

Patients with fistulas should avoid lifting, straining, bending over, or any activity that would "increase the pressure in your head," as all of these will make your symptoms worse and prevent the fistula from healing. You will also want to avoid air pressure changes (for example, using elevators, traveling in the mountains, or flying in airplanes) as these changes will tend to make your symptoms worse.

Coping with Dizziness

You may find that a number of modifications in your daily activities will be necessary so that you can cope with your dizziness. For example, it may be helpful to avoid the circling motions involved in driving on clover-leaf approaches to freeways or in multi-storied parking structures. Or, you may need to have someone shop for you for a while if going up and down supermarket aisles tends to increase your symptoms.

Your condition may make you visually dependent. Because of this, you should take special precautions in situations where clear, normal vision is not available to you. For example, avoid trying to walk through dark rooms and hallways; keep lights or night lights on at all times. Don't drive your car at night or during stormy weather when visibility is poor. And beware of carrying large objects that obstruct your view.

Or, you may find that you are more **proprioception dependent.** That is, your balance and movement are highly dependent on sensations received from your feet, ankles, and legs. Because of this, you should take special precautions in situations where your support surface (what you are standing or walking on) is altered. For example, use great care when walking on soft, deep rugs, loose gravel, highly polished floors, and other uneven surfaces. Make sure your hallways at home are uncluttered and free of obstructions, and toss out all loose throw rugs. Most important, do not place yourself in a situation where you might lose your balance and be at risk for a fall and serious injury; stay off chairs, stools, ladders, roofs, etc. If your balance continues to be a serious problem, you may need to consider using canes or a walker for added safety.

At times you may find it difficult to concentrate or to remember things. You may also notice difficulty with reading, writing, or even speech. These problems are commonly experienced by persons with vestibular disorders. As the condition is brought under control, these symptoms may be expected to improve.

You may feel frustrated, depressed, or even be accused of being "crazy" because, even when you do not feel well, you look just fine to others. Explain to friends and family that you need their patience and understanding while you learn to cope with the symptoms brought on by persistent dizziness.

Chapter 32

Accomplishments in Vestibular Research

Public Health and Education

The National Multipurpose Research and Training Centers, established by the founding legislation of the National Institute on Deafness and Other Communication Disorders (NIDCD), includes two centers, one in Los Angeles, California and one in Baltimore, Maryland, in which research, research training, continuing professional education and public information dissemination on disorders of balance are major components.

In 1993, the NIDCD and the National Aeronautics and Space Administration (NASA) jointly established a multi-institutional center for vestibular research in Chicago, Illinois and Portland, Oregon. Research supported by the center will delineate the selective role of the vestibular sense organs in balance control and construct models of human postural control based on actual physiologic data.

The NIDCD Clearinghouse provides literature searches, information and identifies organizational resources on hearing and balance disorders (as well as those of smell, taste, voice, speech and language) for health professionals, physicians, industry and the public in conjunction with the Combined Health Information Database (CHID).

The NIDCD National Temporal Bone, Hearing and Balance Pathology Resource Registry, established by NIDCD in 1992, provides a

Excerpted from *National Strategic Research Plan*, National Institute on Deafness and Other Communication Disorders, 1994-1995; NIH Pub. No. 97-3217.

database of the temporal bone and brain tissue specimens representing the pathology of hearing and balance disorders held by 22 collaborating laboratories in the United States. Individual investigators can identify and locate all processed temporal bone and brain specimens in the collaborating laboratories by clinical and pathologic diagnosis. The advent of antigen retrieval and DNA extraction techniques greatly enhance the usefulness of these collections for modern molecular biologic research. Furthermore, it provides a nationwide network to acquire new pathologic specimens. As of June 1994, the Registry contains information on over 10,000 temporal bone and brain tissue specimens. The Registry also sponsors training programs in techniques of the study of the pathology of the inner ear, and in conjunction with the Deafness Research Foundation, it disseminates information on temporal bone research to physicians, scientists and the public.

Signal Transduction and Transmission

Electrophysiological and micromechanical studies of hair cells from a variety of species have provided quantitative descriptions of the transduction mechanism, of mechanical adaptation and of voltage-gated ion channels in hair cells. Some molecular constituents of these processes have been identified, including structural proteins, motile elements and ion channels.

The major ion-transport pathways leading to the secretion of potassium by vestibular dark cells have been determined. Several first and second messengers of ion-transport regulation have been identified. First messengers include extracellular potassium and ATP; second messengers include intracellular cAMP, pH and cell volume.

Biophysical and anatomical studies have revealed that the two types of hair cells, type I and type II, have different potassium ionic currents, have different morphologic features and are innervated differently by specialized afferent terminals. These terminals contain different calcium-binding proteins. Type I and type II hair cells and their afferent terminals are aggregated in different places in the neuroepithelium in some end-organs. These studies also have indicated that type I and type II hair cells are actually heterogeneous populations that differ in ultrastructure and morphology of cilia, depending on epithelial location and afferent innervation.

Morphophysiologic experiments have shown that afferent nerve fibers in a particular end-organ differ in their spontaneous discharge and response properties. This response diversity is related to the branching patterns of the afferents, including their location in the sensory epithelium and the types and number of hair cells that they contact.

Information has been obtained about the response of single vestibular afferent fibers to electrical activation of efferent axons originating in the brain stem. Efferent-fiber stimulation can have a predominantly excitatory effect on afferent activity in mammals and fish, but the effect can be both excitatory and inhibitory in other phyla. Efferent neurons contain classical neurotransmitters such as acetylcholine and a variety of neuropeptides and transmitters (metenkephalin and calcitonin-gene related peptide) that may influence receptor cells and afferent fibers in the end-organs.

Considerable progress has been made in identifying the neurotransmitters involved in the vestibular system. The excitatory amino acid, glutamate is the primary hair-cell and eighth cranial nerve neurotransmitter. Some primary afferent vestibular processes may also contain neurofilament proteins, calcium-binding proteins, and/or substance P. Neurons of the vestibular nuclei have been shown to contain a variety of different neurotransmitters, some of which coexist in the same cell. GABA and glycine have been suggested as neurotransmitters of several central vestibular pathways. Calcium-binding proteins, which are usually associated with GABAergic cells, may play a role in neurotransmitter release and/or in buffering intracellular calcium to protect these cells from injury. Receptors for acetylcholine and the opioid peptides are also present on central vestibular neurons. This suggests multiple avenues for the excitatory modulation of vestibular cells.

Development, Aging, Regeneration and Genetics

Normal Development

Considerable progress has been made in identifying transcription factors that mediate inner-ear development. Early development of the vestibular organ apparently depends on very specific genetic foci. Retinoic acid receptors and thyroid hormone receptors, which are zinc-finger transcription factors, have been found to be expressed during specific periods of cellular division and differentiation.

There have been qualitative descriptions of the timing of peripheral synapse formation among hair cells, vestibular afferents, and efferents in a small number of mammalian species, including humans. These studies demonstrate (1) an organized pattern of synapse formation concomitant with receptor differentiation, (2) competition by peripheral processes for synaptic sites on hair cells, and (3) the relatively late formation of efferent connections. Studies in avian and amphibian embryos have taken advantage of distinctive central synaptic morphologies to characterize the time course of synaptogenesis by the central axons of vestibular afferents and to test hypotheses about mechanisms of target selection.

Connections of neurons of the vestibular nerve have been found to depend on trophic factors originating in both the inner ear and brain stem. These trophic factors appear to guide and stabilize synaptic connections. Vestibular and auditory end-organs differ in the timing of susceptibility to these trophic factors.

Recent experiments in the microgravity environment of space flight to assess the development of simple organisms and adaptability of vertebrates have shed light on the predetermined and modifiable aspects of development and plasticity of the vestibular system.

Aging

The age-related decline in vestibular sensors and nerves is now known to exceed age-related declines in other sensory systems. Tests of eye movements and postural control in the elderly have identified age-related decline in the ability to adapt both balance and vestibulo-ocular function to changing environments. Deficits, such as cataracts or arthritis, have been shown to unmask vestibular disorders for which there previously was compensation, thereby resulting in a dramatic increase in vestibular symptoms such as postural instability. There is deterioration in postural equilibrium, gaze and spatial orientation. There are also declining adaptive processes that might otherwise restore declining function. These findings have demonstrated progressive disequilibrium with increasing age to be a major health problem that needs further scientific investigation.

Regeneration

Finding methods to regenerate hair cells from stem cells or supporting cells is a major goal for reversing deficits caused by hair cell death. Currently, some regeneration of vestibular hair cells following damage from aminoglycoside has been observed. Trophic factors that stimulate regeneration are being identified. Investigators are still a long way from regenerating hair cells, but there is a concerted effort to do so and great excitement that it may ultimately be possible.

Genetic Disorders

The gene defective in neurofibromatosis (type 2)—an autosomal dominant disease causing bilateral vestibular schwannomas in one of every 40,000 individuals—was recently located on chromosome 22. A novel type of tumor-suppressor gene has been identified and sequenced. Inactivation of this gene may be responsible for spontaneous vestibular schwannomas. If proven, this exciting possibility would have important implications for treatment.

The genes for Ushers syndrome (type I)—causing vestibular deficits along with deafness and blindness—has been mapped to chromosomes 11 and 14. Additionally, families with vestibular deficits as the major disorder have been identified. New genetic methods are accelerating the identification of disease genes in humans. These methods will be applied to preventing vestibular deficits.

Genes are inserted into nondividing cells such as neurons using recently developed techniques for gene therapy. These gene therapy techniques should be applicable to the inner ear. Additionally, gene therapy developed to kill brain tumors is entering clinical trials. Related techniques may be applicable to vestibular schwannomas.

Control of Posture and Balance

Over the last several years, new models of postural control have suggested new research directions regarding the environmentally dependent and task-dependent roles of vestibular function in the control of equilibrium and orientation.

The patterns of muscle activation in the limbs, trunk and neck evoked by natural vestibular stimulation have been described in animal models and in humans, as have the ways they vary with context. There have been studies characterizing the kinematics and kinetics of posture and movement in normal and in vestibular-deficient animals as well as normal and vestibular-deficient humans.

Automatic postural responses have been shown to be sensitive to prior experience, instruction and intention, initial biomechanical conditions, practice, attention and level of anxiety, as well as to the convergence of sensory inputs signaling disequilibrium.

Vestibular information has been shown to be more critical for coordinating complex, multisegmental body movements than simple, quiet stance. The earliest stabilizing responses of the body to destabilization have now been shown to be triggered by somatosensory information, when available, rather than by vestibular information.

Although individuals with profound vestibular loss may have normal balance reactions in some conditions, their motor repertoire may be extremely limited.

The effects of vestibular stimulation on posture and balance have been demonstrated to depend on actual somatosensory inputs as well as on perceived illusions of somatosensory state. This suggests a common internal map for the perception of self-motion and automatic postural orientation. The use of somatosensory and visual inputs for postural orientation can be altered as individuals compensate for vestibular disorders. This finding may explain context-dependent instability in some individuals. For example, immediately after a vestibular lesion, individuals may become overly dependent on vision for posture and are likely to fall in confusing, visual environments.

Static and dynamic posturography, which quantifies an individual's ability to balance, can now be used to differentiate types of balance disorders. A new rehabilitative approach to improving balance testing posturography combined with biofeedback is under investigation.

The sense of touch has recently been shown to be as powerful as vision in providing postural stabilization. This discovery has important implications for vestibular rehabilitation and supports the use of a cane to reduce gait instability.

Head stability has been shown to be affected by loss of vestibular function for some tasks and directions but not in others. In individuals with vestibular loss, poor head stability may be the basis for poor motor coordination as well as postural instability.

Postural coordination has been shown to be better in individuals who have experienced vestibular loss during childhood, rather than in adulthood.

Using optimal control theory, scientists have developed robust, computational models of postural biomechanics. These models help differentiate biomechanical from sensorineural constraints on postural motor behavior. They may eventually be able to predict why certain postural movements require otolithic organ and/or semicircular canal information.

There has been further progress in understanding the circuitry that underlies vestibular control of posture and movement, particularly control of head position. Projections from semicircular canal and otolithic organ receptors to a variety of vestibulospinal neurons, as well as otolithic organ-semicircular canal convergence, have been characterized. There is new evidence about the relative role of the vestibulospinal and reticulospinal tracts in head stability and balance control. In contrast to previous concentration on supraspinal pathways, recent experiments with natural stimulation have begun to study the potential contribution of spinal interneurons to vestibulocollic and other vestibulospinal mechanisms.

There has been further investigation of higher level neural control of vestibular reflexes. This work includes modulation of these reflexes by the locus coeruleus, an autonomic region of the brain stem, by the cerebellum and by the motor cerebral cortex.

There has been continued research on the pharmacology and biophysics of neurons in vestibular reflex pathways. Cholinergic pathways to the cerebellum have been identified. *In vitro* preparations have provided considerable information about pharmacology of neurons in the vestibular nuclei and about their membrane properties.

Control of Gaze

Over the past several years, considerable progress has been made in characterizing the relationships among vestibular inputs, their central processing and integration with other sensory and motor signals, the distribution of these signals to motor-output pathways, adaptive plastic processes that maintain the vestibular reflexes, and the behavior of the vestibular reflexes themselves.

The dynamic and three-dimensional spatial transformations that occur in vestibulo-ocular and vestibulocollic reflexes were described. The patterns of muscle activation that result have also been described, and models have been advanced that successfully predict the muscle patterns that underlie gaze control.

Information has been obtained on vestibulo-ocular reflexes, eye/head coordination and interactions with vision in response to linear acceleration. Eye-movement control has been shown to involve interactions among otolithic organ, visual and contextual (target distance, position and motion) influences. Further understanding of these control mechanisms should yield quantitative clinical tests of otolithic organ function.

Progress has been made in uncovering and characterizing the neural connections that mediate gaze-stabilizing reflexes and in associating the structural and physiological attributes of their neural elements. Efforts have revealed a complexity of interactions among vestibular, visual and proprioceptive inputs relevant to spatial orientation.

The structure and function of vestibulo-ocular relay neurons (that form the middle portion of three-neuron vestibulo-ocular reflex arcs) have been described. These descriptions are in sufficient detail to reveal how convergent labyrinthine inputs to these neurons and their divergent projections to multiple motor pools could contribute to reflex transformations. Neural models that explore these possibilities in a formal way continue to evolve and provide insight into possible roles for neural elements in vestibular pathways.

Identification of the more complex indirect pathways that contribute to gaze reflexes has been fruitful. This investigation has included important regulatory roles of the cerebellum.

Research has begun to define the biophysics and pharmacology of neurons in vestibular reflex pathways. This could lead to new medications to treat vestibular disorders.

Studies of synaptic function are revealing new information on cellular transmission in vestibular pathways. For example, afferents with different response characteristics have been shown to influence and modulate central pathways linked to different reflex functions selectively.

Information is emerging about the higher level cortical control of gaze, and how and where sensory and motor information from multiple sources is combined and processed in specific cortical neuronal structures.

The vestibular and balance control systems have the remarkable ability to maintain useful function in many novel motion environments and to adapt to abnormal function of one or more of their components. Continuing advances in vestibular health care, particularly rehabilitation, rely on progress based upon sound scientific concepts. The significance of central nervous system phenomena associated with the adaptive process (such as modulation of neuropharmacologic sensitivity, reactive synaptogenesis and modification of synaptic transmission), which are thought to play important roles in adaptive control, must be measured. These processes must be correlated systematically with behavior.

In the normal function of the vestibular system, the essential role of adaptive plasticity has been recognized. This system is not static, but is constantly changing in response to changes in the environment or internal elements (for example, inner-ear or central nervous system diseases).

New understanding is emerging about the neural changes that accompany recovery from unilateral labyrinthectomy, including both recalibration of the magnitude of vestibular reflex responses and the balance between vestibular inputs from the two sides (vestibular compensation). Neuronal structures have been identified that participate in compensation and adaptive recalibration. Cellular and molecular alterations underlying these important processes are being explored. Experimental and modeling efforts are applied to identifying potential sites and mechanisms of adaptive plasticity, both in the brain stem and cerebellum.

Perception of Spatial Orientation and Autonomic Control

A critical use of vestibular information is in spatial orientation and motion perception. For many years, vestibular responses were conceived as being automatic reflexes and not subject to conscious control. Recent research has shown, however, that people can use conscious information from vestibular receptors during movement. The information includes the position where they started and information about how far they have moved. Individuals can also use the imagined location of targets to adjust gaze and balance movements. Thus, the cognitive processing of vestibular information is important for perceiving spatial orientation and also for the automatic control of gaze and balance.

Considerable evidence suggests that many brain-stem neurons that regulate the cardiovascular and respiratory systems receive vestibular inputs. Vestibular signals assist in the rapid countering of changes in blood pressure that can occur during unexpected postural changes. A better understanding of the vestibular contribution to these autonomic functions could lead to improved control of the symptoms and signs of motion sickness, including nausea, hyperventilation and pallor.

New computer models of motion sickness suggest that this syndrome is a byproduct of the process of adaptation to conflicting sensory inputs or between expected and actual sensory input. It has been demonstrated that individuals have a remarkable ability to adapt to unusual motion conditions, although this process of adaptation is often associated with motion sickness. When adaptation is finally achieved, the vertigo and/or motion sickness disappears.

Recent studies provide a better understanding of the effects of microgravity on adaptive vestibular function. Research conducted in space flights has shown alterations in perception of spatial orientation as well as in eye movement and postural control. These adaptations occurred during flight and after return to Earth. It appears that the plasticity of vestibular reflexes, for the most part, permits adaptation during the first few days of microgravity. However, there is some concern about the effect of degraded neurovestibular performance after long microgravity exposures. Areas of intense current

283

research include the study of the precise characteristics of adaptive plasticity in this unique environment as well as the aspects of vestibular function involved in readaption to Earth's gravity after long-duration exposure to space. Increased alteration in vestibular control of gaze and postural equilibrium following space flight has begun to clarify the maladaptive consequences of sudden changes in environment.

Diagnosis

Advances in modern technology have made the evaluation of individuals with vestibular disorders a quantitative science. Since the vestibular control of eye movements is the best understood, most direct and most easily quantified vestibular reflex, scientists and clinicians have emphasized eye movements to develop tests of vestibular function. The recording of eye movements in response to vestibular as well as other sensory stimuli is part of the standard vestibular test battery, owing in part to advances in the understanding of ocular motor control in general. These tests have contributed as well to the ability of investigators to locate vestibular lesions and diagnose vestibular disorders. They also help quantify the natural history as well as the response to therapy of individuals with vestibular disorders. The advent of small, but powerful, desktop computers and simple devices for stimulating and recording vestibular responses have made such testing batteries widely available to individuals with vestibular disorders.

Although the caloric test is still the time-honored mainstay of the clinical vestibular testing battery, vestibular diagnosis has been advanced by the use of more natural stimuli. These include self-generated rotations of the head and new mechanical devices that can precisely measure and control the motion of the body. For example, rotational testing is helpful in diagnosing bilateral peripheral vestibular loss in elderly individuals with unexplained disequilibrium. By their very nature, rotational and translational stimuli always stimulate both labyrinths. Recent studies have shown, however, that by positioning the head appropriately and using stimuli that stress the limits of performance of the labyrinth, rotational tests can be used to help diagnose both unilateral and bilateral peripheral vestibular disorders. Galvanic stimulation, which uses a weak electrical current to excite the vestibular nerve in one labyrinth at a time, has recently shown to be better tolerated than previously thought in both experimental animal models as well as in human beings. These new tests are relatively easy to use, take little time and will be valuable in the diagnosis of both vestibulo-ocular and vestibulospinal dysfunction.

More than these advances in technology, however, have improved vestibular testing. Recent physiologic studies have exposed some of the limits of the ability of vestibular sensors to respond to unusual stimuli, for example, those of extremely high speed and acceleration. When vestibular responsivity is asymmetric, as in certain vestibular diseases, these limitations have been exploited to improve bedside diagnosis, both in objective tests (for example, head-shaking nystagmus) and subjective responses (for example, blurred vision). Important new physiologic concepts, such as the central mechanism that improves the low-frequency response of the semicircular canals (so-called, velocity storage), have been applied in the interpretation of clinical testing results. These considerations have helped in the differentiation of peripheral labyrinthine from central vestibular disorders.

In the last few years, knowledge and appreciation of otolithic organ influences on vestibular reflexes have been applied to the evaluation and testing of individuals, in an attempt to meet the long standing need for a clinical test of otolithic organ function. Otolithic organs respond to linear acceleration, both the force of gravity and linear motion (translation) of the head. New clinical tests are being developed to test normal and disordered otolithic organ function. Rotation of a subject's head about a vertical or nonvertical axis when the axis of rotation is off-center relative to the labyrinth alters the forces acting on the otolithic organs. The vestibulo-generated eye movements made in response to these modes of rotation are currently being investigated as measures of otolithic organ function. Furthermore, the perception of verticality during rotational motion may provide information on the functional status of the otolithic organs. These represent situations in which linear and angular motion are combined. Measurement of the otolith-ocular reflex in response to pure linear motion has been conducted on parallel swings or in linear sleds. Furthermore, realization of the influence of viewing distance on the otolith-ocular reflex, the direction of the line of sight and the state of convergence of the eyes has led to important conceptual and technical advances in the way that otolith-ocular reflexes should be tested.

The quantitative evaluation of balance also has improved with the use of platforms that compute movement of the individual's center of mass with sensitive force transducers under different conditions of sensory (visual, somatosensory and labyrinthine) inputs. Posturography now includes measures of both static and dynamic balance. Both the orientation of the body to altered visual and surface conditions and the automatic postural responses to surface perturbations lend new insights into the functional basis of balance disorders. This can contribute to assessment of the central and peripheral components of postural instability. Methods are being developed to quantify balance during active movements and reactions to perturbation during movements. Such tests are critical to the evaluation of the effects of physical therapy and to understanding compensation for vestibular disorders.

In the last few years, high-resolution magnetic resonance imaging has been shown to be a useful way to locate lesions in individuals with acute peripheral vestibulopathies. Even the individual sensors of the vestibular labyrinth can be imaged and shown to be spared or involved by a pathological process. A beginning also has been made in more reliably diagnosing inner-ear autoimmune disease by measuring antibody responses to specific ear antigens.

Treatment

Medical Therapy

Following advances made in the diagnosis of specific vestibular disorders, the use of specific pharmacotherapeutic agents for the treatment of peripheral and central disorders continues to evolve. The prevalence of human immunodeficiency virus (HIV) and other immune system disorders has increased and, owing to the improved diagnostic methods available, there has been improved early detection and treatment of these disorders. The role of nutrition, diuretics, vasodilators and aminoglycosides in the management of Meniere's disease continues to be explored. Although little is directly known about the etiology and pathophysiology of neurolabyrinthitis, including vestibular neuronitis, clinicians are forced to continue to treat this spectrum of disorders in an empiric manner. Similarly, with improved diagnostic methods, central vestibular disorders such as vertebrobasilar artery insufficiency, vestibular migraine, familial ataxia syndromes and psychophysiologic dizziness are being treated with specific pharmacotherapeutic agents. Recent improvement in the pharmacologic control of the panic and anxiety disorders often associated with these vestibular disorders is encouraging. These agents are broadly characterized as anticholinergic, antihistaminic, antidopaminergic, tranquilizing and histaminic in nature. Although many of the drugs are helpful in relieving these symptoms, the side effects of drowsiness, altered mental alertness and dry mouth and eyes can adversely affect the lives of individuals in terms of safety (falls, work-related injuries or motor vehicle accidents) and quality of life.

In addition to receiving specific therapy, most individuals with vestibular disorders are currently treated with more broadly acting symptomatic therapy to diminish the sensations of vertigo and dizziness and autonomic dysfunction, such as nausea and vomiting.

Vestibular damage secondary to medication side effects may soon be prevented due to a better understanding of the mechanisms of ototoxicity. It may soon be possible to reduce the ototoxic effect of drugs without altering their therapeutic effects.

The application of cellular and molecular methods has resulted in the identification of probable neurotransmitters and receptors in the peripheral and central regions of the vestibular system. However, a detailed understanding of the neurochemistry subserving vestibular function remains to be completed before specific agonist and antagonist therapeutic agents can be developed. Also needed are further studies of the mechanisms of action of currently used drugs and the distribution of their receptors in the peripheral and central regions of the vestibular system.

Surgical Therapy

Strategies for treating peripheral vestibular disorders surgically include unilateral labyrinthine denervation, selective unilateral elimination of posterior semicircular canal function, repair of perilymph fistulas, endolymphatic sac shunting and vestibular nerve vascular decompression. Improvement in diagnostic capabilities, rehabilitation therapy, intraoperative cranial nerve electrophysiologic monitoring and better diagnostic criteria have decreased the morbidity associated with many surgical procedures. However, the efficacy of many of these procedures remains to be proven. These treatment methods represent a significant financial commitment in the United States. Further research in these areas is needed.

Unilateral labyrinthine denervation may be divided into ablative and nonablative procedures. Ablative procedures include labyrinthectomy (transcanal or transmastoid), which is a short and relatively safe procedure, although all residual hearing is lost. Selective chemical "labyrinthectomy" utilizes the vestibulotoxicity of aminoglycosides to ablate vestibular receptors unilaterally. Intratympanic instillation of gentamicin is a promising method; however, minimizing the complication of cochlear ototoxicity by means of delivery systems or absorption methods remains to be investigated. The instillation of the highly vestibulotoxic agent streptomycin into the labyrinth showed early promise in unilateral vestibular ablation for the treatment of

Meniere's disease; however, the results of a recent multicenter prospective study of this method have raised serious questions regarding efficacy. If there is useful hearing in a unilaterally affected ear, selective vestibular neurectomy by means of a middle cranial fossa (MCF) retrolabyrinthine (RL) or posterior fossa (PF) approach is currently the accepted procedure. The MCF approach is technically more difficult; however, advances in the intraoperative monitoring of auditory and facial nerve function may prove to decrease the incidence of facial paralysis and hearing loss associated with this approach.

Selective transection of the posterior ampullary (singular) nerve was developed based on a clear understanding of the pathophysiology of benign paroxysmal positional vertigo and has been successful in more than 90 percent of the small subset of individuals with the disabling chronic form of this disorder. The development of the posterior canal occlusion procedure, which is technically much easier, shows promise for the surgical management of this disorder. In addition, the success of canal-repositioning maneuvers and the application of rehabilitation therapy appears to be reducing the number of individuals requiring surgery.

Recent advances in diagnostic methods such as transtympanic endoscopy and use of perilymphatic protein or dye markers are encouraging as methods for detecting perilymph fistulas. Although these studies have lowered the frequency with which surgical repair of round or oval window fistulas is undertaken, demonstration of surgical efficacy is still necessary.

Another nonablative procedure theoretically designed to correct the pathologic endolymphatic fluid metabolism in Meniere's disease is the shunting of the endolymphatic sac. The efficacy of this once extremely popular procedure was brought into question as a result of a small prospective, double-blinded study performed in Denmark over a decade ago. However, a resurgence in interest in this procedure is currently under way in the United States and Europe. Nevertheless, demonstration of efficacy is still necessary.

Rehabilitative Therapy

The use of specific exercises to reduce vertigo and to improve gaze and postural stability in elderly persons at risk for falling and in individuals with vestibular disorders has become a standard of treatment. Vestibular rehabilitation is focused on (1) facilitating central neural compensation, (2) reducing vertigo with habituation, (3) improving balance, coordinated movement and mobility, (4) improving gaze stabilization, and (5) improving physical conditioning. Therapeutic exercises are based on results of animal research demonstrating that motor experience can increase the rate and extent of recovery following vestibular dysfunction or loss. This research demonstrates that limiting sensorimotor experience can delay and permanently retard recovery. Research to determine the efficacy/effectiveness of vestibular rehabilitation is showing that exercises designed specifically for each individual's functional deficits can be effective in improving balance, reducing vertigo, increasing mobility and speed of locomotion and in reducing head instability. In fact, although both vestibular rehabilitation and vestibular suppressant medication reduce vertigo, balance improves more through the use of exercise. Outcome measures of treatment efficacy/effectiveness now include questionnaires assessing the functional limitations of vertigo, static and dynamic posturography, eye-movement tests and kinematic quantification during locomotion and other activities.

The most significant advance in the rehabilitation of one specific, but common, peripheral vestibular disorder (benign paroxysmal positional vertigo) is the canal-repositioning maneuver. Preliminary experience with this maneuver suggests that it may be effective in relieving the condition, sometimes immediately. The underlying pathophysiologic mechanism is believed to be either a repositioning of displaced otoconia away from the involved posterior semicircular canal or it is a form of central nervous system habituation or suppression of the abnormal vestibular signals.

Despite advances in many areas, significant gaps in understanding the scientific basis of vestibular rehabilitation remain. The physiologic basis for relief of vertigo through positioning exercise needs to be clarified. The usefulness of pre- and postoperative rehabilitation protocols to facilitate compensation and full recovery has not been tested. Functional outcome measures to assess functional limitations and disability are needed. Identification of those diagnoses with the best rehabilitation outcomes is also lacking. The effect of age on improvement or recovery of function needs further delineation, as do the other factors that retard compensation. Finally, new methods need to be developed to habituate to visual motion cues.

Part Four

Disorders of the Nose and Sinuses

Chapter 33

You and Your Stuffy Nose

Nasal congestion, stuffiness, or obstruction to nasal breathing is one of man's oldest and most common complaints. While it may be a mere nuisance to some people, to others it is a source of considerable discomfort, and it detracts from the quality of their lives.

Medical writers have classified the causes of nasal obstruction into four categories, recognizing that overlap exists between these categories and that it is not unusual for a patient to have more than one factor involved in his particular case.

Infections

An average adult suffers a common "cold" two to three times per year, more often in childhood and less often the older he gets as he develops more immunity. The common "cold" is caused by any number of different viruses, some of which are transmitted through the air, but most are transmitted from hand-to-nose contact. Once the virus gets established in the nose, it causes release of the body chemical histamine, which dramatically increases the blood flow to the nose—causing swelling and congestion of nasal tissues—and which stimulates the nasal membranes to produce excessive amounts of mucus. Antihistamines and decongestants help relieve the symptoms of a "cold," but time alone cures it.

©1996. American Academy of Otolaryngology–Head and Neck Surgery, Inc., One Prince Street, Alexandria, VA 22314-3357. For more information, visit our home page at http://www.entnet.org.

During a virus infection, the nose has poor resistance against bacterial infections, which explains why bacterial infections of the nose and sinuses so often follow a "cold." When the nasal mucus turns from clear to yellow or green, it usually means that a bacterial infection has taken over and a physician should be consulted.

Acute sinus infections produce nasal congestion, thick discharge, and pain and tenderness in the cheeks and upper teeth, between and behind the eyes, or above the eyes and in the forehead, depending on which sinuses are involved.

Chronic sinus infections may or may not cause pain, but nasal obstruction and offensive nasal or postnasal discharge is often present. Some people develop polyps (fleshy growths in the nose) from sinus infections, and the infection can spread down into the lower airways leading to chronic cough, bronchitis, and asthma. Acute sinus infection generally responds to antibiotic treatment; chronic sinusitis usually requires surgery.

Structural Causes

Included in this category are deformities of the nose and the nasal septum, which is the thin, flat cartilage and bone that separates the nostrils and nose into its two sides. These deformities are usually due to an injury at some time in one's life. The injury may have been many years earlier and may even have been in childhood and long since forgotten. It is a fact that 7 percent of newborn babies suffer significant nasal injury just from the birth process; and, of course, it is almost impossible to go through life without getting hit on the nose at least once. Therefore, deformities of the nose and the deviated septum should be fairly common problems—and they are. If they create obstruction to breathing, they can be corrected with surgery.

One of the most common causes for nasal obstruction in children is enlargement of the adenoids: tonsil-like tissues which fill the back of the nose up behind the palate. Children with this problem breath noisily at night and even snore. They also are chronic mouth breathers, and they develop a "sad" looking face and sometimes dental deformities. Surgery to remove the adenoids and sometimes the tonsils may be advisable.

Other causes in this category include nasal tumors and foreign bodies. Children are prone to inserting various objects such as peas, beans, cherry pits, beads, buttons, safety pins, and bits of plastic toys into their noses. Beware of one-sided foul smelling discharge, which can be caused by a foreign body. A physician should be consulted.

Allergy

Hay fever, rose fever, grass fever, and "summertime colds" are various names for allergic rhinitis. Allergy is an exaggerated inflammatory response to a foreign substance which, in the case of a stuffy nose, is usually a pollen, mold, animal dander, or some element in house dust. Foods sometime play a role. Pollens may cause problems in spring (trees), summer (grasses) or fall (weeds), whereas house dust allergies are often most evident in the winter. Molds may cause symptoms year-round. Ideally the best treatment is avoidance of these substances, but that is impractical in most cases.

In the allergic patient, the release of histamine and similar substances results in congestion and excess production of watery nasal mucus. Antihistamines help relieve the sneezing and runny nose of allergy. Many antihistamines are now available without a prescription. The most familiar brands include Chlortrimeton®, Benadryl® and Dimetane® (although most are also available in generic forms). Newer, non-sedating antihistamines, which require a prescription, include Seldane®, Hismanal® and Claritin®. Decongestants shrink congested nasal tissues. Examples include ENTex®, Guaifed®, Deconsal® and Sudafed® (which is available without a prescription in several generic forms). Combinations of antihistamines with decongestants are also available. All these preparations have potential side effects, and patients must heed the warnings of the package or prescription insert. This is especially important if the patient suffers from high blood pressure, glaucoma, irregular heart beats, difficulty in urination, or is pregnant.

- **Warning:** Patients who get sleepy from antihistamines should not drive an automobile or operate dangerous equipment after taking them. Also, decongestants stimulate the heart and raise the pulse and blood pressure; they should be avoided by patients who have high blood pressure, irregular heart beats, glaucoma or difficulty in urination.

Pregnant patients should consult their obstetrician before taking *any* medicine.

Cortisone-like drugs (corticosteroids) are extremely potent. These are often administered as nasal sprays for allergy, rather than as pills or by injection, to minimize the risk of serious side effects associated with these other dosage forms. Patients using steroid nasal sprays should closely follow their physician's instructions, and should consult their physician immediately if they develop nasal bleeding and crusting, nasal pain, or changes in vision.

Allergy shots are the most specific treatment available, and they are highly successful in allergic patients. Skin tests or at times blood tests are used to make up treatment vials of substances to which the patient is allergic. The physician determines the best concentration for initiating the treatment. These treatments are given by injection. They work by forming blocking antibodies in the patient's blood stream, which then interfere with the allergic reaction. Injections are typically given for a period of three to five years.

Patients with allergies have an increased tendency to develop sinus infections and require treatment as discussed in the previous section.

Vasomotor Rhinitis

"Rhinitis" means inflammation of the nose and nasal membranes. "Vasomotor" means blood vessel forces. The membranes of the nose have an abundant supply of arteries, veins, and capillaries, which have a great capacity for both expansion and constriction. Normally these blood vessels are in a half-constricted, half-open state. But when a person exercises vigorously, his hormones of stimulation (i.e., adrenaline) increase. The adrenaline causes constriction or squeezing of the nasal blood vessels, which shrinks the nasal membranes so that the air passages open up and the person breaths more freely.

The opposite takes place when an allergic attack or a "cold" develops. The blood vessels expand, the membranes become congested (full of excess blood), and the nose becomes stuffy or blocked.

In addition to allergies and infections, other events can also cause nasal blood vessels to expand, leading to vasomotor rhinitis. These include psychological stress, inadequate thyroid function, pregnancy, certain anti-high blood pressure drugs, overuse or prolonged use of decongesting nasal sprays, and irritants such as perfumes and tobacco smoke.

In the early stages of each of these disorders, the nasal stuffiness is temporary and reversible. That is, it will improve if the primary cause is corrected. However, if the condition persists for a long enough period, the blood vessels lose their capacity to constrict. They become somewhat like varicose veins. They fill up when the patient lies down and when he lies on one side, the lower side becomes congested. The congestion often interferes with sleep. So it is helpful for stuffy patients to sleep with the head of the bed elevated two to four inches-accomplish this by placing a brick or two under each castor of the bedposts at the head of the bed. Surgery may offer dramatic and long time relief.

Summary

Stuffy nose is one symptom caused by a remarkable array of different disorders, and the physician with special interest in nasal disorders will offer treatments based on the specific causes. Additional information and suggestions can be found in the AAO-HNS pamphlets "Hay fever, Summer Colds and Allergies" and "Antihistamines, Decongestants and 'Cold' Remedies."

What is Otolaryngology–Head and Neck Surgery? (Ear, Nose, and Throat Specialist)

An otolaryngologist is a physician concerned with the medical and surgical treatment of the ears, nose, throat, and related structures of the head and neck.

The American Academy of Otolaryngology–Head and Neck Surgery, Inc. represents more than 7,500 ear, nose, and throat specialists. For more information or a list of otolaryngologists practicing in your area, please contact the Academy.

Chapter 34

Sinusitis

You're coughing and sneezing and tired and achy. You think that you might be getting a cold. Later, when the medicines you've been taking to relieve the symptoms of the common cold are not working and you've now got a terrible headache, you finally drag yourself to the doctor. After listening to your history of symptoms and perhaps doing a sinus X-ray, the doctor says you have sinusitis.

Sinusitis simply means inflammation of the sinuses, but this gives little indication of the misery and pain this condition can cause. Chronic sinusitis, sinusitis that recurs frequently, affects an estimated 32 million people in the United States. Americans spend millions of dollars each year for medications that promise relief from their sinus symptoms.

Sinuses are hollow air spaces, of which there are many in the human body. When people say, "I'm having a sinus attack," they usually are referring to symptoms in one or more of four pairs of cavities, or spaces, known as *paranasal sinuses*. These cavities, located within the skull or bones of the head surrounding the nose, include the frontal sinuses over the eyes in the brow area, the *maxillary sinuses* inside each cheekbone, the *ethmoids* just behind the bridge of the nose and between the eyes, and behind them, the *sphenoids* in the upper region of the nose and behind the eyes.

Each sinus has an opening into the nose for the free exchange of air and mucus, and each is joined with the nasal passages by a continuous

From http://www.niaid.nih.gov/factsheets/sinusitis.htm; National Institute of Allergy and Infectious Diseases, August 1996.

mucous membrane lining. Therefore, anything that causes a swelling in the nose—an infection or an allergic reaction—also can affect the sinuses. Air trapped within an obstructed sinus, along with pus or other secretions, may cause pressure on the sinus wall. The result is the sometimes intense pain of a sinus attack. Similarly, when air is prevented from entering a paranasal sinus by a swollen membrane at the opening, a vacuum can be created that also causes pain.

Symptoms

Sinusitis has its own localized pain signals, depending upon the particular sinus affected. Headache upon awakening in the morning is characteristic of sinus involvement. Pain when the forehead over the frontal sinuses is touched may indicate inflammation of the frontal sinuses. Infection in the maxillary sinuses can cause the upper jaw and teeth to ache and the cheeks to become tender to the touch. Since the ethmoid sinuses are near the tear ducts in the corner of the eyes, inflammation of these cavities often causes swelling of the eyelids and tissues around the eyes and pain between the eyes. Ethmoid inflammation also can cause tenderness when the sides of the nose are touched, a loss of smell, and a stuffy nose. Although the sphenoid sinuses are less frequently affected, infection in this area can cause earaches, neck pain, and deep aching at the top of the head.

Other symptoms of sinusitis can include fever, weakness, tiredness, a cough that may be more severe at night, and runny nose or nasal congestion. In addition, drainage of mucus from the sphenoids down the back of the throat (postnasal drip) can cause a sore throat and can irritate the membranes lining the larynx (upper windpipe).

Causes

Viruses can enter the body through the nasal passages and set off a chain reaction resulting in sinusitis. For example, the nose reacts to an invasion by viruses that cause infections such as the common cold, flu, or measles by producing mucus and sending white blood cells to the lining of the nose, which congest and swell the nasal passages. When this swelling involves the adjacent mucous membranes of the sinuses, air and mucus are trapped behind the narrowed openings of the sinuses. If the sinus openings become too narrow to permit drainage of the mucus, then **bacteria**, which normally are present in the respiratory tract, begin to multiply. Most apparently healthy people harbor bacteria, such as *Streptococcus pneumoniae* and *Haemophilus influenzae*, in their upper respiratory tracts with no ill effects until the body's defenses are weakened or drainage from the sinuses is blocked by a cold or other viral infection. The bacteria that may have been living harmlessly in the nose, throat, or sinus area can multiply and cause an acute sinus infection.

Medicines, too, can set off a nasal reaction with accompanying sinusitis. For example, intolerance to aspirin and other related non-steroidal anti-inflammatory medications, such as ibuprofen, can be associated with sinusitis in patients with asthma or nasal polyps (small growths on the mucous membrane lining of the sinuses).

Sometimes, **fungal infections** can cause acute sinusitis. Although these organisms are abundant in the environment, they usually are harmless to healthy people, indicating that the human body has a natural resistance to them. Fungi, such as *Aspergillus* and *Curvularia*, can cause serious illness, in people whose immune systems are not functioning properly. Some people with fungal sinusitis have an allergic-type reaction to the fungi.

Chronic inflammation of the nasal passages (rhinitis) also can lead to sinusitis. **Allergic rhinitis** or hay fever (discussed below) is the most common cause of chronic sinusitis and is a frequent cause of acute sinusitis. **Vasomotor rhinitis**, caused by humidity, cold air, alcohol, perfumes, and other environmental conditions, also can result in a sinus infection.

Chronic Sinusitis

Chronic sinusitis refers to inflammation of the sinuses that continues for weeks, months, or even years.

As noted above, allergies are the most common cause of chronic sinusitis. Inhalation of airborne allergens (foreign substances that provoke an allergic reaction), such as dust, mold, and pollen, often set off allergic reactions (allergic rhinitis) that, in turn, may contribute to sinusitis. People who are allergic to fungi can develop a condition called "allergic fungal sinusitis." As body cells react against these inhaled substances, they release chemical compounds, such as histamine, at the mucosal surface. These chemicals then cause the nasal passages to swell and block drainage from the sinuses, resulting in sinusitis.

Damp weather, especially in northern temperate climates, or pollutants in the air and in buildings also can affect people subject to chronic sinusitis.

Chronic sinusitis can be caused by structural abnormalities of the nose, such as a deviated septum (the bony partition separating the two nasal passages), or by small growths called nasal polyps, both of which can trap mucus in the sinuses.

Diagnosis

Although a stuffy nose can occur in other conditions, like the common cold, many people confuse simple nasal congestion with sinusitis. A cold, however, usually lasts about seven days and disappears without treatment. Acute sinusitis lasts longer than a week and usually does not go away on its own. A doctor can diagnose sinusitis by medical history, physical examination, X-rays, and if necessary, MRIs or CT scans (magnetic resonance imaging and computed tomography).

Treatment

After diagnosing sinusitis and identifying a possible cause, a doctor can prescribe a course of treatment that will clear up the source of the inflammation and relieve the symptoms.

Sinusitis is treated by re-establishing drainage of the nasal passages, controlling or eliminating the source of the inflammation, and relieving the pain. Doctors generally recommend decongestants to reduce the congestion, antibiotics to control a bacterial infection, if present, and pain relievers to reduce the pain.

Most patients with sinusitis that is caused by bacteria can be treated successfully with antibiotics used along with a nasal or oral decongestant.

Over-the-counter and prescription decongestant nose drops and sprays, however, should not be used for more than a few days. When used for longer periods, these drugs can lead to even more congestion and swelling of the nasal passages.

For many years, the combination of allergic disease and infectious sinusitis has been considered the most difficult form of sinus disease to treat. The patient with uncontrolled nasal allergies frequently experiences a lot of congestion, swelling, excess secretions, and discomfort in the sinus areas. Therefore, the patient should work with a doctor who understands the diagnosis and treatment of allergic diseases to pinpoint the cause of the allergies and follow an allergy care program to help alleviate sinusitis.

Doctors often prescribe steroid nasal sprays, along with other treatments, to reduce the congestion, swelling, and inflammation of sinusitis. Because steroid nasal sprays have no serious side effects, they can be used for long-term treatment. In some people, however, they irritate the nasal passages.

For patients with severe chronic sinusitis, a doctor may prescribe oral steroids, such as prednisone. Because oral steroids can have significant side effects, they are prescribed only when other medications have not been effective.

Although sinus infection cannot be cured by home remedies, people can use them to lessen their discomfort. Inhaling steam from a vaporizer or a hot cup of water can soothe inflamed sinus cavities. Another treatment is saline nasal spray, which can be purchased in a pharmacy. A hot water bottle; hot, wet compresses; or an electric heating pad applied over the inflamed area also can be comforting.

In treating patients with severe sinusitis, a physician may use special procedures. One technique requires the patient to lie on his back with his head over the edge of the examining table. A decongestant fluid is placed in the nose, and air is suctioned out of the nose so that the decongestant fluid can shrink the sinus membranes sufficiently to permit drainage. Or, a thin tube can be inserted into the sinuses for washing out entrapped pus and mucus.

Sometimes, however, surgery is the only alternative for preventing chronic sinusitis. In children, problems often are eliminated by removal of adenoids obstructing nasal-sinus passages. Adults who have had allergic and infectious conditions over the years sometimes develop polyps that interfere with proper drainage. Removal of these polyps and/or repair of a deviated septum to ensure an open airway often provides considerable relief from sinus symptoms. The most common surgery done today is **functional endoscopic sinus surgery**, in which the natural openings from the sinuses are enlarged to allow drainage.

Prevention

Although people cannot prevent all sinus disorders—any more than they can avoid all colds or bacterial infections—they can take certain measures to reduce the number and severity of the attacks and possibly prevent sinusitis from becoming chronic. Appropriate amounts of rest, a well-balanced diet, and exercise can help the body function at its most efficient level and maintain a general resistance to infections. Eliminating environmental factors, such as climate and pollutants, is not always possible, but they can often be controlled.

Many people with sinusitis find partial relief from their symptoms when humidifiers are installed in their homes, particularly if room air is heated by a dry forced-air system. Air conditioners help to provide an even temperature, and electrostatic filters attached to heating and air conditioning equipment are helpful in removing allergens from the air.

A person susceptible to sinus disorders, particularly one who also is allergic, should avoid cigarette smoke and other air pollutants. Inflammation in the nose caused by allergies predisposes a patient to a strong reaction to all irritants. Drinking alcohol also causes the nasal-sinus membranes to swell.

Sinusitis-prone persons may be uncomfortable in swimming pools treated with chlorine, since it irritates the lining of the nose and sinuses. Divers often experience congestion with resulting infection when water is forced into the sinuses from the nasal passages.

Air travel, too, poses a problem for the individual suffering from acute or chronic sinusitis. A bubble of air trapped within the body expands as air pressure in a plane is reduced. This expansion causes pressure on surrounding tissues and can result in a blockage of the sinuses or the eustachian tubes in the ears. The result may be discomfort in the sinus or middle ear during the plane's ascent or descent. Doctors recommend using decongestant nose drops or inhalers before the flight to avoid this difficulty.

People who suspect that their sinus inflammation may be related to dust, mold, pollen, or food—or any of the hundreds of allergens that can trigger a respiratory reaction—should consult a doctor. Various tests can determine the cause of the allergy and also help the doctor recommend steps to reduce or limit allergy symptoms.

Chapter 35

Tricks to Treating Sinus Problems

"Tension . . . pressure . . . pain!" With these words and pictures of a twisting coil, a tightening vise, and a lightning bolt imposed on a sufferer's skull, television commercials for over-the-counter (OTC) pain relievers once sought to capture the miseries of sinus trouble. Through the years, Madison Avenue has ransacked a torture chamber full of such props ("including hammers pounding anvils, tightening nooses, and throbbing masses of tissue) to express one of the most common afflictions.

In addition to the symptoms celebrated by advertisers, sinus-nasal congestion can have many unpleasant indirect effects. Difficulty breathing through the nose can cause loss of sleep, or at least snoring. Postnasal drip trickling down the throat can cause nausea. Worse, sinuses clogged for a long time seem to invite infection, sometimes producing lengthy sequences of colds.

More than 31 million people in the United States suffer from sinus complaints, making over 16 million visits annually to their doctors. Many others resign themselves to routine discomfort. What can they do about it?

The common complaint that "I have sinus" shows that sinus illness is widely misunderstood. Everybody has sinuses, cavities hollowed in the bone structure of the skull. The problem is sinusitis, inflammation of these cavities due to viral, bacterial and fungal infections or allergic reactions, or sometimes rhinitis, irritation of the

FDA Consumer, October 1992.

lining inside the nose. Inflammation may invite infection, which aggravates the problem.

Any bone cavity is a sinus, but the culprits in sinusitis are the eight facial cavities grouped around the nose, the paranasal sinuses. Some anatomists theorize that these enhance the resonance of the voice, warm and moisten inhaled air, and relieve the skull of the excessive weight solid bone would impose. Others believe that the sinuses form simply because the facial bones of the skull of a newborn must grow faster than the cranium above to help the infant breathe and eat better.

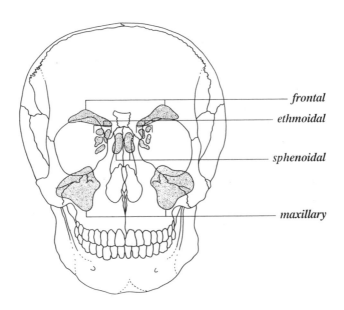

Figure 35.1. The Paranasal Sinuses. The frontal sinuses are located above the eyes. The ethmoidal sinuses, located between the eyes and behind the nose, are thought to be the critical point of sinus disease. According to one theory, if these sinuses can be cleared, the other ones will drain through them. The sphenoidal sinuses are located on either side at the top of the nose, about where glasses might pinch. The maxillary sinuses, beneath the eye in the cheek area, are the largest. Because of their closeness to the teeth, pressure here can be mistaken for a toothache.

Plumbing Problems

The function of sinuses in the plumbing system of the skull is even more problematical. The word sinus is Latin for bay, though these sinuses drain into the "river" of the nose, rather than the other way around. A membrane of mucus lines the system to screen impurities. However, these areas may be too small or poorly positioned to handle the volume of mucus some people produce, particularly those susceptible to allergies. If its passages are not clear, the system can clog as solidly as an icy Hudson Bay in February.

Mucus is a thick, opaque fluid produced to protect sensitive parts of the system. In the facial sinuses and nose it filters the air we breathe, trapping smoke or other irritants before they can pollute the lungs. When excessive irritants produce overabundant mucus, even a sinus well formed and positioned for drainage can be overwhelmed, with a growing pressure inside producing pain and a sense of swelling. Overflow may clog the nose or flush it, by "sniffles."

Its position may allow an affected sinus to misdirect pain to another area that shares a common nerve. For example, pressure in a maxillary sinus (beneath the eye) might send throbs of pain down the cheek toward the mouth, producing a kind of toothache. The eyes may also feel irritated from pressure in a maxillary sinus. A chameleon disease with symptoms mimicking those of other conditions, sinusitis may combine with chronic rhinitis, particularly in response to allergens. Breathing through the nose may become impossible. On the other hand, nasal stuffiness and headaches from other causes are often wrongly blamed on sinusitis.

Sinusitis may go away in time. Otherwise, at best it produces discomfort, at worst, grave medical consequences. Different treatments suit different degrees of severity.

Even a simple practice like drinking abundant fluids can assist sinus drainage by moistening and thinning mucus. Vaporizers, sometimes fortified with menthol or eucalyptus preparations can enhance this process. Some people report that home remedies like chewing horseradish root or imbibing soups made with garlic provide short-term decongestion.

Over-the-Counter Relief

The Federal Trade Commission regulates the advertising of OTC medications, while the Food and Drug Administration is responsible for ensuring their safety and effectiveness. Many OTC drug products enjoy long records of successfully relieving occasional sinus congestion. Antihistamines block the effect on nasal tissue of histamine, a chemical mediator triggering allergic reactions. While antihistamines reduce itching and sneezing, they may be less effective against swelling and excessive mucus. They may produce dry mouth, dizziness, drowsiness, and other side effects.

Decongestants may be taken orally or as nasal sprays or drops. They reduce the swelling that clogs airways. Nervousness, irritability, and insomnia are potential side effects. Individuals with high blood pressure, heart disease, diabetes mellitus, or hyperthyroidism should not take oral nasal decongestants without the advice of a physician, since such drugs can aggravate these conditions. Taking certain other drugs, such as monoamine oxidase inhibitors (a type of prescription drug for depression), at the same time as such decongestants can produce dangerous effects such as elevated blood pressure.

OTC topical decongestants such as nasal sprays or nose drops work quickly through ingredients active up to 12 hours and are quite safe to use for up to three days—always note the cautions on the packaging—but can cause temporary stinging, irritation, or drying up of nasal mucosa. Tolerance may develop quickly, so patients risk a rebound effect harder to remedy than the original congestion if they use such products for more than three consecutive days.

Many oral OTC products combine both an antihistamine and a nasal decongestant. They reduce itching and sneezing as well as relieve congestion; however, users may experience the side effects of both drugs.

When nasal and sinus congestion is more severe, as on rainy days or early in the morning, faster-acting products may work well; generalized discomfort may call for the longer-acting products.

When sinus illness persists, OTC drug products may become less effective and should be used more cautiously. Regular users may develop a "drug tolerance" for OTC nasal decongestants and antihistamines that renders them less and less effective. Simply switching products with different ingredients from time to time may work, but the continued need for these products could indicate chronic sinusitis, calling for more aggressive treatments.

Stronger Medicine

When is sinus trouble serious enough to warrant medical attention? Chronic sinusitis demands the attention of a physician.

Sinusitis that interferes with routine daily activities, forcing naps or cancellation of plans, may signal serious chronic trouble. Rebound congestion may mean it's time to-look beyond OTC stopgap remedies to more comprehensive doctor-prescribed courses of treatment. Repeated absence from work or school is another likely sign. Frequent colds, stubborn earaches, or other infections may be harbingers of sinus infection. Since many people get so used to sinus pain that they take it for granted, it's important to note any serious impact on health and lifestyle.

Allergies are common triggers of nose and sinus inflammation, so one way to alleviate sinusitis is by targeting the causes of allergy. (See Minimizing Allergies at end of chapter.)

Antibiotics to control infection may be necessary in both acute and chronic sinusitis. Clogged nasal passages and filled sinuses readily become infected. Because of their proximity to such sensitive areas as the eye muscles and the brain, infected sinuses can have serious consequences, including meningitis (inflammation of brain membranes). Complications of untreated sinus infection can be fatal. Antibiotics are used to kill the bacteria that cause infection. If antibiotic therapy fails, surgery may be necessary.

Determined Doctor

Claudia Gaffey, M.D., a medical officer with FDA's Center for Devices and Radiological Health, was a long-time sinus sufferer. Like the title character in the recent film "The Doctor," she learned that, in the role of patient, even a physician may not be taken seriously.

Like many chronic sinus sufferers, Gaffey found that even medical colleagues thought her complaints exaggerated. She was told her symptoms were not related to sinus disease because conventional x-ray film did not show abnormalities. Frustrated, she drew on her medical background to review the latest research in otolaryngology (ear, nose and throat medicine), even though as a pathologist she had not been trained in that specialty.

She learned that sinusitis, though a potentially debilitating problem, is only now being recognized as one of the most frequently overlooked and misunderstood of common respiratory diseases. Physicians commonly dismissed sinus patients as chronic complainers (if not hypochondriacs) until the superior diagnostic tools of the last decade penetrated the previously inaccessible ethmoid complex (the region between the eyes and behind the nose), now thought to be a critical point of sinus disease. Otolaryngologists today are working to educate other doctors about diagnosis and treatment of all forms of sinusitis.

Using state-of-the-art methods, physicians at Johns Hopkins University assessed Gaffey's serious sinus condition and corrected it through a course of antibiotic therapy, which she says was longer and more intense than is conventionally prescribed by U.S. physicians. This relieved her condition without surgery. She says that better control of her allergies led to complete resolution of her sinus problems.

When Surgery Is Necessary

Very few cases today require surgical treatment. Yet when sinus trouble is chronic and severe and when medication fails to relieve it, surgery may be needed, not just to relieve discomfort but to protect against serious consequences.

Though it's uncommon, polyps can develop in the facial sinuses. Benign cysts that retain mucus may build harmlessly, especially in the large maxillary or frontal sinuses under and over the eye. More intrusive or malignant growths must be removed.

To detect and assess sinus disease, physicians most often order plain film x-ray examinations of the sinuses to look for fluid, masses, or swelling of normal tissue. If more detail is required, or if the difficulty lies in the ethmoid region, computerized tomography (CT or CAT) scanning or magnetic resonance imaging (MRI) can supply it. Sometimes these procedures are used to assess accurately the structure of the sinuses, since anatomic abnormalities may be responsible for repeated sinus infections. An endoscope (a fiber-optic device tiny enough to be inserted up the nose) is another tool important for evaluating the sinuses that allows physicians to look directly into some sinuses for diagnosis or for surgery. FDA regulates all these devices.

Sinus surgery ranges from simple to elaborate, and like all invasive surgery it can be traumatic for the patient. A sub-surgical procedure called irrigation works by blasting encrusted matter out of the sinus with a stream of warm salt water, either through the natural opening or by needle, the way one might clean out the backyard grill with a garden hose. A "scrubbing" does the same by means of instruments.

Surgery can reshape the sinuses and nasal passages to allow proper drainage. A deviated septum (the wall of cartilage and bone, down the middle of the nose when skewed off center) may be straightened to allow proper air-passage or pierced to create alternative airways. Bloated tissue blocking passages can be removed. Small receptors in the nose can be reconfigured or eliminated. Individual sinuses may be reshaped and their outlets enlarged. In some cases, sinus walls may be obliterated surgically without harm.

Not all major sinus operations require skin incisions or breaking facial bones. Many medical centers now have considerable experience with endoscopic sinus surgery. A major advantage to this kind of surgery is that it permits resection only of affected areas in the sinuses, preserving as much normal functioning mucosa as possible. One current theory is that if the ethmoid sinus area can be cleared, the other sinuses will drain naturally through it. In many cases, the surgeon will be able to operate here through the nose. The endoscope, so useful in diagnosing sinus problems, also makes this operation possible, since surgeons can use it to see what they are doing in a previously inaccessible area. Since this sinus adjoins sensitive areas, the delicate procedure involves a slight risk of damage to eye muscles or seepage of brain fluids.

Laser surgery is used by otolaryngologists when feasible. These new procedures are far less bloody and shocking to the system than traditional methods.

In simple cases, laser surgery is done on an outpatient basis. There is no need for bandages or wadding in the nose afterward. A disadvantage is that, because they are in early development, laser techniques may pose slightly higher risk of eye or brain damage, though those risks are still quite low. Properly performed, sinus surgery has a very high success rate, freeing many people from daily miseries and allowing them to breathe properly for the first time in years.

With so many medical tools at hand, there seems no reason now for anyone to be resigned to a lifetime of sinus discomfort. Moreover, clogged sinuses invite infection that can become quite dangerous, so nobody should tolerate it too long. A lifetime of discomfort isn't inevitable if one takes sinus trouble seriously.

Minimizing Allergies

Doctors use alternative options, often in combination, to help a patient with allergies. One option is to instruct the patient to avoid the allergen (substance causing the allergy); the other is to treat the allergic reaction. Testing to determine what substances a person is allergic to has become less uncomfortable in recent years, and increasingly precise with the introduction of standardized allergenic extracts.

Once the substances that trigger one's allergies are identified, one can readily avoid eating certain foods or wearing certain fabrics. Special cleansers can remove molds from walls and woodwork. Pets may have to find other homes.

For people with multiple allergies or allergies to substances commonly present in the air, avoidance is more difficult. Pollens from grass, trees, and weeds and other airborne allergens may force people sensitive to them to remain indoors with the air conditioner running on many summer days. Although the effectiveness of many air filter devices has yet to be demonstrated by scientific studies, many individuals feel that they benefit from them.

When avoidance is not feasible, prescription products, some of them relatively new, can provide significant relief of symptoms. Although they too have potential side effects, the controlled dosages in which they should be taken minimize risk.

Cromolyn sodium inhalers prevent release of histamine in the body to prevent allergic responses and forestall nasal/sinus symptoms. However, they can cause mild irritation of the nasal mucus membranes. The medication seeks to prevent allergic responses but may have to be taken for a couple of weeks before it is fully effective.

Inhaled corticosteroid nasal sprays suppress irritants, reduce inflammation of swollen membranes, and relieve sneezing, itching and congestion. The doses metered by precision dispensers in the United States are small enough to avoid harmful effects.

Prescription oral antihistamines and antihistamine-decongestant combinations are generally stronger than their OTC counterparts. They require caution, because their potential side effects are stronger, too. They can disturb coordination and cause dizziness. Adhering to the prescribed instructions is essential.

Two non-sedating prescription antihistamines, Seldane (terfenadine) and Hismanal (astemizole), pose serious heart problems for certain patients under some conditions.

If a patient has allergic reactions throughout the year, allergen desensitization may be a helpful alternative. Allergy shots are subcutaneous injections that seek to increase a patient's tolerance by exposure to increasing doses of the allergens. Depending on the patient's sensitivity and environment, months of periodic injections, followed perhaps by less frequent maintenance injections, may be necessary to build immunity. When immunization succeeds, it may produce permanent relief without need for further shots. Like all therapeutic agents, immunotherapy does not work for everybody, and it may be inconvenient, uncomfortable and costly. For many people, however, it is literally "worth a shot."

—by S. J. Ackerman

S. J. Ackerman is a writer in Washington, D.C., who is breathing easier after recent sinus surgery.

Chapter 36

Allergic and Non-Allergic Rhinitis

Do you suffer from a runny or stuffy nose much of the time? You may not have given it much thought because it typically is not a serious condition. It can, however, be quite annoying. This condition is known as rhinitis. Approximately 40 million people in the U.S. suffer to one degree or another from rhinitis. Although hay fever, or seasonal allergic rhinitis, is the condition that most people are familiar with, there are different types of rhinitis. This fact sheet reviews these conditions and current treatments.

Classification

Many physicians use the following classification for chronic rhinitis:

Atopic Rhinitis

There are three types of atopic (associated with allergic-like symptoms) rhinitis.

1. **Seasonal Allergic Rhinitis (also known as hay fever).**
    This is triggered by allergy to pollens, including trees in
    spring, grasses in summer and weeds in fall. Symptoms in-
    clude sneezing, itching, tickling in the nose, runny or stuffy
    nose and watery or itchy eyes. Seasonal rhinitis is diagnosed
    primarily by your medical history. Skin testing is not always
    indicated, especially if your symptoms are mild.

2. **Perennial Rhinitis (year-round) with Allergic Triggers.**
    These triggers include indoor allergens such as mold, house
    dust mite, cockroach and animal dander. Symptoms are the
    same as seasonal allergic rhinitis but are experienced
    throughout the year. The physician makes the diagnosis for
    perennial rhinitis by your medical history and positive skin
    tests to relevant allergens.

3. **Perennial Rhinitis with Non-Allergic Triggers.** This type of
    rhinitis is not well understood. Although not triggered by allergy,
    it's an allergic-like condition with increased eosinophils (a special
    type of white blood cell associated with allergy) in the lining and
    secretions of the nose. Symptoms are the same as perennial
    rhinitis with allergic triggers. Diagnosis is determined from
    negative skin tests and a nasal smear test positive for eosino-
    phils. Nasal polyps can be a complication of this condition.

Idiopathic Non-Allergic Rhinitis

This is also known as vasomotor rhinitis. A person with this type
reacts to temperature and humidity changes, smoke, odors and emotional upsets. Symptoms are primarily nasal congestion and postnasal drip. Diagnosis comes after negative skin tests and nasal smear
negative for eosinophils.

Infectious Rhinitis

This can occur as an acute viral respiratory infection (cold) which
may clear rapidly or continue with symptoms up to six weeks. Some
people develop the complication of an acute or chronic bacterial sinus infection, usually associated with blocked sinus drainage. Symptoms of infectious rhinitis are an increased amount of colored
(yellow-green) and thickened nasal discharge and nasal congestion.
The diagnosis of an acute or chronic sinus infection is confirmed by
an abnormal sinus X-ray or CT scan.

Other Types

1. **Rhinitis Medicamentosa.** This type is associated with long-term use of decongestant nasal sprays or recreational use of cocaine. Symptoms typically are nasal congestion and postnasal drip. A person who has taken a decongestant nasal spray for months or years is using this treatment inappropriately. These medications are intended for short-term use only. Overuse can cause rebound congestion, which leads to increased nasal obstruction. It is very important for a person with rebound congestion to work closely with a physician to gradually withdraw the nasal spray.

2. **Mechanical Obstruction.** This is most often associated with a deviated septum or enlarged adenoids. If you have chronic nasal obstruction that is one-sided, a medical evaluation is recommended.

3. **Hormonal.** This is generally associated with pregnancy or untreated hypothyroidism.

Diagnosis

Often a person may have more than one type of rhinitis. In making the diagnosis, an evaluation by your doctor may include:

1. **History.** Specific symptoms and when they occur, family history and work history.

2. **Physical exam.**

3. **Nasal smears.** Microscopic exam of nasal secretions, especially eosinophils.

4. **Allergy testing.** Skin testing by a board-certified allergist is generally indicated for someone with recurrent symptoms. A positive skin test indicates the presence of IgE antibody which can react with specific substances to produce an allergic reaction. In most cases, an allergic person will react to more than one substance.

5. **Sinus X-ray.** About 40 percent of persons with perennial rhinitis will have changes on the sinus X-ray. This can indicate the presence of sinusitis (inflammation of the sinuses) with or without infection or nasal polyps.

Complications

Complications of **seasonal allergic rhinitis** are rare. The condition may be associated with bronchial asthma, but evidence that rhinitis specifically predisposes you to asthma is not convincing. Two epidemiologic studies in the U.S. found that asthma followed allergic rhinitis in 1 to 10 percent of the cases, which suggests that the subsequent development of asthma in rhinitis sufferers may be only slightly more common than in the overall population. In childhood, bronchial asthma may precede the onset of allergic rhinitis. Persons with rhinitis are prone to recurrent respiratory, sinus and ear infections.

Treatment of Rhinitis

Environmental Control

Avoidance of triggers is clearly the most important treatment for allergic rhinitis. Although total avoidance is usually not possible (except for family pets), you can take a few steps to significantly reduce your exposure to allergens.

Keep your doors and windows closed. The use of central air conditioning dramatically reduces the level of indoor pollen and can also lessen indoor humidity. Lower humidity reduces both mold and dust mite allergen concentrations. Pollen and mold counts can vary throughout the day. Peak times are:

1. **grass**—afternoon and early evening

2. **ragweed**—early midday

3. **mold spores**—some types peak during warm, dry, windy afternoons; other types occur at high levels during periods of dampness and rain and peak in the early morning hours.

Molds

It may help to limit your outdoor activities during the times of highest pollen and mold counts. Mold can grow in damp areas of your home, such as the kitchen, bathroom or basement. If you are allergic to mold, take measures to lessen mold growth. These include:

1. Ventilate these areas well.

2. Clean damp areas frequently, using a weak, chlorine bleach solution as needed.

3. Use a humidifier with caution because frequent use increases growth of mold and dust mites within your home. Clean your humidifier routinely as it can become a source for mold and bacteria growth.

4. Consider a dehumidifier if your basement is damp, or if you live in a very humid climate.

Dust Mites

If you are allergic to house dust mites and live in a humid area:

1. Cover your mattress and box spring in plastic encasings.

2. Wash your pillows, sheets and blankets weekly in hot water. Mites will survive lukewarm water.

Pets

Dander from pets, particularly cats and dogs, is a major year-round allergen. If you are allergic to your pet, the obvious recommendation is removal of the pet from your home. If you choose to keep it, completely exclude the animal from your bedroom, and keep the doors and heating ducts closed. Keep in mind that the more restricted the area in which the pet is allowed, the less allergic exposure you will have.

Irritants

Many irritants (non-allergenic substances) in the environment can also trigger rhinitis symptoms. Reducing exposure to irritants is recommended for persons with allergic or non-allergic rhinitis. Cigarette smoke is a strong respiratory irritant and it is important that no one smoke in your home. You may also need to avoid aerosol sprays, perfumes, dusty or polluted environments, strong cleaning products and other sources of strong odors.

Commonly Used Medication for Rhinitis

The goal of medical treatment is to reduce symptoms and use medications with few or no side effects.

Antihistamines

These oral (tablet/syrup) medications are effective for the itching, sneezing and nasal discharge associated with allergic rhinitis. They also relieve itchy and watery eyes, but are not effective in reducing nasal congestion.

- **Over-the-counter medications:** Many preparations are available such as chlorpheniramine and brompheniramine. Side effects can include drowsiness, dry mouth and urinary retention.

- **Prescription medications:** A newer class of antihistamines does not cause drowsiness, but is more expensive than other preparations. Terfenadine (Seldane®)—taken two times a day. Astemizole (Hismanal®)—taken once a day.

Decongestants

These medications are effective in reducing nasal obstruction and are available as oral (tablet/syrup) preparations and as nasal sprays. Commonly used oral preparations are pseudoephedrine and phenyl-propanolamine. Side effects: shaking, restlessness and urinary retention. There are also combination antihistamine and decongestant preparations:

- **Over-the-counter medications:**
  - Dimetapp®
  - Drixoral®

- **Prescription medications:**
  - Seldane®
  - Tavist-D®

Decongestant nasal sprays should be limited to three to 10 days' use because rebound congestion can develop with prolonged administration. Rebound congestion can cause increased nasal congestion, which leads to more frequent use of the nasal spray. Commonly available brands: Afrin®, Neo-Synephrine® and Dristan®.

Nasal Corticosteroids

These prescription nasal sprays are typically the most effective medications for all types of rhinitis. They decrease nasal inflammation and mucus production, lessen nasal obstruction and promote normal sinus drainage. These prescription nasal sprays are preventive medications and do not immediately relieve symptoms. Because there is little absorption of the medication into the bloodstream, the risk of steroid side effects is extremely low. Side effects: sensations of nasal burning or irritation and mild nosebleeds.

- Available **prescription medications:**
  - Beclomethasone (Beconase AQ®, Vancenase AQ®)
  - Flunisolide (Nasalide®)
  - Triamcinolone (Nasacort®)

Nasal Cromolyn

This prescription nasal spray reduces milder symptoms of nasal discharge and sneezing. This is also a preventive medication and does not relieve symptoms immediately. The recommended dose is one spray per nostril four to six times a day. It is available as Nasalcrom®. Side effects: sensations of nasal burning or irritation and sneezing.

Atrovent®

This prescription medication occasionally benefits those with non-allergic rhinitis. It is available in an inhaler for lung conditions, but is also used as a nasal spray to reduce watery nasal discharge.

Oral Corticosteroids

These prescription tablet/syrup preparations are very effective in treating and preventing symptoms of rhinitis. However, the side effects of oral steroids, especially with long-term use, limit their use. Your doctor may prescribe a short course (three to seven days) for more severe symptoms. It is important to note that the corticosteroids used in respiratory treatment are not the same as the anabolic steroids used by athletes.

Nasal Wash

A saltwater wash is helpful in removing mucus from the nose. It temporarily reduces symptoms of nasal obstruction and postnasal drainage.

- **Nasal Wash Method.** Purchase saline (saltwater) through any pharmacy, or make a new solution every day. Use one teaspoon table salt in one pint warm water with a pinch of baking soda. Prepare the solution in a clean glass or plastic bottle with a screw-on cap. To use:

- **Method 1.** Pour some saline into the palm of your hand and "snuff" it up your nose, one nostril at a time. Spit it out of your mouth and blow your nose lightly afterward. The procedure is best done with your head down, bent far over the sink.

- **Method 2.** Purchase a large all-rubber ear syringe at any drugstore. Fill it completely with saline solution. Lean way over the sink with your head down. Insert the syringe tip in one nostril, just enough to keep the solution from running out of your nose. Gently squeeze the bulb and release several times to swish the solution around in your nose, then squeeze the bulb hard enough to make the saline go up and over the palate in the roof of your mouth and run out. Repeat for your other nostril.

- The nose should be cleaned several times per day by one of these methods. If you have yellow or green discharge from the nose, perform nasal irrigations even more often. Use at least one cupful of saline each time. Nasal washes are done before putting other medication in the nose.

Immunotherapy

Immunotherapy ("allergy shots") consists of a series of injections containing the allergens believed to be triggering allergy symptoms. The objective is to reduce your sensitivity to these allergens so that you experience fewer symptoms. Treatment usually begins with injections of a weak solution given once or twice a week, with the strength gradually increasing. When the strongest dosage is reached, the injection is then usually given once a month.

Immunotherapy has proven effective against the following allergens:

- grass pollen
- ragweed pollen
- birch pollen
- mountain cedar pollen
- house dust mite
- cat and dog dander
- Alternaria mold spores

320

Skin testing, or RAST testing, can identify your specific allergens. Immunotherapy is specific against only the allergens used in the treatment. For example, if someone with allergy to both ragweed pollen and grass pollen is treated for ragweed only, this person will continue to experience rhinitis triggered by grass pollen.

Physicians generally recommend immunotherapy for allergic rhinitis in someone with clear-cut allergy to very specific allergens who responds poorly to treatment or whose symptoms persist over several seasons or throughout the year. Doctors at National Jewish recommend that allergy testing and immunotherapy be done by a board-certified allergist.

Chapter 37

Post-Nasal Drip

What Is Post-Nasal Drip?

Post-nasal discharge, also called post-nasal drip (PND), describes the sensation of mucous accumulation in the throat or a *feeling* that mucus is dripping downward from the back of the nose. PND can be caused by excessive or thick secretions or throat muscle and swallowing disorders.

Normally, the glands lining the nose and sinuses produce one to two quarts of thin mucus a day. On the surface of this mucous membrane lining, the rhythmic beat of invisible cilia (which look like tiny hairs under the microscope) thrust the mucus backward. Then it is swallowed unconsciously. This mucus lubricates and cleanses the nasal membranes, humidifies air, traps and clears inhaled foreign matter, and fights infection. Mucus production and clearance is regulated by a complex interaction of nerves, blood vessels, glands, muscles, hormones, and cilia.

Abnormal Secretions

Increased thin clear secretions can be due to colds and flu (upper respiratory viruses), allergies, cold temperatures, bright lights, certain foods and spices, pregnancy and hormonal changes, various drugs (including birth control pills and especially high blood pressure medications), and structural abnormalities, such as a deviated or irregular nasal septum. (The septum is the cartilage and bony partition which divides the nose into its two sides, beginning at the nostrils and extending to the back of the nasal cavity.)

Vasomotor rhinitus describes a nonallergic "hyperirritable nose" which may feel congested, blocked or wet.

Increased thick secretions are frequently caused by wintertime low humidity in homes and buildings heated without adding moisture to the air. They can also result from sinus or nose infections and some allergies, especially to certain foods such as dairy products. If the secretions of a common cold become thick and green or yellow it is likely that a bacterial sinus infection is developing. Also, particularly in children, they can signify a foreign body in the nose (such as a bean, wadded paper, piece of toy, etc.).

Decreased secretions may be caused by any of the following:

- Long-term exposure to environmental irritants (such as cigarette smoke, industrial pollutants, and automobile fumes), which can dry and damage nasal mucous membranes. When secretions are reduced, they are usually thicker than normal and produce the false sensation of increased mucus.

- Structural abnormalities (such as nasal septal irregularities) which alter air currents may then dry surrounding membranes. (Thus, depending on their type, structural problems can increase or decrease secretions.)

- Age. Mucous membranes commonly shrink and dry with age, causing reduced mucus that is thicker than normal which the elderly perceive as PND.

- Other less common disorders of the tissues lining the nose and sinuses can alter mucous production or flow.

Swallowing Problems

Swallowing is a complicated process by which food and fluid go from the mouth into the esophagus (tube connecting the throat to the stomach). It requires coordinated nerve and muscle interaction in the mouth, throat, and esophagus. Swallowing problems may result in accumulation of solids or liquids in the throat, which can spill into the voice box (larynx) and breathing passages (trachea and bronchii) causing hoarseness, throat clearing, or cough.

Several factors contribute to swallowing problems:

- With **age**, swallowing muscles often lose strength and coordination. Thus, even normal secretions may not pass smoothly into the stomach.

- During **sleep**, swallowing occurs much less frequently, and secretions may accumulate. Coughing and vigorous throat clearing are often needed when awakening.

- At any age, **nervous tension** or **stress** can trigger throat muscle spasms, resulting in a sensation of a lump in the throat. Frequent throat clearing, which usually produces little or no mucus, can make the problem worse by increasing irritation.

- **Growths or swellings** in the food passages may slow or prevent the passage of liquids and/or solids.

- Swallowing dysfunction may be caused by **gastroesophageal reflux,** which is a return of stomach contents and acid into the esophagus or into the throat. Heartburn, indigestion, and sore throat are common symptoms, which may be aggravated while lying down (especially following eating). Hiatal hernia, a pouch-like structure at the junction of the esophagus and stomach, often contributes to the reflux.

Chronic Sore Throat

Post-nasal drip often leads to a sore, irritated throat. Usually, throat cultures will not show strep or other infections, but the tonsils and other glandular tissues in the throat may swell, causing discomfort or a feeling of a throat lump. Successful treatment of the post nasal drip will usually clear up these throat symptoms.

Before treatment is started, a diagnosis must be made. This requires a detailed ear, nose, and throat exam and possible laboratory, endoscopic, and x-ray studies.

Treatment

Bacterial infection is treated with antibiotics, but these drugs may provide only temporary relief. In cases of chronic sinusitis, surgery to open the blocked sinuses or drainage pathways may be required.

Allergy is managed by avoiding the cause where possible. Antihistamines and decongestants, cromolyn and steroid (cortisone type) nasal sprays, various other forms of steroids, and hyposensitization (allergy shots) may be used. However, some antihistamines may dry and thicken secretions even more; decongestants can aggravate high blood pressure, heart, and thyroid disease (these drugs commonly are found in nonprescription medications for colds). Steroid sprays generally may be used safely for years under medical supervision. Oral and injectable steroids rarely produce serious complications in short term use. Because significant side effects can occur, they must be monitored very carefully if used for prolonged periods.

Gastroesophageal reflux is treated by elevating the head of the bed six to eight inches, avoiding late evening meals and snacks and eliminating alcohol and caffeine. Antacids (e.g. Maalox®, Mylanta®, Gaviscon®) and drugs that block stomach acid production (e.g. Zantac®, Tagamet®, Pepcid®) may be prescribed. A trial of treatment may be suggested before x-rays and other diagnostic studies are performed.

Structural abnormalities may require surgical correction. A septal deviation can prevent normal drainage from the sinuses and contribute to the development of chronic sinusitis. A septal spur (sharp projection) can cause irritation and abnormal secretions. A septal perforation (hole) can cause crusting. Enlarged or deformed nasal turbinates (the structures on the side walls of the nasal cavity which regulate and humidify airflow) and/or polyps (i.e. outgrowths of nasal membrane resulting from infection, allergy or irritants) may cause similar problems.

It is not always possible to determine whether an existing structural abnormality is causing the post-nasal drip or if some other condition is to blame. If medical treatment fails, the patient must then decide whether to undergo surgery in an attempt to relieve the problem.

In some cases, no specific cause can be found for PND. When no correctable disease is present, attention is usually directed to thinning secretions so they can pass more easily. This is particularly true for the elderly, who often have inadequate fluid intake. These patients should drink eight glasses of water a day, eliminate caffeine, and avoid diuretics (fluid pills) if possible. Mucous thinning agents such as guaifenesin or organic iodine may be employed. Guaifenesin (e.g. Humibid®, Robitussin®) rarely produces significant side effects. In the rare instances when organic iodine (Organidin®) causes swelling of the saliva glands or a rash, the drug must be discontinued.

Nasal irrigations may alleviate thickened or reduced secretions. These can be performed two to six times a day either with a nasal douche device or a Water Pik® equipped with a special nasal irrigation nozzle (purchased separately). Warm water with baking soda or salt (½ tsp. to the pint) or Alkalol®, a non-prescription irrigating solution (full strength or diluted by half with warm water), may be helpful. Finally, use of simple saline non-prescription nasal sprays (e g. Ocean®, Ayr®, Nasal®,) to moisten the nose is often very helpful.

Chapter 38

Should I Take Antihistamines?

Drugs for stuffy nose, sinus trouble, congestion, and the common cold constitute the largest segment of the over-the-counter market for America's pharmaceutical industry. When used wisely, they provide welcome relief for at least some of the discomforts that affect almost everyone at one time or another and that affect many people chronically. Drugs in these categories are useful for relief of symptoms from allergies, upper respiratory infections (i.e., sinusitis, colds, flu), and vasomotor rhinitis (a chronic stuffy nose caused by such unrelated conditions as emotional stress, thyroid disease, pregnancy, and others). These drugs do not cure the allergies, infections, etc.; they only relieve the symptoms, thereby making the patient more comfortable.

Antihistamines

Histamine is an important body chemical that is responsible for the congestion, sneezing, and runny nose that a patient suffers with an allergic attack or an infection. Antihistamine drugs block the action of histamine, therefore reducing the allergy symptoms. For the best result, antihistamines should be taken before allergic symptoms get well established.

The most annoying side effect that antihistamines produce is drowsiness. Though desirable at bedtime, it is a nuisance to many people who need to use antihistamines in the daytime. To some people, it is even hazardous. These drugs are not recommended for daytime use for people who may be driving an automobile or operating equipment that could be dangerous. The first few doses cause the most sleepiness; subsequent doses are usually less troublesome.

Typical antihistamines include Benadryl®, Chlor-Trimetron®, Claritin®, Dimetane®, Hismanal®, Nolahist®, PBZ®, Polaramine®, Seldane®, Tavist®, Teldrin®, Zyrtec®, etc. Some of these antihistamines may be available over-the-counter without a prescription. **Read labels carefully, and use only as directed.**

Decongestants

Congestion in the nose, sinuses, and chest is due to swollen, expanded, or dilated blood vessels in the membranes of the nose and air passages. These membranes have an abundant supply of blood vessels with a great capacity for expansion (swelling and congestion). Histamine stimulates these blood vessels to expand as described previously.

Decongestants, on the other hand, cause constriction or tightening of the blood vessels in those membranes, which then forces much of the blood out of the membranes so that they shrink, and the air passages open up again.

Table 38.1. Antihistamines and Decongestants

Medicine	Symptoms Relieved	Side Effects
Antihistamines	Sneezing Runny Nose Stuffy Nose Itchy Eyes Congestion	Drowsiness Dry Mouth & Nose
Decongestants	Stuffy Nose Congestion	Stimulation Insomnia Rapid Heart Beat
Combinations of Above	All of Above	Any of Above (more or less)

Decongestants are chemically related to adrenaline, the natural decongestant, which is also a type of stimulant. Therefore, the side effect of decongestants is a jittery or nervous feeling. They can cause difficulty in going to sleep, and they can elevate blood pressure and pulse rate. Decongestants should not be used by a patient who has an irregular heart rhythm (pulse), high blood pressure, heart disease, or glaucoma. Some patients taking decongestants experience difficulty with urination. Furthermore, decongestants are often used as ingredients in diet pills. To avoid excessively stimulating effects, patients taking diet pills should not take decongestants.

Typical decongestants are phenylephrine (Neo-Synephrine®, phenylpropanolamine (Dura-Vent®, Exgest®, Entex®, Propagest®), and pseudoephedrine (Novafed®, Sudafed®, etc.) Again, some of these decongestants may be available over-the-counter without a prescription. Read labels carefully, and use only as directed.

Combination Remedies

Theoretically, if the side effects could be properly balanced, the sleepiness caused by antihistamines could be canceled by the stimulation of decongestants. Numerous combinations of antihistamines with decongestants are available: Actifed®, A.R.M.®, Chlor-Trimeton D®, Claritin D®, Contac®, CoPyronil 2®, Deconamine®, Demazin®, Dimetapp®, Drixoral®, Isoclor®, Nolamine®, Novafed A®, Ornade®, Sudafed Plus®, Tavist D®, Triaminic®, and Trinalin®, to name just a few. Remember, some of these combination remedies may be available over-the-counter without a prescription. **Read labels carefully, and use only as directed.**

A patient may find one preparation quite helpful for several months or years but may need to switch to another one when the first loses its effectiveness. Since no one reacts exactly the same as another to the side effects of these drugs, a patient may wish to try his own ideas on adjusting the dosages. One might take the antihistamine only at night and take the decongestant alone in the daytime. Or take them together, increasing the dosage of antihistamine at night (while decreasing the decongestant dose) and then doing the opposite for daytime use.

"Cold" Remedies

Decongestants and/or antihistamines are the principal ingredients in "cold" remedies, but drying agents, aspirin (or aspirin substitutes)

331

and cough suppressants may also be added. The patient should choose the remedy with ingredients best suited to combat his own symptoms. If the label does not clearly state the ingredients and their functions, the consumer should ask the pharmacist to explain them.

Nose Sprays

The types of nose sprays that can be purchased without a prescription usually contain decongestants for direct application to nasal membranes. They can give prompt relief from congestion by constricting blood vessels. However, direct application creates a stronger stimulation than decongestants taken by mouth. It also impairs the circulation in the nose, which after a few hours, stimulates the vessels to expand to improve the blood flow again. This results in a "bounce-back" effect. The congestion recurs. If the patient uses the spray again, it starts the cycle again. Spray—decongestion—rebound—and more congestion.

In infants, this rebound rhinitis can develop in two days, whereas in adults, it often takes several more days to become established. An infant taken off the drops for 12 to 24 hours is cured, but well-established cases in adults often require more than a simple "cold turkey" withdrawal. They need decongestants by mouth, sometimes corticosteroids, and possibly (in patients who have used the sprays for months and years continuously) a surgical procedure to the inside of the nose. For this reason, the labels on these types of nose sprays contain the warning **"Do not use this product for more than three days."** Nose sprays should be reserved for emergency and short term use.

(The above description and advice does not apply to the type of prescription anti-allergy nose sprays that may be ordered by your physician.)

Chapter 39

Nose Sprays

Direct Relief for Congestion and Irritation

It could be your first summer cold. Or maybe it's the air conditioning, a recent visit from your neighbor's pet or your freshly mown grass. Any of these irritants can cause mucous membranes in your nose and sinuses to become inflamed and swollen. The result: a stuffy or runny nose.

With a cold, the congestion usually goes away in a few days. But if you have allergies or another nasal problem, congestion can seem never-ending.

Cortisone shots, decongestants and antihistamines have been used to relieve congestion, sneezing and itchy, watery eyes for more than 40 years. Within the past 10 years, however, medicated nose sprays have proven just as effective. Because sprays deliver the medication directly to your nasal membranes, they also cause fewer side effects.

When a Spray Can Help

A nose spray can help control symptoms caused by these conditions:

Allergic Rhinitis

This response is an overreaction by your immune system to an otherwise harmless substance (allergen). Delicate tissues in your nose

Reprinted from June 1995 *Mayo Clinic Health Letter* with permission of Mayo Foundation for Medical Education and Research, Rochester, Minnesota 55905. For subscription information, call 1-800-333-9038.

become inflamed and release histamine, an irritating chemical that can cause sneezing, a stuffy or runny nose and itchy, watery eyes.

Allergens such as molds, house dust and tiny particles from an animal's skin or hair can trigger symptoms year-round (perennial rhinitis). The effect of seasonal pollens varies by geographical location.

Nonallergic Rhinitis

Sneezing and a runny or stuffy nose may develop for unknown reasons and persist year-round. Typically, temperature changes, air conditioning, fatigue, alcohol, fumes and dust trigger or worsen symptoms.

In nonallergic rhinitis, swollen nasal and sinus membranes may also secrete excess mucus to clear the irritation. Backward flow of mucus into your throat can lead to postnasal drip.

Polyps

Sometimes, a runny or stuffy nose is related to development of pea-size noncancerous nasal tumors. If polyps enlarge enough, they can block nasal passages and make breathing difficult.

Dry Nose

Allergies, dry air or a cold can dry nasal tissues, causing irritation.

The Best Approach

The ideal way to manage allergies and other nasal problems is to avoid the source of your irritation. In addition, the following information shows the types of nose sprays available to help control your symptoms.

Note on decongestant sprays: use sparingly. Using a decongestant spray for more than five to seven days commonly has a rebound effect. When you stop using the drug, your symptoms return and worsen. Continued use can lead to chronic congestion and irritation called rhinitis medicamentosus.

All Nose Sprays Are Not the Same

A nose spray can be part of your defense against nasal congestion and irritation. Here are the four types and how to use them.

334

Corticosteroid

Availability. Available by prescription as beclomethasone (such as Beconase, Vancenase), budosonide (Rhinocort), flunisolide (Nasalide), fluticasone (Flonase) and triamcinolone (Nasacort).

Indications. Most effective for relieving congestion caused by allergic and nonallergic rhinitis and nasal polyps.

How to use. Daily, instead of sporadically when symptoms develop. Takes at least a week to become fully effective.

Side effects. Fewer side effects than steroid pills or injections. May cause sneezing, an itchy, burning nose or an unpleasant taste in your mouth.

Cromolyn sodium

Availability. Available by prescription as Nasalcrom.

Indications. Works best to prevent sneezing and itchy runny nose caused by mild to moderate allergies.

How to use. Start using four to six weeks before the start of allergy season. Use at least four times a day.

Side effects. Rarely, it can cause sneezing or nasal irritation.

Decongestant

Availability. Available over-the-counter as oxymetazoline (Afrin, Dristan), phenylephrine (Neo-Synephrine, Nostril) and xylometazoline (Otrivin).

Indications. For acute relief of congestion due to a cold. Don't use for chronic symptoms caused by allergic and nonallergic rhinitis.

How to use. Use for no more than three days, if at all.

Side effects. Can become habit-forming or aggravate high blood pressure. In rare cases, can cause an irregular heartbeat.

Saline

Availability. Available over-the-counter as Afrin Saline, Ayr, Breathe Free, Dristan Saline, Humist, NaSal, Ocean Nasal Mist, SalineX and Seamist.

Indications. Relieves mild congestion, loosens mucus and prevents crusting caused by allergies and other irritations.

How to use. As needed until symptoms improve.

Side effects. None.

Chapter 40

When Smell and Taste Go Awry

Minutes after a sudden April shower, the rich, earthy scent of spring permeates the air. A whiff from a backyard grill evokes cherished images from childhood, and a crisp autumn day has its own aroma.

Imagine a spicy slice of pizza, or freshly brewed coffee, and your mouth waters in anticipation. But for 2 million people in the United States, the senses of smell and taste are dulled, distorted, or gone altogether. Many more of us get some idea of their plight when these senses are temporarily stifled by the sniffles.

Compared to the loss of hearing or sight, being unable to taste or smell normally may seem more an oddity than an illness. But those with such ailments would probably disagree.

There are several reasons why knowledge about how the "chemical senses" of taste and smell work lags behind what we know about the other senses. One reason is that a problem with taste or smell often is not perceived as a serious medical condition.

"These disorders are not associated with significant morbidity and mortality, and affect fewer than 5 percent of the population, so it is not a major public health concern," says Lucinda Miller, Pharm.D., in the division of family medicine at the Baylor College of Medicine in Houston. She adds that this attitude translates into skimpy research funding. In some situations, however, a poor or lacking sense of smell can be dangerous. Robert Henkin, M.D., Ph.D., of the Taste

FDA Consumer, November 1991.

and Smell Clinic in Washington, D.C., recalls one patient who died in a house fire because he did not smell the smoke in time to escape.

Another hindrance to learning more about smell and taste is that the physical bases of these senses are difficult to study in a laboratory. Taste buds, for example, cannot easily be grown outside of the body, as can visual tissue such as rod and cone cells. And, more often than not, laboratory animals cannot stand in for humans because their tastes differ. Consider sugars. We humans love sucrose (table sugar), but armadillos, hedgehogs, lions, and sea gulls do not respond to it.

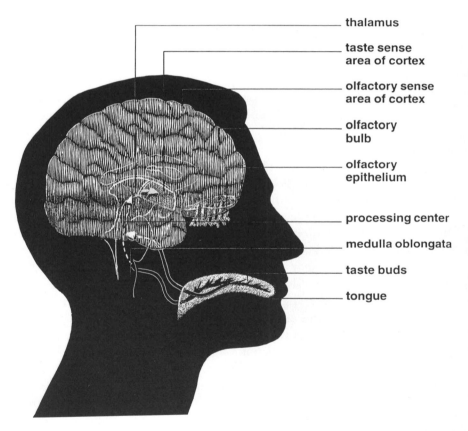

thalamus

taste sense area of cortex

olfactory sense area of cortex

olfactory bulb

olfactory epithelium

processing center

medulla oblongata

taste buds

tongue

Figure 40.1. The senses of smell and taste begin with detection by receptors in the tongue (taste buds) and receptors high in the nose (olfactory epithelium). Nerve impulses generated here travel through the medulla oblongata, processing center, and thalamus to the taste and smell areas of the brain's cortex that interpret the messages as smell and taste.

Opossums love lactose (milk sugar) but rats avoid it, and chickens hate the sugar xylose, while cattle love it and we are indifferent. These diverse tastes in the animal kingdom help ensure that there is enough food to go around.

Despite these hurdles, research into smell and taste is starting to open up. An exciting recent discovery, by Linda Buck, Ph.D., and Richard Axel, Ph.D., of Columbia University in New York, was that hundreds of genes are responsible for the sense of smell. This explains the capacity of the human nose to detect thousands of distinct odors.

Many non-scientists have also helped explain our sense of smell. In September 1986, 1.5 million readers of *National Geographic* magazine scratched six scented patches in their issues, sniffed them, and sent the results identifying the aromas to biopsychologists Avery N. Gilbert, Ph.D., and Charles Wysocki, Ph.D., of the Monell Chemical Senses Center in Philadelphia. Although the investigators are still wading through the data, in preliminary results on a sample of 26,200 respondents published in the October 1987 issue of the magazine, the researchers said that two-thirds of the readers report temporarily losing their ability to smell at one time or another, and that 1 percent could not smell three or more of the sample scents.

Biology of the Senses

All senses work in basically the same way. Special nerve cells bearing sense receptors collect information from the environment. When these receptors are stimulated they send a message to the brain, where the cerebral cortex forms a perception, a person's particular view of the stimulus.

The ability to detect the strong scent of a fish market, the antiseptic odor of a hospital, the aroma of a ripe melon—and thousands of other smells—is possible thanks to a yellowish patch of tissue the size of a quarter high up in the nose. This fabric of sensation is actually a layer of 12 million specialized cells. The end of each cell sports 10 to 20 hairlike growths called cilia. Each cilium has a receptor that binds an odorant molecule—a bit of that fish or melon. The binding triggers a nerve impulse, and the message travels along the nerve cell, through a hole in the skull, to a part of the brain called the olfactory bulb. Although scientists do not know exactly how, the brain interprets the pattern receptors send it to register "hospital smell" or "cantaloupe."

The expert nose of the bloodhound is due to its 4 billion olfactory cells. Still, the human sense of smell is nothing to sneeze at—people can detect one molecule of green pepper smell in a gaseous sea of 3 trillion other molecules. Our 12 million smell cells and their many million more receptors allow us to discern some 10,000 scents. But, without air, there is nothing to smell, as astronauts can attest. In the vacuum of space, odorant molecules cannot reach their senses, and eating in space is a rather tasteless—and some would say joyless—experience.

Most of what we call taste is really smell. We usually realize this when a cold hits our nasal passages. Even though the taste buds aren't blocked, the smell cells are, and this dulls much of food's flavor.

"Smell and taste are two distinct neurophysiological systems. The sense of taste is only sweet, sour, salty, and bitter. Other components of flavor are mediated by the olfactory system," says Beverly Cowart, Ph.D., director of the taste and smell clinic at Jefferson University

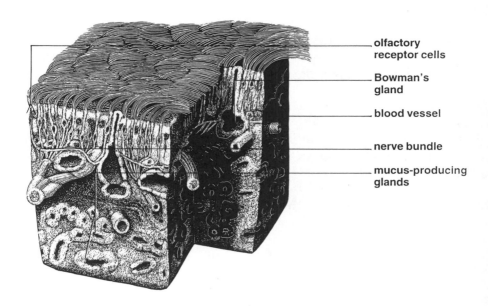

olfactory receptor cells

Bowman's gland

blood vessel

nerve bundle

mucus-producing glands

Figure 40.2. The sense of smell begins in a patch of tissue the size of a quarter, high in the nose, sketched here greatly magnified. In this tissue, the olfactory receptor cells are stimulated by odorant molecules dissolved in the mucus produced by surrounding glands, including the Bowman's gland. The receptor cells collect into bundles beneath the surface, forming the olfactory nerve, which leads to a region in the brain called the olfactory bulb.

Hospital in Philadelphia. A third sensory system delivers information to the brain about a food's texture, temperature, and chemical irritancy.

Taste comes from 10,000 taste buds, which are clusters of cells resembling the sections of an orange. Taste buds are found on the tongue, cheeks, throat, and the roof of the mouth. Each taste bud houses 60 to 100 receptor cells. These cells bind food molecules dissolved in saliva, and alert the brain to interpret them. Cattle, with 25,000 taste buds, are the bloodhound equivalent in the taste department.

The body regenerates taste buds about every three days. Although the tongue is often depicted as having regions in which taste buds specialize in a particular sensation—the tip tastes sweetness, the front saltiness, the sides sour, and the back bitter—researchers find that taste buds with all specificities are scattered everywhere. In fact, a single taste bud can have receptors for all four general types of tastes, says Henkin, who carried out much of the work describing the distribution of taste buds on the tongue.

Individual Differences

One person loves liver and onions; another gags at the thought. Of the 68 percent of women who can detect armpit odor (a chemical called androstenone), 72 percent report disliking it; of the 57 percent of men who can smell androstenone, only 50 percent dislike it. What accounts for these individual palates and noses? To some extent, what you taste or smell is in your genes. For example, the ability to smell a squashed skunk or freesia flowers is inherited.

Linda Bartoshuk, Ph.D., of the Yale University School of Medicine in New Haven, Conn., is fascinated by "why different people do not have the same experience when they eat." She and others have recently expanded upon a classical bit of genetic lore. It has been known for many years that 7 in 10 people inherit the ability to taste a bitter chemical called PTC (phenylthiocarbamide). PTC is a harmless chemical not found in food, but impregnated into paper strips for use in laboratory teaching experiments. Bartoshuk finds that PTC "tasters" can detect many bitter substances that are tasteless to others.

"For example, tasters don't like the taste of saccharin, but non-tasters don't mind it. Potassium chloride [a salt substitute] tastes nasty to tasters, like salt to others. Table sugar, too, is sweeter if you are a PTC taster," she says. Bartoshuk also finds that the protein in milk tastes different to tasters and non-tasters, making cheese, for example, pleasantly tart to some, but bitter to others.

341

The ability to detect bitter tastes can show up very early in life, when smell and taste are particularly acute. "We believe the possibility should be checked that some babies who fail to gain weight may be responsive to this bitter taste in milk," Bartoshuk adds.

Treating Disorders

Because there are several steps to smelling and tasting, there are plenty of ways for things to go awry. The direct connection between the outside environment and the brain makes the sense of smell very vulnerable to damage. Smell and taste disorders can be triggered by colds and flu, allergies, nasal polyps (swollen mucus membrane inside the nose), a head injury, chemical exposure, a nutritional or metabolic problem, or a drug or disease. In many cases, a cause cannot be identified.

Taste or smell, or both, can be absent, diminished, heightened, or distorted (see table 40.3). Interestingly, Richard Mattes, Ph.D., and co-workers at Monell find that while those with taste or smell loss eat to compensate and gain weight, those with distorted smell or taste find eating so disturbing that they lose weight.

It is difficult to imagine how greatly enjoyment of life can be affected by a loss in the senses of smell and taste. Judith Birnberg, of Long Island, N.Y., wrote about her plight in the March 21, 1988, "My Turn" column in *Newsweek* magazine. Birnberg spent a year sneezing inexplicably, and was suddenly left with the ability to sense only the texture and temperature of food. She was unable to smell or taste. For years, Birnberg lived on her memories of smelling piping hot coffee and peeled oranges. Her condition, attributed to "allergy and infection," mysteriously comes and goes. When taste and smell are intact, she rushes off to the nearest restaurant—but more often than not, her sensory acuity fades before the food arrives.

Birnberg had blood and urine tests galore, CAT scans, and biopsies, had her sinuses drained, and took zinc supplements. Nothing worked. Finally, she found relief with prednisone. This strong steroid drug reduces swelling of the mucous membranes in the nose, and may therefore improve the sense of smell, but its efficacy as a treatment for smell disorders has not been proven.

Feeling better, Birnberg went about smelling everything. "I inhaled all odors, good and bad, as if drunk," she wrote. Prednisone, though, suppresses the immune system, so she can only take it intermittently.

Distorted Sensation

A group of 12 travelers touring Peru and Bolivia prepared for a day of hiking in the Andes mountains. A day before, three of them had begun taking acetazolamide (Diamox), a drug that prevents acute mountain sickness, which each had previously suffered. The headache, nausea, weakness, and shortness of breath of acute mountain sickness typically begins when one reaches 5,900 feet elevation, and can progress to severe respiratory problems by 9,000 feet. These hikers planned an expedition to 12,000 feet. All went well, but the night after the climb, the group went out for beer. To three of the people, the brew tasted unbearably bitter, and a drink of cola to wash away the taste was equally offensive. At fault: acetazolamide.

The taste distortion caused by this particular drug makes biochemical sense. The drug inhibits an enzyme that normally dismantles bitter-tasting carbonic acid before it has a chance to register on the taste buds.

"The drug stirs up anything with carbonation, enabling the person to taste the terribly bitter taste of carbonic acid," says Baylor College of Medicine's Miller. She has studied the drug's temporary effects on taste and believes the problem is more widespread than drug manufacturers realize. "People are scared, because it is a strange taste. Some people may not report it, and may not make the connection to the drug. They blame it on altitude sickness," she adds.

Acetazolamide isn't the only drug to alter the chemical senses. "Drugs can alter taste and smell in many potential ways, affecting cell turnover, the neural conduction system, the status of receptors, and changes in nutritional status," says Monell's Mattes.

Drugs containing sulfur atoms are notorious for squelching taste. They include the anti-inflammatory drug penicillamine, the anti-hypertensive captopril (Capoten), and transdermal (patch) nitroglycerin to treat chest pain. The antibiotics tetracycline and metronidazole (Flagyl) cause a metallic taste.

Cancer chemotherapy and radiation treatment often alter taste and smell, but this is rarely reason to change therapy. "A taste and smell problem is probably not life-threatening, and treating something like cancer is the first priority," Mattes says.

Exposure to toxic chemicals can affect taste and smell, too. A 45-year-old woman from Altoona, Pa., suddenly found that once-pleasant smells had become offensive. Her doctor, Joseph Silverman, M.D., traced her problem to inhaling a paint stripper. Hydrocarbon solvents in the product—toluene, methanol, and methylene chloride—were the culprits responsible for her "cacosmia," the association of an odor of decay with normally inoffensive stimuli. She said she was helped by an antidepressant medication. However, since this type of drug is not approved for treating such disorders, this was an experimental use of the drug.

Taste distortions can be very upsetting. "It's easier for people to understand losing a sense than to suddenly have everything twisted. Since smell mediates a lot of food's flavor, when you don't smell at all, food tastes bland. You can perk it up by adding salt, sugar, lemon juice or spices. But for dysosmics, food is actively unpleasant," says Cowart.

Sometimes a foul taste can persist with no food involved. This is a "taste phantom," a sensation that comes out of nowhere, says Bartoshuk. The condition is fairly common among women past menopause. At Yale, Bartoshuk helps pinpoint the source of phantom tastes. "Is it caused by a molecule in the mouth that shouldn't be there, or is brain stimulation abnormal? We can tell the difference by using anesthesia, which is a nerve inhibitor," she says.

If she anesthetizes the mouth and the bad taste goes away, then it's due to molecules there. If, following anesthesia, the patient gets worse, this points to the brain as the cause of the problem.

There are a number of special centers where people with absent or distorted senses of smell and taste can seek help. These include: Monell, facilities at Yale University, the State University of New York Health Science Center in Syracuse, the Hospital of the University of Pennsylvania in Philadelphia, Georgetown University in Washington, D.C., the University of Colorado in Denver, and the University of Connecticut Health Center at Farmington.

Table 40.3. Types of Smell and Taste Disorders

These are the terms that doctors are likely to use when discussing taste and smell disorders.

	Smell	Taste
loss of sensation	anosmia	ageusia
diminished sensation	hyposmia	hypogeusia
heightened sensation	hyperosmia	hypergeusia
distorted sensation	dysosmia	dysgeusia

With researchers' increasing understanding of the complex interplays between the environment and our nervous systems that provide the nonessential but intensely enjoyable senses of smell and taste, it's likely that more and more sufferers of deficits in these systems will be identified and helped. Those of us with healthy senses can appreciate the complex neural connections that enable us to fully experience that April rain, July barbecue, and October's fragrant fallen leaves, and the myriad taste combinations that make dining so pleasurable.

A Lifetime of Smell and Taste

We can smell and taste from birth. Regina M. Sullivan, Ph.D., and co-workers at the University of California at Irvine Medical Center in Irvine recently studied day-old infants to determine their ability to connect an odor with a pleasant experience.

Half the group of 66 newborns received citrus odors and simultaneous stroking several times for a day. The other 33 babies experienced the odor alone, stroking alone, or stroking followed by the odor. The next day, all the infants were exposed to the odor five times, for 30-second periods. The only babies who turned toward the odor were those who received the odor during stroking, thereby associating the citrus smell with touch.

Taste buds are most numerous in children under 6, which may explain why youngsters are such picky eaters. Recognizing that children's heightened sense of taste might account for compliance problems in giving antibiotic medication, Michael E. Ruff, M.D., and co-workers in the departments of pediatrics and pharmacy at Tripler Army Medical Center in Honolulu asked 30 adults to rank the pleasantness of the taste of the active ingredients in the 14 most often prescribed pediatric antibiotic suspensions. If parents, with their diminished sense of taste compared to their offspring, find a particular antibiotic distasteful, then perhaps drug manufacturers can be alerted to those products that need work in the palatability department—a major task when a medicine must contain a naturally bad-tasting substance. In this taste test, cephalosporins tasted best, and penicillins the worst.

Taste and smell hold up remarkably well with age, probably because the body frequently replaces receptor-bearing cells, even in the elderly. Monell researchers concluded from the *National Geographic* Smell Survey that "detection ability remains near youthful levels well into the seventh decade," but they found that ability to detect the intensity of odors and to describe odors wanes with time. These deficits may reflect changes in thought processing, such as taste and smell recognition, rather than in the sense organs, suggests Richard Mattes, Ph.D., of Monell.

One disturbing finding is that older people are less likely to find the smell of chemicals called mercaptans offensive than are younger people. Mercaptans are added to odorless natural gas to serve as a warning if gas is escaping from an oven, for example.

Disease and drugs can affect smell and taste and may also account for the lessened acuity of these senses in older people, according to James Weiffenbach, Ph.D., sensory psychologist at the National Institute of Dental Research in Bethesda. "Among the participants in the Baltimore Longitudinal Study of Aging of the National Institute of Aging, we found that whether you are healthy or not is a more powerful determinant of taste complaints than whether you are younger or older. So maybe older people report more taste complaints because they are more likely to have medical problems," he says.

Weiffenbach also mentions a telling "overlooked point": that of senior citizens living in retirement centers where the food really isn't as tasty as the home-cooked cuisine they may have been used to. "They know the food doesn't taste as good as it did 10 years ago, because it really doesn't," he says.

—by Ricki Lewis, Ph.D.

Ricki Lewis, a writer in Scotia, N.Y., has a Ph.D. in genetics and is the author of a college biology text.

Chapter 41

When Food Loses Its Flavor

The aroma of freshly baked cinnamon buns. . .a pot of coffee brewing on the stove. . . steak grilling on the barbecue. Everyone knows the pleasures of such scents. And anyone with a head cold knows the frustration of missing out on them. Fortunately, such lapses are usually temporary and generally clear up on their own.

But about half of adults over age 65 have some degree of chronic smell (olfactory) impairment. Because the sense of smell contributes more to the perception of flavor than any other sense—including taste—such deficits can seriously limit the enjoyment of food. Severe olfactory impairment can lead to malnutrition, depression, and other problems that may affect health and safety.

When the underlying cause of olfactory impairment can be identified and treated, the ability to smell can sometimes be restored. If not, lifestyle measures can help compensate for the loss. But the disorders that adversely affect smell are frequently difficult to diagnose. And because olfactory impairment is almost never life-threatening, physicians are sometimes inclined to dismiss it without attempting a diagnosis or offering advice.

What Accounts for Taste?

The flavor of food depends on information gleaned from the taste buds, olfactory receptors, and trigeminal nerve endings, all of which send sensory impulses to the brain. Inflammation in and around these structures can impair taste and smell.

What Goes Wrong?

The flavor of a particular food depends primarily on four properties: taste, odor, texture, and temperature. This information is obtained from three sources:

Taste buds. Located mostly on the tongue, taste buds are sensitive to four basic qualities: salty, sour, bitter, and sweet.

Olfactory receptors. Found inside the top of the nose, olfactory receptors respond to many different odors. Researchers estimate that the sense of smell is 4,000 times more sensitive than the sense of taste. Three-quarters of a particular flavor depends on information obtained from olfactory receptors. Unlike most nerve cells, olfactory receptors continually regenerate every three or four months.

Trigeminal nerve endings. Located on the membranes lining the lips, mouth, and nose, trigeminal nerve endings respond to texture, temperature, and pain. Trigeminal nerve endings are responsible for the burning sensation associated with hot pepper and the cooling sensation associated with peppermint.

Nearly all temporary and about one-quarter of permanent smell problems are caused by chronic inflammation of the mucous membranes lining the nose (rhinitis) or sinuses (sinusitis); this blocks the nasal passages and prevents odors from reaching the olfactory receptors.

The most frequent causes of inflammation are allergies and infections. Sufferers typically experience a gradual loss of smell, with periods of decline followed by periods of improvement. Because inflammation does not usually damage the olfactory receptors, deficits caused by this problem generally are reversible.

Much less frequently, the olfactory receptors become damaged. If the receptors cannot regenerate, sensory loss is permanent. In adults, the most frequent causes of permanent impairment are viral infection, head trauma, and neurological disorders such as Parkinson's disease or Alzheimer's disease.

Smell can also be impaired by drugs (especially the anticancer medication methotrexate); exposure to environmental pollutants used in mining, manufacturing, and other work-related environments; and brain tumor.

Finally, although olfactory impairment can result in depression, in about 10% of patients depression is the underlying cause. Patients with depression-related deficits sometimes complain about scent distortion. Rather than experiencing an absence of smell, everything these patients sniff or eat seems to have a putrid or foul odor.

Solving the Problem

When inflammation is the underlying cause of olfactory impairment, smell can nearly always be restored with a one-week course of a systemic corticosteroid such as prednisone. If an allergy is suspected, inhaled steroids may also be required; if bacterial infection is present, antibiotics are necessary; if depression is the underlying cause, counseling and antidepressant medications can help.

If the olfactory receptors are damaged and do not regenerate on their own, no treatment can help. Fortunately, however, all is not lost because the taste buds and trigeminal nerves usually remain intact. Thus, most patients can continue to enjoy food by:

- using flavor enhancers (including vinegar, lemon, menthol, cayenne, hot pepper, and other spices) and fruit-based sweeteners;
- varying food textures and taste sensations (e.g., alternating sweet and sour, or crunchy and soft);
- avoiding cigarettes, caffeine, and food that is very hot or very cold;
- eating slowly;
- displaying food attractively;
- brushing teeth after meals rather than before, because toothpaste can mask food flavors.

Coping with a Severe Deficit

Severe, irreversible olfactory impairment can lead to serious problems, including malnutrition and depression. Other potential problems include food poisoning because sufferers are insensitive to odors that may indicate spoilage; poor personal hygiene because body odors that prompt washing are not perceived; and a decline in personal safety because sufferers are oblivious to smoke, gas leaks, and other

349

potential hazards. Incorporating the following lifestyle measures can help decrease these risks:

- Challenge taste buds with spices and flavorings.

- Eat regular, planned meals.

- Dine with other people as often as possible.

- Label stored foods with a throwaway date; visually inspect foods for signs of spoilage.

- Install smoke and carbon monoxide detectors.

- Ask someone to inspect your; home periodically for unusual odors.

- Wash often and on a regular schedule (at least twice a week).

For More Information

Davidson T.M., et al. *Postgraduate Medicine*. 1995: vol. 98, p. 107–18.

Evans, W.J., et al. *Patient Care*. 1994: September 30, p. 41–64.

Chapter 42

Care and Prevention of Nose Bleeds

Care and Prevention

Most nosebleeds are mere nuisances; but some are quite frightening, and a few are even life threatening. Physicians classify nosebleeds into two different types.

1. **Anterior Nosebleed:** The nosebleed that comes from the front part of the nose and begins with a flow of blood out one or the other nostril if the patient is sitting up or standing.

2. **Posterior Nosebleed:** The nosebleed that comes from deep in the nose and flows down the back of the mouth and throat even if the patient is sitting up or standing.

Obviously, if the patient is lying down, even the anterior nosebleeds seem to flow in both directions, especially if the patient is coughing or blowing his nose.

Nevertheless, it is important to try to make the distinction since posterior nosebleeds are often more severe and almost always require the physician's care. Posterior nosebleeds are more likely to occur in older people, persons with high blood pressure, and in cases of injury to the nose or face.

Nosebleeds in children are almost always of the anterior type. Anterior nosebleeds are common in dry climates or during the winter months when the dry air parches the nasal membranes so that they crust, crack, and bleed. This can be prevented if you will place a bit of lubricating cream or ointment about the size of a pea on the end of your fingertip and then rub it up inside the nose, especially on the middle portion (the septum).

Many physicians suggest any of the following lubricating creams or ointments. They can all be purchased without a prescription: A and D Ointment®, Mentholatum®, Vicks Vaporub®, and Vaseline®. Up to three applications a day may be needed, but usually every night at bedtime is enough.

If the nosebleeds persist, you should see your doctor, who may recommend cautery to the blood vessel that is causing the trouble.

To Stop an Anterior Nosebleed

If you or your child has an anterior nosebleed, you may be able to care for it yourself using the following steps:

1. Pinch all the soft parts of the nose together between your thumb and two fingers.

2. Press firmly toward the face—compressing the pinched parts of the nose against the bones of the face.

3. Hold it for 5 minutes (timed by a clock).

4. Keep head higher than the level of the heart—sit up or lie with head elevated.

5. Apply ice (crushed in a plastic bag or washcloth) to nose and cheeks.

To Prevent Re-bleeding After Bleeding Has Stopped

1. Do not pick or blow nose (sniffing is all right).

2. Do not strain or bend down to lift anything heavy.

3. Keep head higher than the level of the heart.

If Re-bleeding Occurs

1. Clear nose of all blood clots by sniffing in forcefully.

Care and Prevention of Nose Bleeds

2. Spray nose four times on both sides with decongestant spray (such as Afrin®, Duration®, Neo-Synephrine®, etc.).

3. Pinch and press nose into face again.

4. Call your doctor.

When to Call the Doctor or Go to a Hospital Emergency Room

- If bleeding cannot be stopped or keeps reappearing.
- If bleeding is rapid or if blood loss is large.
- If you feel weak or faint, presumably from blood loss.
- If bleeding begins by going down the back of the throat rather than the front to the nose.

Chapter 43

Understanding Rhinoplasty: Nasal Surgery

Every year, half a million people who are interested in improving the appearance of their noses seek consultation with facial plastic surgeons. Some are unhappy with the noses they were born with, and some with the way aging has changed their nose. For others, an injury may have distorted the nose, or the goal may be improved breathing. But one thing is clear: nothing has a greater impact on how a person looks than the size and shape of the nose. Because the nose is the most defining characteristic of the face, a slight alteration can greatly improve one's appearance.

If you have wondered how nose surgery, or rhinoplasty, could improve your looks, self-confidence, or health, you need to know how rhinoplasty is performed and what you can expect. This chapter cannot answer all your concerns, but can provide answers to many of the questions you may have.

Successful facial plastic surgery is a result of good rapport between patient and surgeon. Trust, based on realistic expectations and exacting medical expertise, develops in the consulting stages before surgery. Your surgeon can answer specific questions about your specific needs.

Is Rhinoplasty for You?

As with all facial plastic surgery, good health and realistic expectations are prerequisites. Understanding nose surgery is also critical.

Since there is no ideal in rhinoplasty, the goal is to improve the nose aesthetically, making it harmonize better with other facial features.

Skin type, ethnic background, and age are important factors to be considered in discussions with your surgeon prior to surgery. Before the nose is altered, a young patient must reach full growth, usually around age fifteen or sixteen. Exceptions are cases in which breathing is severely impaired.

Before deciding on rhinoplasty, ask your facial plastic surgeon if any additional surgery might be recommended to enhance the appearance of your face. Many patients have chin augmentation in conjunction with rhinoplasty to create a better balance of features.

Making the Decision for Rhinoplasty

Whether the surgery is desired for functional or cosmetic reasons, your choice of a qualified facial plastic surgeon is of paramount importance. Many facial plastic surgeons are trained in both ear, nose, throat, and facial cosmetic surgery, which provides you, the patient, with the highest level of training and expertise. Your surgeon will examine the structure of your nose, both externally and internally, to evaluate what you can expect from rhinoplasty. Your surgeon will also discuss factors that may influence the outcome of the surgery, such as skin type, ethnic background, age, degree of deformity, and degree of function of nasal structures.

You can expect a thorough explanation of the surgeon's expectations and the risks involved in surgery. Following a joint decision by you and your surgeon to proceed with rhinoplasty, the surgeon will take photographs of you and discuss the options available. Your surgeon will explain how the nasal structures, including bone and cartilage, can be sculpted to reshape the nose and indicate how reshaping the chin, for example, could enhance the desired results.

After conducting a thorough medical history, your surgeon will offer information regarding anesthesia, the surgical facility to be used, and the costs for the procedure.

Understanding the Surgery

The definition of rhinoplasty is, literally, shaping the nose. First, incisions are made and the skin of the nose is lifted from its underlying bone and cartilage support system. The majority of incisions are made inside the nose, where they are invisible. In some cases, an incision is made in the area of skin separating the nostrils. Next, certain amounts of underlying bone and cartilage are removed or rearranged to provide a newly shaped structure. For example, when the tip of the nose is too large, the surgeon can sculpt the cartilage in this area to reduce it in size. The angle of the nose in relation to the upper lip can be altered for a more youthful look or to correct a distortion.

The skin is then redraped over the new frame and the incisions are closed. A splint is applied to the outside of the nose to help retain the new shape while the nose heals. Soft, absorbent material may be used inside the nose to maintain stability along the dividing wall of the air passages called the septum. Risk factors in rhinoplasty are generally minor, and your facial plastic surgeon will discuss these prior to surgery.

What to Expect After the Surgery

Immediately after surgery, a small splint will be placed on your nose to protect it and to keep the structure stable for at least five to eight days. If packing is placed inside the nose during surgery, it is removed the morning following the surgery. Your face will feel puffy, especially the first day after surgery. Pain medication may be required. Your surgeon will advise you to avoid blowing your nose for seven days after surgery. In the immediate days following surgery, you may experience bruising and minor swelling in the eye area. Cold compresses often reduce the bruising and discomfort. Absorbable sutures are usually used that do not have to be removed. Nasal dressing and splints are usually removed six or seven days after surgery.

It is crucial that you follow your surgeon's directions, especially instructions to keep your head elevated for a certain period after surgery. Some activities will be prohibited in the weeks after the procedure. Sun exposure, exertion, and risk of injury must be avoided. If you wear glasses, special arrangements must be made to ensure that the glasses do not rest on the bridge of the nose. Tape and other devices are sometimes used to permit wearing glasses without stressing the area where surgery was performed.

Follow-up care is vital for this procedure to monitor healing. Obviously, anything unusual should be reported to your surgeon immediately. It is essential that you keep your follow-up appointments with your surgeon.

Insurance does not generally cover surgery that is purely for cosmetic reasons. Surgery to correct or improve nasal function or surgery for major deformity or injury may be reimbursable in whole or in part. It is the patient's responsibility to check with the insurance carrier for information on the degree of coverage.

Facial Plastic Surgery

American Academy of Facial Plastic and Reconstructive Surgery, Inc.
1110 Vermont Avenue, N.W., Suite 220
Washington, D.C. 20005-3522
(202) 842-4500

The American Academy of Facial Plastic and Reconstructive Surgery, Inc. (AAFPRS) is the world's largest association of facial plastic and reconstructive surgeons—those physicians performing cosmetic and reconstructive surgery of the face, head, and neck. The Academy's bylaws provide that AAFPRS fellows be board-certified surgeons with training and experience in facial plastic surgery and be fellows of the American College of Surgeons.

Part Five

Disorders of the Throat

Chapter 44

Sore Throats:
Causes and Cures

What Causes a Sore Throat?

Sore throat is one symptom of an array of different medical disorders. Infections cause the majority of sore throats, and these are the sore throats that are contagious (can be passed from one person to another). Infections are caused by either viruses (such as the flu, the common cold, mononucleosis), or bacteria (such as strep, mycoplasma or hemophilus).

The most important difference between viruses and bacteria is that bacteria respond well to antibiotic treatment, but viruses do not.

Viruses

Most viral sore throats accompany the flu or a cold. When a stuffy-runny nose, sneezing, and generalized aches and pains accompany the sore throat, it is probably caused by viruses. These are highly contagious and spread quickly in a community, especially in the winter. The body cures itself of a viral infection by building antibodies that destroy the virus, a process that takes about a week.

Sore throats accompany other viral infections such as measles, chicken pox, whooping cough, and croup. Canker sores and fever blisters in the throat also can be very painful.

©1996. American Academy of Otolaryngology–Head and Neck Surgery, Inc., One Prince Street, Alexandria, VA 22314-3357. For more information, visit our home page at http://www.entnet.org.

One special viral infection takes much longer than a week to be cured: infectious mononucleosis or "mono." This virus lodges in the lymph system, causing massive enlargement of the tonsils (with white patches on their surface) and swollen glands in the neck, armpits, and groin. It creates a severely sore throat, sometimes causes serious difficulties breathing, and can affect the liver, leading to jaundice (yellow skin and eyes). It also causes extreme fatigue that can last six weeks or more.

"Mono" is a severe illness in a teenager or young adult, but it is less severe in a child. Since it can be transmitted by saliva, it has been nicknamed the "kissing disease." However, it can also be transmitted from mouth-to-hand to hand-to-mouth or by sharing of towels and eating utensils.

Bacteria

Strep throat is an infection caused by a particular strain of streptococcus bacteria. This infection can also case damage to the heart valves (rheumatic fever) and kidneys (nephritis). Streptococcal infections can also cause scarlet fever, tonsillitis, pneumonia, sinusitis, and ear infections.

Because of these possible complications, a strep throat should be treated with an antibiotic. Strep is not always easy to detect by examination, and a throat culture may be needed.

A newly developed strep test detects a streptococcal infection in about 15 minutes. These tests, when positive, influence the physician to prescribe antibiotics. However, strep tests might not detect a number of other bacteria that can also cause severe sore throats that deserve antibiotic treatment. For example, severe and chronic cases of tonsillitis or tonsillar abscess may be culture negative. Similarly, negative cultures are seen with diphtheria, and infections from oral sexual contacts will escape detection with strep culture tests.

Tonsillitis is an infection of the lumpy tissues on each side of the back of the throat. In the first two to three years of childhood, these tissues "catch" infections, sampling the child's environment to help develop his immunities (antibodies). Healthy tonsils do not remain infected. Frequent sore throats from tonsillitis suggest the infection is not fully eliminated between episodes. A medical study has shown that children who suffer from frequent episodes of tonsillitis (such as 3 to 4 times each year for several years) were healthier after their tonsils were surgically removed.

Infections in the nose and sinuses can also cause sore throats because mucus from the nose drains down into the throat and carries the infection with it.

The most dangerous throat infection is epiglottitis, caused by bacteria that infect a portion of the larynx (voice box) and cause swelling that closes the airway. This infection is an emergency condition that requires prompt medical attention. Suspect it when swallowing is extremely painful (causing drooling), when speech is muffled, and when breathing becomes difficult. A strep test may miss this infection and be negative.

Allergy

Hay fever and allergy sufferers can get an irritated throat during an allergy attack the same way they get a stuffy, itchy nose, sneezing, and post nasal drip. The same pollens and molds that irritate the nose when they are inhaled also may irritate the throat. Cat and dog danders and house dust are common things that can cause sore throats for people with allergies to them.

Irritation

During the cold winter months, dry heat may create a recurring, mild sore throat with a parched feeling, especially in the mornings. This often responds to humidification of bedroom air and increased liquid intake. Patients with a chronic stuffy nose, causing mouth breathing, also suffer with a dry throat. They need examination and treatment of the nose.

An occasional cause of morning sore throat is regurgitation of stomach acids up into the back of the throat where they are extremely irritating. This can be avoided if you tilt your bedframe so that the head is elevated four to six inches higher than the foot. You should also avoid eating and drinking for one to two hours before retiring. You might find antacids helpful. If these fail, see your doctor.

Industrial pollutants and chemicals in the air can irritate the nose and throat, but by far the most common and pervasive air pollutant is tobacco smoke. It cannot be tolerated by many persons who are either allergic or over sensitive to its contents. Other irritants include smokeless tobacco, alcoholic beverages, and spicy foods.

A person who strains his voice (yelling at a sports event, for example) gets a sore throat not only from muscle strain, but also from the rough treatment of his throat membranes. Well-trained, experienced public speakers and singers learn to produce loud voices by taking deep breathes and using their chest and abdominal muscles.

363

Tumors

Tumors of the throat, tongue, and larynx (voice box) are usually (but not always) associated with long time use of tobacco and alcohol. Sore throat and difficult swallowing—sometimes with pain radiating to the ear—may be symptoms of such a tumor. More often the sore throat is so mild or so chronic that it is hardly noticed. Other important symptoms include hoarseness, a lump in the neck, unexplained weight loss and/or spitting up blood in the saliva or phlegm.

How Can I Treat My Own Sore Throat?

A mild sore throat associated with cold or flu symptoms can be made more comfortable with the following remedies:

- Increase your liquid intake. (Warm tea with honey is a favorite home remedy.)
- Use a steamer or humidifier in your bedroom.
- Gargle with warm salt water several times daily: ¼ tsp salt to ½ cup water.
- Take mild pain relievers such as acetominophen (Tylenol®, Datril®, Tempra®), ibuprophen (Advil®), etc.

When Should I See a Doctor?

Whenever a sore throat is severe, persists longer than the usual five to seven day duration of a cold or flu, and is not associated with an avoidable allergy or irritation, you should seek medical attention. The following signs and symptoms should alert you to see your physician:

- Severe and prolonged sore throat
- Difficulty breathing
- Difficulty swallowing
- Difficulty opening the mouth
- Joint pain
- Earache
- Rash
- Fever (over 101°)
- Blood in saliva or phlegm
- Frequently recurring sore throat
- Lump In neck
- Hoarseness lasting over 2 weeks

When Should I Take Antibiotics?

Antibiotics are drugs that kill or impair bacteria. Penicillin or erythromycin (well-known antibiotics) are prescribed when the physician suspects streptococcal or other bacterial infection that will respond to them. However, a number of bacterial throat infections do not respond to penicillin, but require other categories of antibiotics instead. Antibiotics do not cure viral infections, but viruses do lower the patient's resistance to bacterial infections. When such a combined infection occurs, antibiotics may become necessary.

When an antibiotic is prescribed, it should be taken—as the physician directs—for the full course (usually 10 days). Otherwise the infection will probably be suppressed rather than eliminated, and it can return.

What If My Throat Culture Is Negative?

A strep culture tests only for the presence of streptococcal infections. Many other infections, both bacterial and viral, will yield negative cultures and sometimes so does a streptococcal infection. Therefore, when your culture is negative, your physician will base his decision for treatment on the severity of your symptoms and the appearance of your throat on examination. Do not discontinue your medications unless your physician instructs you to do so.

Should Other Family Members Be Treated or Cultured?

When strep throat is proven by test or culture, many experts recommend treatment of other family members, because streptococcal infections are so highly contagious. Others recommend treating only the family members with sore throats and culturing the others. So be sure you tell your physician how other family members are feeling. Practice good sanitary habits; avoid close physical contact and sharing of napkins, towels, and utensils with the infected person. Handwashing makes good sense.

The advice in this pamphlet is for general information. But remember, the best advice for your specific case is the advice you get from your physician who hears your symptoms and examines your throat.

Chapter 45

Cough:
The Common and the
Complex

Coughing is one of the most common reasons patients see a doctor, and doctors write more prescriptions for cough than for any other symptom. In most instances, coughing is caused by an upper respiratory infection known as the common cold. But coughing can also be a symptom of other chronic medical conditions, most often postnasal drip syndrome (PNDS), asthma, and gastroesophageal reflux disease (GERD). In a recent study published in the *Archives of Internal Medicine*, these three conditions accounted for 92% of all persistent coughs among a total of 88 subjects who did not have colds.

Other causes of coughing include acute bronchitis (an infection of the air passages in the lungs), chronic obstructive pulmonary disease (COPD), cancer of the lung and throat structures, and congestive heart failure (CHF). And there is another frequently overlooked possibility, according to a recent study in the *Journal of the American Medical Association*. Examining the records of 307 adults suffering from a persistent, unexplained cough, researchers found that whooping cough (pertussis) was the cause in 12% of cases. Despite the availability of an effective vaccine, the incidence of this common childhood infection is on the rise in young and old alike.

Some coughs can be treated without a doctor's care, while others require professional attention. The characteristics of a given cough—whether it's loose or tight, for example, and the time of day it occurs—

can help identify the underlying cause. Yet, the *Archives of Internal Medicine* study suggests that relying on these characteristics is not enough to ensure an accurate diagnosis. Other symptoms must be noted, and in some instances laboratory tests or imaging studies may be needed. Knowing when to see a doctor can make the difference between a speedy recovery and continued discomfort. In those rare instances when a serious illness is the cause, it may even be lifesaving.

When to Go It Alone

Coughing is a reflex that keeps the lungs and airways free of phlegm (excess mucus) and foreign objects (such as food) that might interfere with breathing. A cough can be voluntary or involuntary, and it may be brought on by a variety of stimuli including inflammation of the airways due to a cold, acute bronchitis, or PNDS; chemical irritants, such as cigarette smoke or toxic fumes; and breathing in very hot or very cold air.

Coughs come in two basic forms: productive (a wet, loose cough characterized by excessive phlegm) and nonproductive (a dry cough with little or no phlegm). The productive cough associated with a cold accelerates recovery by clearing the airways of accumulated phlegm. But there's no benefit to a scratchy, nonproductive cough, which can cause throat irritation and interrupt sleep. Both types of cough may persist for several weeks, usually because of complications such as PNDS or acute bronchitis.

Because all colds are viral infections, they do not respond to antibiotic treatment (see "When to Use Antibiotics" at end of this chapter). But coughing and other symptoms can be relieved with home remedies and over-the-counter products. Coughs associated with colds usually clear up on their own in one to two weeks. Self-treatment is appropriate, provided there are no other symptoms such as persistent fever, headache, sore throat, blood in the phlegm, or chest pain. For a productive cough, drinking plenty of water and other clear fluids to thin phlegm is the most effective remedy. Loosened phlegm can be spit out, but there is no harm in swallowing it. Don't bother with over-the-counter (OTC) "expectorant" cough medicines. Virtually all of them contain guaifenesin, which is less effective than water. Cough drops can be used to soothe the throat, but hard candy, tea with lemon, and chicken soup are just as effective.

In contrast, OTC cough "suppressants" (antitussives) can be helpful for an irritating unproductive cough, especially at night. Antitussives contain dextromethorphan, a non-narcotic chemical variant of morphine.

Dextromethorphan suppresses the part of the brain that controls the cough reflex. But because cough suppression can lead to phlegm build-up, antitussives should be used sparingly, and drinking more water is still important. If an antitussive is necessary, choose single ingredient products such as Benylin DM, Delsym, Hold, and Sucrets Cough Control Formula. Avoid multiple-ingredient preparations, which may contain antitussive and expectorant combinations along with an antihistamine or decongestant. These ingredients may work against each other. For example, antihistamines dry up secretions, while expectorants loosen them. Also, the dosages used in multiple-ingredient products may be ineffective. Avoid codeine-based suppressants unless they're recommended by a doctor; improper use can worsen the cough and lead to dependency if the drug is taken for too long.

When to Get Help

A doctor's care is advised for any cough that continues to worsen after about a week. In such cases, the cough may have qualities that, together with other symptoms, point toward medical problems such as:

Postnasal Drip Syndrome

The most common complication of a cold, PNDS is characterized by inflammation of the sinuses (sinusitis) or the lining of the nose (rhinitis), along with a discharge that flows into the throat. A PNDS-associated cough can be productive or nonproductive, and it may be either viral or bacterial. Treatment is with antihistamines or decongestants, and sometimes inhaled corticosteroids. If the infection does not clear up within about a week, an antibiotic may be prescribed.

Acute Bronchitis

Unlike chronic bronchitis, which is usually associated with cigarette smoking, acute bronchitis comes on suddenly and is generally preceded by a cold. Wheezing, breathlessness, fever, tightness behind the breastbone, and a persistent, productive cough are characteristic. Antibiotics are not generally necessary, either because the infection is viral (and not responsive to antibiotics) or because it's bacterial and may clear up without them. Pain relievers, such as aspirin and acetaminophen (Tylenol), can be used as needed for fever and aches, and bronchodilators (such as albuterol) may be prescribed to break up congestion. Most cases resolve in a week or two.

Asthma

This chronic condition, a narrowing of the small airway passages (bronchioles) in the lungs, usually develops by adulthood. The symptoms, including wheezing, breathlessness, and chest tightness, often worsen at night. Over time, lung tissue may be permanently damaged. Treatment is with bronchodilators and inhaled corticosteroids. Proper therapy is important because, in addition to bringing relief, it can prevent lung damage.

Gastroesophageal Reflux Disease

Chronic heartburn, or GERD, is often associated with a cough, hoarseness, and discomfort when swallowing. Symptoms frequently worsen when the sufferer is lying down. Treatment is with antacids and other medications known as H2-blockers, proton pump inhibitors, and prokinetic drugs. Other measures include a high-protein, low-fat diet and avoiding meals for at least two hours before lying down. Sometimes a biopsy or an imaging study (endoscopy) of the throat may be required. If left untreated, GERD occasionally leads to chronic inflammation of the esophagus (esophagitis) or, in rare instances, esophageal cancer. Symptoms may take up to six months to go away.

Pertussis

A bacterial infection, pertussis is characterized by a hacking, explosive cough that may end in a high-pitched inspiratory "whoop." The cough often worsens at night, and patients are frequently listless and have a low-grade fever. Pertussis can be diagnosed through a blood test or a nasal swab culture. Treatment is with erythromycin (an antibiotic), along with adequate nutrition and fluids. Erythromycin is most effective when taken early in the course of the illness. Codeine may be used to decrease coughing. Those who have pertussis should avoid crowds, infants, and children in order to decrease the likelihood of transmission. Vaccination is recommended for all children, but there is as yet no consensus on immunization or re-immunization for older adults.

Special Precautions for Smokers

While the following three conditions can occur in anyone, they're more likely in a smoker or ex-smoker who develops a persistent, unexplained cough:

Chronic Obstructive Pulmonary Disease

This term usually refers to emphysema (inflammation and thinning of the tiny air sacs called alveoli in the lungs) or chronic bronchitis (bronchial inflammation lasting three months or more), which frequently occur together. COPD-associated coughs tend to be productive. Diagnosis is usually through pulmonary function testing, a procedure that measures the volume of exhaled air. Treatment is important to prevent progressive lung damage. The most important step is to stop smoking. Therapy may involve inhaled bronchodilators, corticosteroids, supplementary oxygen, and antibiotics, depending on the extent and nature of the problem.

Cancer

Coughs associated with cancer often appear suddenly and may be accompanied by weight loss, blood in the phlegm (lung cancer), or hoarseness (certain throat cancers). Microscopic examination of the phlegm and imaging studies (including chest x-ray and endoscopy) are frequently recommended. Treatment may involve some combination of surgery, chemotherapy, and radiation.

Congestive Heart Failure

This condition occurs when the heart can no longer keep up with its workload. It can be caused by many underlying problems, including high blood pressure and COPD. Coughs associated with CHF are usually nonproductive; they tend to worsen when patients are lying on their back and lessen when they sit upright. Diagnosis is through chest x-ray and cardiac studies. Treatment depends on the underlying cause.

Medications That Can Cause a Cough

Angiotensin-converting enzyme (ACE) inhibitors such as captopril (Capoten), enalapril (Vasotec), and lisinopril (Prinivil and Zestril) are often prescribed for high blood pressure because they generally produce fewer side effects than many other antihypertensive drugs. But they cause a dry cough in up to one-quarter of people who take them. If you take an ACE inhibitor and develop a cough, tell your doctor. It may be possible to change medications.

Other drugs that occasionally cause a cough are beta-blockers such as metoprolol (Lopressor) and propranolol (Inderal) and, ironically, the corticosteroids and bronchodilators that are sometimes used to treat coughs. Such problems can usually be avoided by changing medications or using a metered-dose inhaler to help deliver the proper dosage.

When to Use Antibiotics

In many instances of cough, antibiotics are unnecessary. If bacterial, the infection may clear up without them. If viral, it will not respond. But because identifying the underlying cause may require costly and time-consuming laboratory tests, physicians sometimes prescribe antibiotics without a clear indication that they will be effective. Unfortunately, this practice has led to the development of antibiotic-resistant bacteria that are difficult to cure. To discourage this problem, infectious-disease experts recommend using antibiotics only for illnesses caused by bacteria that will not clear up, or for the prevention of secondary infections in certain patients, such as those who are frail or elderly. Thus, antibiotics generally should be limited to coughs associated with pertussis, persistent sinusitis, or chronic bronchitis, and for those who have these problems along with other medical complications.

For More Information

Mello, C.J. *Archives of Internal Medicine*. 1996: vol. 156, p. 997.

Nenning, M.E. *Journal of the American Medical Association*. 1996: vol. 275, p. 1672.

Chapter 46

Cough:
Practical Approaches to a
Nagging Problem

To cough is normal. Most people cough once or twice an hour while awake and may not even realize it.

But when a nagging cough disrupts your sleep, embarrasses you or bothers others, getting rid of that cough becomes a priority. Although some coughs need your doctor's attention, many respond to simple self-care and the right medicine.

Coughing Is a Line of Defense

Your respiratory system works nonstop to defend against irritants. Defenses include trapping irritants in nasal hairs and mucus, carrying mucus upward and outward on cilia (tiny hair-like structures lining air passages in your lungs) and coughing.

A cough isn't as simple as it seems. It's a carefully coordinated reflex involving your brain and several muscles and organs in your throat, chest and abdomen. In a fraction of a second, a sequence of steps builds to a release of compressed air at speeds greater than 100 miles per hour.

The Cough Reflex

A cough begins when an irritant reaches one of the cough receptors in your nose, throat or chest. The receptor sends a message to

Reprinted from November 1994 *Mayo Clinic Health Letter* with permission of Mayo Foundation for Medical Education and Research, Rochester, Minnesota 55905. For subscription information, call 1-800-333-9038.

the cough center in your brain, signaling your body to cough. After you inhale, your epiglottis and vocal cords close tightly, trapping air within your lungs. Your abdominal and chest muscles contract forcefully, pushing against your diaphragm. Finally, your vocal cords and epiglottis open suddenly, allowing trapped air to explode outward.

It's Usually an Irritation

There are many reasons why you may cough. Here are typical irritations that can be short-lived or become prolonged:

- Infection—Cold and flu (influenza) are the most common causes of cough.

- Post-nasal drip—An overproduction of mucus can occur with some allergies and sinusitis (inflamed mucous membranes within sinuses). The slow trickling of mucus from the back of your nose down into your throat causes irritation.

- Environment—Irritants include smog, dust, home aerosol sprays, and cold or dry air. Cigarette smoke irritates the airways of both smokers and nonsmokers. If you smoke, nicotine paralyzes the movement of cilia. When cilia can't help clear away excess mucus, it builds up and causes coughing.

- Asthma—A new cough can result from undiagnosed mild asthma (inflammation and constriction in air passages).

- Gastroesophageal reflux—Coughing that seems worse when you're lying down may be caused by backup of stomach acid into your esophagus or, in rare cases, your lungs. Gastroesophageal reflux may also make a cough associated with asthma worse.

- Medications—Coughing can be a side effect of inhaled medications, such as corticosteroids. Coughing can also occur with use of beta blockers and ACE (angiotensin-converting enzyme) inhibitors prescribed for high blood pressure and heart disease.

- Coughing—Sometimes there's no medical explanation for a cough. Some people cough to release nervous tension, gain attention or express anger. Whatever the reason, one cough can irritate your throat and lead to another, setting up a vicious cycle.

Finding Relief

The best ways to control a simple cough depend on what kind it is:

374

Halt a Dry, Hacking Cough

A dry cough doesn't produce mucus. Generally, one that's associated with a cold will go away within a week or two.

But if a persistent cough irritates your throat, suck on hard candy or cough drops. Or drink tea sweetened with honey.

If a cough disrupts your sleep, raise the head of your bed 6 to 8 inches. This may prevent coughing due to gastroesophageal reflux.

To temporarily reduce the frequency of your cough, take an over-the-counter cough suppressant.

Codeine has long been considered the most effective suppressant. But in most states, cough formulas containing codeine are available only by prescription because codeine is a narcotic.

Dextromethorphan (deks-tro-muth-OR-fan) is nearly as effective as codeine with less risk of side effects. It's often used in longer-acting cough medicines, such as Robitussin-DM and Vicks Formula 44, to provide overnight relief.

Water Down a Productive Cough

A cough that brings up mucus helps remove irritants from your lungs and air passages. To thin mucus and make it easier to cough up, drink plenty of water. Using a humidifier or vaporizer may also help loosen mucus.

Cough medicines called expectorants are intended to thin mucus associated with a productive cough. But studies show they don't work any better than drinking liquids or breathing warm moist air.

If your cough is productive, it's best not to suppress it. On the other hand, if it continually disrupts your sleep, you can take just enough cough suppressant to decrease the frequency and severity of your cough, but not to get rid of it altogether.

When you have a cough combined with a runny nose, aches, pain and general discomfort, you'll find an array of preparations designed to relieve multiple symptoms. Some products, such as Benadryl, Genahist and Benylin, contain diphenhydramine (di-fen-HI-druh-mene), an antihistamine with suppressant action.

Antihistamines may help dry up secretions associated with allergies, sinusitis and post-nasal drip. But the high dose needed to control your cough can cause sedation. Don't take diphenhydramine when you need to stay alert or in combination with tranquilizers or alcohol.

For just a cough, a cough suppressant is all you need and is less expensive than a combination product.

375

For Serious Coughs

If your cough lasts longer than 2 to 3 weeks, see your doctor. Managing a chronic cough requires careful evaluation and identification of a specific cause.

Home Humidifiers—Help or Hazard?

When breathing dry indoor air makes you cough, increase the humidity. But don't let the remedy to one problem create another.

Dirty portable humidifiers can be a source of unhealthful bacteria and fungi. To minimize growth, the U.S. Consumer Product Safety Commission suggests:

Change the water every day. Empty the tank and dry surfaces with a soft towel. Refill with clean water. Note: Some products recommend use of distilled water. Tap water contains minerals that can create bacteria-friendly deposits. When released into the air, these minerals often appear as white dust on your furniture.

Sanitize every 1 to 2 weeks. Empty the tank and fill with a solution of 1 teaspoon bleach to 1 gallon water. Let the solution soak for 20 minutes. Rinse until you can no longer smell bleach.

Keep humidity between 30 and 50 percent. Levels higher than 60 percent may create a build-up of moisture. When moisture condenses on surfaces, bacteria and fungi can grow. Periodically check humidity with a hygrometer, available at your local hardware store.

Chapter 47

Hoarseness: Prevention and Treatment Tips

What Is Hoarseness?

Hoarseness is a general term which describes abnormal voice changes. When hoarse, the voice may sound breathy, raspy, strained, or there may be changes in volume (loudness) or pitch (how high or low the voice is). The changes in sound are usually due to disorders related to the vocal folds which are the sound producing parts of the voice box (larynx) (see Figure 47.1.A). While breathing, the vocal folds remain apart (see Figure 47.2.B). When speaking or singing, they come together (see Figure 47.2.C), and as air leaves the lungs, they vibrate, producing sound. The more tightly the vocal folds are held and the smaller the vocal folds, the more rapidly they vibrate. More rapid vibration makes a higher voice pitch. Swelling or lumps on the vocal folds prevent them from coming together properly, which makes a change in the voice.

What Are the Causes?

There are many causes of hoarseness. Fortunately, most are not serious and tend to go away in a short period of time. The most common causes are **acute laryngitis** which usually occurs due to swelling from a common cold, upper respiratory tract viral infection, or

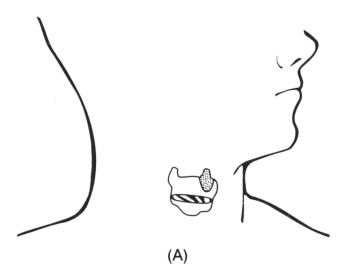

(A)

Figure 47. 1. A. The vocal cords.

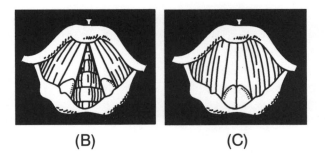

(B)   (C)

Figure 47. 2. B. Breathing; *C.* Speaking or singing.

irritation caused by excessive voice use such as screaming at a sporting event or rock concert.

More prolonged hoarseness is usually due to using your voice either too much, too loudly, or improperly over extended periods of time. These habits can lead to **vocal nodules** (singers nodes), which are callous-like growths, or may lead to polyps of the vocal folds (more extensive swelling). Vocal nodules are common in children and adults who raise their voice in work or play. Uncommonly, polyps or nodules may lead to cancer.

A common cause of hoarseness in older adults is **gastroesophageal reflux**, when stomach acid comes up the swallowing tube (esophagus) and irritates the vocal folds. Many patients with reflux-related changes of voice do not have symptoms of heartburn. Usually, the voice is worse in the morning and improves during the day. These people may have a sensation of a lump in their throat, mucous sticking in their throat or an excessive desire to clear their throat.

Smoking is another cause of hoarseness. Since smoking is the major cause of throat cancer, if smokers are hoarse, they should see an otolaryngologist.

Many unusual causes for hoarseness include **allergies, thyroid problems, neurological disorders, trauma to the voice box** and occasionally the **normal menstrual cycle.** Many people experience some hoarseness with **advanced age.**

Who Can Treat My Hoarseness?

Hoarseness due to a cold or flu may be evaluated by family physicians, pediatricians and internists (who have learned how to examine the larynx). When hoarseness lasts longer than two weeks or has no obvious cause, it should be evaluated by an otolaryngologist–head and neck surgeon (ear, nose and throat doctor). Problems with the voice are best managed by a team of professionals who know and understand how the voice functions. These professionals are otolaryngology–head and neck surgeons, speech/language pathologists, and teachers of singing, acting, or public speaking. Voice disorders have many different characteristics which may give professionals a clue to the cause.

When Should I See an Otolaryngologist (ENT Doctor)?

- If hoarseness lasts longer than 2-3 weeks
- If hoarseness is associated with:

1. Pain not from a cold or flu
2. Coughing up blood
3. Difficulty swallowing
4. A lump in the neck

- Complete loss or severe change in voice lasting longer than a few days

How Is Hoarseness Evaluated?

An otolaryngologist will obtain a thorough history of the hoarseness and your general health. Your doctor will usually look at the vocal folds with a mirror placed in the back of your throat. Occasionally a very small lighted flexible scope (fiberoptic tube scope) may need to be passed through your nose (or in some cases, a rigid scope may be used which is placed in the back of your mouth) in order to view your vocal folds. Videotaping the examination may also help with the analysis.

These procedures are not uncomfortable and are well tolerated by most patients. In some cases, special tests (known as acoustic analysis) designed to evaluate the voice may be recommended. These measure voice irregularities, how the voice sounds (acoustic content), airflow and other characteristics that are helpful in establishing a diagnosis and guiding treatment.

How Are Vocal Disorders Treated?

The treatment of hoarseness depends on the cause. Most hoarseness can be treated by simply resting the voice or modifying how it is used. The otolaryngologist may make some recommendations about voice use behavior, refer the patient to other voice team members, and in some instances recommend surgery if a discreet lesion, such as a nodule or polyp, is identified. Avoidance of smoking or exposure to secondhand smoke (passive smoking) is recommended to all patients. Drinking fluids is also helpful.

Specialists in speech/language pathology are trained to assist patients in behavior modification which may help eliminate some voice disorders. Sometimes, patients have developed bad habits, such as smoking or overuse of their voice by yelling and screaming, which may cause the voice disorder. The speech/language pathologist may teach patients to alter their method of speech production to improve the sound of the voice and to resolve problems, such as vocal nodules.

When a patient's problem is specifically related to singing, a singing teacher may help improve the patients' singing techniques.

What Can I Do to Prevent and Treat Mild Hoarseness?

- If you smoke, quit
- Avoid agents which dehydrate the body, such as alcohol and caffeine
- Avoid secondhand smoke
- Drink plenty of water
- Humidify your home
- Watch your diet—avoid spicy foods and alcohol
- Try not to use your voice too long or too loudly
- Seek professional voice training
- Avoid speaking or singing when your voice is injured or hoarse (this is similar to not walking on a sprained ankle)

Chapter 48

Tonsils and Adenoids

Tonsils and adenoids are masses of tissue that are similar to the lymph nodes or "glands" found in the neck, groin, and armpits. Tonsils are the two masses on the back of the throat. Adenoids are high in the throat behind the nose and the roof of the mouth (soft palate) and are not visible through the mouth without special instruments.

Tonsils and adenoids are near the entrance to the breathing passages where they can catch incoming germs, which cause infections. They "sample" bacteria and viruses and can become infected themselves. Scientists believe they work as part of the body's immune system by filtering germs that attempt to invade the body, and that they help to develop antibodies to germs.

This happens primarily during the first few years of life, becoming less important as we get older. Children who must have their tonsils and adenoids removed suffer no loss in their resistance.

What Affects Tonsils and Adenoids?

The most common problems affecting the tonsils and adenoids are recurrent infections (throat or ear) and significant enlargement or obstruction that causes breathing and swallowing problems.

Abscesses around the tonsils, chronic tonsillitis, and infections of small pockets within the tonsils that produce foul-smelling, cheese-

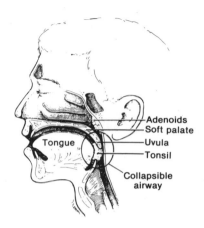

Figure 48.1. *Tonsils and adenoids, side view.*

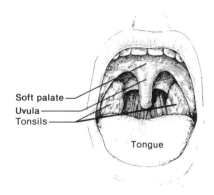

Figure 48.2. *Location of the tonsils, front view.*

like formations can also affect the tonsils and adenoids, making them sore and swollen. Tumors are rare, but can grow on the tonsils.

When Should I See My Doctor?

You should see your doctor when you or your child suffer the common symptoms of infected or enlarged tonsils or adenoids.

What Should I Expect at the Exam?

Your physician will ask about problems of the ear, nose, and throat and examine the head and neck. He will use the small mirror or a flexible lighted instrument to see these areas.

Cultures/strep tests are important in diagnosing certain infections in the throat, especially "strep" throat.

X-rays are sometimes helpful in determining the size and shape of the adenoids. Blood tests can determine problems such as mononucleosis.

The Exam

The primary methods used to check tonsils and adenoids are:

- Medical history
- Physical examination
- Throat cultures/Strep tests
- X-rays
- Blood tests

How Are Tonsil and Adenoid Diseases Treated?

Bacterial infections of the tonsils, especially those caused by streptococcus, are first treated with antibiotics. Sometimes, removal of the tonsils and/or adenoids may be recommended. The two primary reasons for tonsil and/or adenoid removal are (1) recurrent infection despite antibiotic therapy and (2) difficulty breathing due to enlarged tonsils and/or adenoids.

Such obstruction to breathing causes snoring and disturbed sleep that leads to daytime sleepiness in adults and behavioral problems in children. Some orthodontists believe chronic mouth breathing from large tonsils and adenoids causes malformations of the face and improper alignment of the teeth.

Chronic infection can affect other areas such as the eustachian tube—the passage between the back of the nose and the inside of the ear. This can lead to frequent ear infections and potential hearing loss.

Recent studies indicate adenoidectomy may be a beneficial treatment for some children with chronic earaches accompanied by fluid in the middle ear (otitus media with effusion).

In adults, the possibility of cancer or a tumor may be another reason for removing the tonsils and adenoids.

In some patients, especially those with infectious mononucleosis, severe enlargement may obstruct the airway. For those patients, treatment with steroids (e.g., cortisone) is sometimes helpful.

Tonsillitis and Its Symptoms

Tonsillitis is an infection in one or both tonsils. One sign is swelling of the tonsils. Other signs or symptoms are:

- Redder than normal tonsils
- A white or yellow coating on the tonsils
- A slight voice change due to swelling
- Sore throat
- Uncomfortable or painful swallowing
- Swollen lymph nodes (glands) in the neck
- Fever
- Bad breath

Enlarged Adenoids and Their Symptoms

If you or your child's adenoids are enlarged, it may be hard to breathe through the nose. Other signs of constant enlargement are:

- Breathing through the mouth instead of the nose most of the time
- Nose sounds "blocked" when the person speaks
- Noisy breathing during the day
- Recurrent ear infections
- Snoring at night
- Breathing stops for a few seconds at night during snoring or loud breathing (sleep apnea)

Surgery

Your Child

Talk to your child about his/her feelings and provide strong reassurance and support throughout the process. Encourage the idea that the procedure will make him/her healthier. Be with your child as much

386

as possible before and after the surgery. Tell him/her to expect a sore throat after surgery. Reassure your child that the operation does not remove any important parts of the body, and that he/she will not look any different afterward. If your child has a friend who has had this surgery, it may be helpful to talk about it with that friend.

Adults and Children

For at least two weeks before any surgery, the patient should refrain from taking aspirin or other medications containing aspirin. (**WARNING:** Children should never be given aspirin because of the risk of developing Reye's syndrome).

- If the patient or patient's family has had any problems with anesthesia, the surgeon should be informed. If the patient is taking any other medications, has sickle cell anemia, has a bleeding disorder, is pregnant, has concerns about the transfusion of blood, or has used steroids in the past year, the surgeon should be informed.

- A blood test and possibly a urine test may be required prior to surgery.

- Generally, after midnight prior to the operation, nothing (chewing gum, mouthwashes, throat lozenges, toothpaste, water) may be taken by mouth. Anything in the stomach may be vomited when anesthesia is induced, and this is dangerous.

When the patient arrives at the hospital or surgery center, the anesthesiologist or nursing staff may meet with the patient and family to review the patient's history. The patient will then be taken to the operating room and given an anesthetic. Intravenous fluids are usually given during and after surgery.

After the operation, the patient will be taken to the recovery area. Recovery room staff will observe the patient until discharged. Every patient is special, and recovery times vary for each individual. Many patients are released after 2-10 hours. Others are kept overnight. Intensive care may be needed for select cases.

Your ENT specialist will provide you with the details of pre-operative and post-operative care and answer any other questions you may have.

After Surgery

There are several post-operative symptoms that may arise. These include (but are not limited to) swallowing problems, vomiting, fever, throat pain, and ear pain. Occasionally, bleeding may occur after surgery. If the patient has any bleeding, your surgeon should be notified *immediately*.

Any questions or concerns you have should be discussed openly with your surgeon, who is there to assist you.

Chapter 49

Swallowing Disorders

Difficulty in swallowing (dysphagia) is common among all age groups, especially the elderly. The term dysphagia refers to the feeling of difficulty passing food or liquid from the mouth to the stomach. This may be caused by many factors, most of which are not threatening and temporary. Difficulties in swallowing rarely represent a more serious disease, such as a tumor or a progressive neurological disorder. When the difficulty does not clear up by itself, in a short period of time, you should see an otolaryngologist–head and neck surgeon.

How You Swallow

People normally swallow hundreds of times a day to eat solids, drink liquids, and swallow the normal saliva and mucus that the body produces. The process of swallowing has four stages:

1. The first is *oral preparation*, where food or liquid is manipulated and chewed in preparation for swallowing.

2. During the *oral stage*, the tongue propels the food or liquid to the back of the mouth, starting the swallowing response.

3. The *pharyngeal stage* begins as food or liquid is quickly passed through the pharynx (the canal that connects the mouth with the esophagus) into the esophagus or swallowing tube.

4. In the final, *esophageal stage*, the food or liquid passes through the esophagus into the stomach.

Although the first and second stages have some voluntary control, stages three and four occur by themselves, without conscious input.

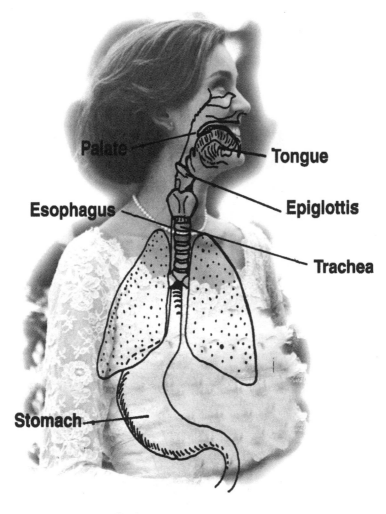

Figure 49.1. *Swallowing*

What Causes Swallowing Disorders?

Any interruption in the swallowing process can cause difficulties. It may be due to simple causes such as poor teeth, ill fitting dentures, or a common cold. One of the most common causes of dysphagia is gastroesophageal reflux. This occurs when stomach acid moves up the esophagus to the pharynx, causing discomfort. Other causes may include: stroke; progressive neurological disorder; the presence of a tracheostomy tube; a paralyzed or unmoving vocal cord; a tumor in the mouth, throat, or esophagus; or surgery in the head, neck, or esophageal areas.

Symptoms

Symptoms of swallowing disorders may include:

- drooling,

- a feeling that food or liquid is sticking in the throat,

- discomfort in the throat or chest (when gastroesophageal reflux is present),

- a sensation of a foreign body or "lump" in the throat,

- weight loss and inadequate nutrition due to prolonged or more significant problems with swallowing, and

- coughing or choking caused by bits of food, liquid, or saliva not passing easily during swallowing, and being sucked into the lungs.

Who Evaluates and Treats Swallowing Disorders?

When dysphagia is persistent and the cause is not apparent, the otolaryngologist–head and neck surgeon will discuss the history of your problem and examine your mouth and throat. This may be done with the aid of mirrors or a small tube (flexible laryngoscope), which provides vision of the back of the tongue, throat, and larynx (voice box). If necessary, an examination of the esophagus, stomach, and upper small intestine (duodenum) may be carried out by the otolaryngologist or a gastroenterologist.

These specialists may recommend X-rays of the swallowing mechanism, called a barium swallow or upper G-I, which is done by a radiologist.

If special problems exist, a speech pathologist may consult with the radiologist regarding a modified barium swallow or videofluroscopy. These help to identify all four stages of the swallowing process. Using different consistencies of food and liquid, and having the patient swallow in various positions, a speech pathologist will test the ability to swallow. An exam by a neurologist may be necessary if the swallowing disorder stems from the nervous system, perhaps due to stroke or other neurologic disorders.

Possible Treatments

Once the cause is determined, swallowing disorders may be treated with:

- Medication
- Swallowing therapy
- Surgery

Many of these disorders can be treated with medication. Drugs that slow stomach acid production, muscle relaxants, and antacids are a few of the many medicines available. Treatment is tailored to the particular cause of the swallowing disorder.

Gastroesophageal reflux can often be treated by changing eating and living habits—for example:

- Eat a bland diet with smaller, more frequent meals,
- Eliminate alcohol and caffeine,
- Reduce weight and stress,
- Avoid food within three hours of bedtime, and
- Elevate the head of the bed at night.

If these don't help, antacids between meals and at bedtime may provide relief.

Many **swallowing disorders** may be helped by direct swallowing therapy. A speech pathologist can provide special exercises for coordinating the swallowing muscles or restimulating the nerves that trigger the swallow reflex. Patients may also be taught simple ways to place food in the mouth or position the body and head to help the swallow occur successfully.

Some patients with swallowing disorders have difficulty feeding themselves. An occupational therapist can aid the patient and family in feeding techniques. These techniques make the patient as independent as possible. A dietician or nutritional expert can determine the amount of food or liquid necessary to sustain an individual and whether supplements are necessary.

Surgery is used to treat certain problems. If a narrowing or stricture exists, the area may need to be stretched or dilated. If a muscle is too tight, it may need to be dilated or even released surgically. This procedure is called a myotomy and is performed by an otolaryngologist–head and neck surgeon.

Many causes contribute to swallowing disorders. If you have a persistent problem swallowing, see an otolaryngologist–head and neck surgeon.

Chapter 50

Salivary Glands: What's Normal, What's Abnormal?

Where Are Salivary Glands?

The glands are located in and around the mouth and throat. The major salivary glands are called the parotid, submandibular and sublingual glands (see Figure 50.1).

They all secrete saliva into the mouth: the parotid through ducts near the upper teeth, submandibular into the front portion under the tongue, and the sublingual through multiple ducts in the floor of the mouth.

In addition to these glands, there are hundreds of tiny glands called minor salivary glands located in the lips, inner cheek area (buccal mucosa) and extensively in other linings of the mouth and throat. Salivary glands produce the saliva used to moisten your mouth, initiate digestion, and help protect teeth from decay.

What Causes Abnormal Glands?

Abnormalities of the salivary glands which cause clinical symptoms can be grouped as follows:

Obstruction. Obstruction to the flow of saliva most commonly occurs in the parotid and submandibular glands, usually due to stone formation. Symptoms typically occur when eating. Saliva production is initiated, but cannot exit the ductal system, leading to swelling of the involved gland and significant pain, sometimes with an infection.

Inflammation. If stones are not totally obstructive, the major glands will swell during eating and then gradually subside after eating, only to enlarge again at the next meal. Infection often develops in the abnormally pooled saliva, leading to more severe pain and swelling in the glands. If untreated long enough, the glands may become abscessed.

In some individuals the duct system of the major salivary glands may be abnormal. These ducts can develop small constrictions which decrease salivary flow, leading to infection and obstructive symptoms.

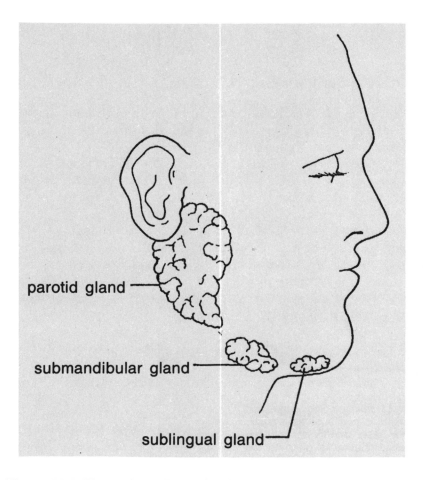

Figure 50.1. *The major salivary glands.*

Infection. The most common salivary gland infection is mumps, which involves the parotid glands. While this is most common in children, it can occur in adults. However, if an adult has swelling in the area of the parotid gland on one side, it is more likely due to an obstruction or a tumor.

Infections occurring because of ductal obstruction or sluggish flow of saliva have already been mentioned.

Secondary infection of salivary glands from adjacent lymph nodes also occurs. These lymph nodes are the glands in the upper neck which often become tender during a common sore throat. Many of these lymph nodes are actually located on, within, and deep in the substance of the parotid gland, near the submandibular glands. When these lymph nodes enlarge through infection, this is noticed by the patient as a red, painful swelling in the area of the parotid or submandibular glands. Lymph nodes also enlarge due to tumors and inflammation.

Tumors. Primary benign and malignant salivary gland tumors usually show up as painless enlargements of these glands. Tumors rarely involve more than one gland and are detected as a growth in the parotid, submandibular area, on the palate, floor of mouth, cheeks, or lips. These enlargements should be checked by an otolaryngologist–head and neck surgeon.

Malignant tumors of the major salivary glands can grow quickly, are painful, and can cause loss of movement of part or all of the affected side of the face. These symptoms should be immediately investigated.

Salivary gland enlargement is also seen in auto-immune diseases, which cause significant inflammation. Patients often have a dry mouth or dry eyes. This may occur with other systemic diseases such as rheumatoid arthritis. Diabetes may cause enlargement of the salivary glands, especially the parotid glands. Salivary gland swelling (usually on both sides) is also seen in alcoholics.

How Does Your Doctor Make the Diagnosis?

The diagnosis of salivary gland disease depends upon a careful history, a physical examination, and laboratory tests. If an obstruction of the major salivary glands is suspected, it may be necessary to anesthetize the opening of the salivary ducts in the mouth, and to probe, and dilate the duct to help an obstructive stone pass. Prior to such instrumentation, dental x-rays may show the location of calcified stones.

If a mass is found in the salivary gland, it is helpful to obtain an x-ray called a CT scan. CT scans will show whether the mass is an actual part of a salivary gland, or an associated lymph node.

In many cases a fine needle aspiration biopsy in the doctor's office is helpful. The accuracy of this test is approximately 80% to 90%. An open biopsy, where a skin incision is made and a small sample of the gland removed, is not usually recommended in the office. This is an incisional biopsy and because of the possibility of injury to underlying nerves within the parotid gland may need to be done in the operating room.

Treatment of Salivary Gland Disease

Treatment of salivary diseases is broadly classified into two categories: medical and surgical. Selection of treatment depends upon the nature of the problem. If it is due to systemic diseases (diseases that involve the whole body, not one isolated area), then the underlying problem process must be treated. This may require consultation with other specialists. If the disease process relates to salivary gland obstruction and subsequent infection, antibiotics are used. Sometimes instrumentation of the ducts will be needed.

If a mass has developed within the salivary gland, removal of the mass may be required. Most masses in the parotid gland area are benign. When surgery is necessary, great care must be taken to avoid damage to the facial nerve which lies within this gland. When malignant masses are present in the parotid gland, it may be possible to surgically remove these masses and preserve most of the facial nerve. Radiation treatment will often be recommended after surgery. This is typically administered four to six weeks after the surgical procedure to allow adequate healing before irradiation.

The same general principles apply to masses in the submandibular area or in the minor salivary glands within the mouth and upper throat. Benign diseases are best treated by surgery alone, whereas malignant diseases may require surgery and postoperative irradiation. If the mass in the vicinity of a salivary gland is a lymph node which has become enlarged due to cancer from another site, then obviously a different treatment plan will be necessary. Such treatment can be very effectively directed by an otolaryngologist–head and neck surgeon.

In summary, salivary gland diseases are due to many different causes. These diseases are treated both medically and surgically. Such treatment is readily managed by an otolaryngologist–head and neck surgeon with experience in this area.

Chapter 51

Snoring:
Not Funny but Not Hopeless

An anonymous wit has said:

> "Laugh and the world laughs with you,
> Snore and you sleep alone."

Some 45 percent of normal adults snore at least occasionally, and 25 percent are habitual snorers. Problem snoring is more frequent in males and overweight persons, and it usually grows worse with age.

More than 300 devices are registered in the U.S. Patent and Trademark Office as cures for snoring. Some are variations on the old idea of sewing a tennis ball on the pajama back—to force the snorer to sleep on his side. (Snoring is often worse when the person sleeps on his back.) Chin and head straps, neck collars, and devices inserted into the mouth are usually disappointing as snoring cures. Many electrical devices have been designed to produce painful or unpleasant stimuli when the patient snores. The presumption was that a person could be trained or conditioned not to snore. Unfortunately, snoring is not under the person's control whatsoever; and if these devices work it is probably because they keep the snorer awake.

What Causes Snoring?

The noisy sounds of snoring occur when there is an obstruction to the free flow of air through the passages at the back of the mouth and nose. This is the collapsible part of the airway (see Figure 51.1.) where the tongue and upper throat meet the soft palate and uvula (the fleshy structure that dangles from the roof of the mouth back into the throat). When these structures strike against each other and vibrate during breathing, that is snoring. Persons who snore have at least one of the following problems:

1. Poor muscle tone (lack of tightness) in the muscles of the tongue and throat. Flabby muscles allow the tongue to fall backwards into the airway or allow the throat muscles to be drawn in from he sides into the airway. This occurs when the person's muscular control is too relaxed from alcohol or from drugs which cause sleepiness. It also happens in some persons when they relax in the deep-sleep stages.

2. Excessive bulkiness of tissues of the throat. Large tonsils and adenoids, for example, commonly cause snoring in children. Overweight persons also have bulky neck tissues. Cysts or tumors could also be present, but they are rare.

3. Excessive length of the soft palate and uvula. A long palate may narrow the opening from the nose into the throat. As it dangles in the airway, it acts as a flutter valve during relaxed breathing, and contributes to the noise of snoring. A long uvula makes matters even worse.

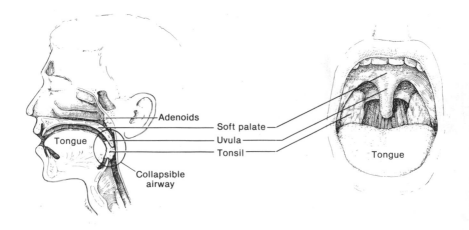

Figure 51.1. *Snoring occurs when there is an obstuction to the free flow of air through the passages at the back of the mouth and nose.*

4. Obstructed nasal airways. When a person has a stuffy or blocked-up nose he must pull hard to inhale air through it. This creates an exaggerated vacuum in his throat, in the collapsible part of the airway, and it pulls together the floppy tissues of the throat. So snoring occurs even in persons who would not snore if they could breathe through the nose properly. This explains why some people snore only during the hay fever season, or when they have a cold or sinus infection. Also, deformities of the nose or nasal septum frequently cause such obstruction. "Deviated septum" is a common term for a deformity inside the nose in the wall that separates one nostril from the other.

Is Snoring Serious?

Socially—yes. It is disruptive to family life. It makes the snorer an object of ridicule and causes other household members sleepless nights and resentfulness. Snorers become unwelcome roommates on vacations or business trips.

And medically—yes. It disturbs the sleeping patterns of the snorer himself, so that he may not sleep restfully. Furthermore, heavy snorers tend to develop high blood pressure at a younger age than nonsnorers.

The most exaggerated form of snoring is known as obstructive sleep apnea, when loud snoring is interrupted by frequent episodes of totally obstructed breathing. This is serious if the episodes last over 10 seconds each and occur more than 7 times per hour. Your physician may recommend a laboratory sleep study as a way of evaluating your symptoms. Apnea patients may experience 30 to 300 obstructed events per night, and many spend as much as half their sleep time with blood oxygen levels below normal. During their obstructive episodes, the heart must pump harder to circulate the blood faster. This can cause irregular heartbeats, and after many years it leads to elevated blood pressure and heart enlargement. The immediate effect of this oxygen starvation is that the person must sleep in a lighter stage and tense his muscles enough to open his airway to get air into his lungs. Since snorers with severe sleep apnea are often unaware of it, laboratory sleep study may be the only way to discover it.

Persons with obstructive sleep apnea may spend little of their night-time hours in the deep-sleep stages that are essential for a good rest. Therefore, they awaken unrefreshed and are sleepy much of the day. They may fall asleep while driving to work or while on the job.

Can Snoring Be Cured?

By far the majority of snorers can be helped. For adults who are mild or occasional snorers, the following self-help remedies are worth trying.

1. Adopt an athletic life-style and exercise daily to develop good muscle tone and lose weight.

2. Avoid tranquilizers, sleeping pills, and antihistamines before bedtime.

3. Avoid alcoholic beverages within 4 hours of retiring.

4. Avoid heavy meals within 3 hours of retiring.

5. Avoid getting overtired; establish regular sleeping patterns.

6. Sleep sideways rather than on the back. Consider sewing a pocket on the pajama back to hold a tennis ball. This helps to avoid sleeping on your back.

7. Tilt the entire bed with the head upwards 4" (place bricks under the bedposts at the bedhead).

8. Allow the nonsnorer to get to sleep first.

Heavy snorers, those who snore in any position they sleep in, and so-called "obnoxious snorers" need more help than the suggestions above.

When snoring becomes disruptive to the life of the snorer or his family, medical advice should be sought, especially if other household members suspect the obstructive sleep apnea problem (very loud snoring with periods when all airflow stops—even though the snorer is trying to breathe).

The heavy snorer deserves a thorough examination of the nose, mouth, palate, throat, and neck. Studies in a sleep laboratory are valuable to determine how serious the snoring is and what effects it has on the snorer's health. Treatment will depend, of course, on the diagnosis. It may be as simple as managing a nasal allergy or infection, surgically correcting a nasal deformity, or removing tonsils and adenoids. Or, snoring/apnea may respond best to surgery on the throat and palate to tighten up flabby tissues and expand the air passages, an operation called UvuloPalatoPharyngoPlasty (UPPP). To the patient it feels like having a tonsillectomy. If surgery is too risky, unwanted or unsuccessful, the patient may sleep every night wearing a nasal mask which delivers air pressure into the throat ("CPAP").

Every chronically snoring child should also be thoroughly examined. Medical evidence suggests a tonsillectomy and adenoidectomy will probably make an important difference in the health and well-being of the child.

Remember, snoring means obstructed breathing, and obstruction can be serious. It's not funny, and it's definitely not hopeless.

Chapter 52

Sleep Apnea

What Is Sleep Apnea?

Sleep apnea is a serious, potentially life-threatening condition that is far more common than generally understood. First described in 1965, sleep apnea is a breathing disorder characterized by brief interruptions of breathing during sleep. It owes its name to a Greek word, apnea, meaning "want of breath." There are two types of sleep apnea: central and obstructive. Central sleep apnea, which is less common, occurs when the brain fails to send the appropriate signals to the breathing muscles to initiate respirations. Obstructive sleep apnea is far more common and occurs when air cannot flow into or out of the person's nose or mouth although efforts to breathe continue.

In a given night, the number of involuntary breathing pauses or "apneic events" may be as high as 20 to 30 or more per hour. These breathing pauses are almost always accompanied by snoring between apnea episodes, although not everyone who snores has this condition. Sleep apnea can also be characterized by choking sensations. The frequent interruptions of deep, restorative sleep often lead to early morning headaches and excessive daytime sleepiness.

Early recognition and treatment of sleep apnea is important because it may be associated with irregular heartbeat, high blood pressure, heart attack, and stroke.

National Heart, Lung and Blood Institute, NIH Pub. No. 95-3798, September 1995.

Who Gets Sleep Apnea?

Sleep apnea occurs in all age groups and both sexes but is more common in men (it may be underdiagnosed in women) and possibly young African Americans. It has been estimated that as many as 18 million Americans have sleep apnea. Four percent of middle-aged men and 2 percent of middle-aged women have sleep apnea along with excessive daytime sleepiness. People most likely to have or develop sleep apnea include those who snore loudly and also are overweight, or have high blood pressure, or have some physical abnormality in the nose, throat, or other parts of the upper airway. Sleep apnea seems to run in some families, suggesting a possible genetic basis.

What Causes Sleep Apnea?

Certain mechanical and structural problems in the airway cause the interruptions in breathing during sleep. In some people, apnea occurs when the throat muscles and tongue relax during sleep and partially block the opening of the airway. When the muscles of the soft palate at the base of the tongue and the uvula (the small fleshy tissue hanging from the center of the back of the throat) relax and sag, the airway becomes blocked, making breathing labored and noisy

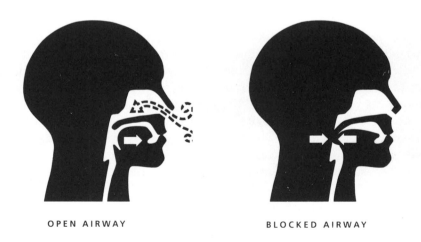

OPEN AIRWAY   BLOCKED AIRWAY

Figure 52.1. Airflow in open and blocked airways.

and even stopping it altogether. Sleep apnea also can occur in obese people when an excess amount of tissue in the airway causes it to be narrowed. With a narrowed airway, the person continues his or her efforts to breathe, but air cannot easily flow into or out of the nose or mouth. Unknown to the person, this results in heavy snoring, periods of no breathing, and frequent arousals (causing abrupt changes from deep sleep to light sleep). Ingestion of alcohol and sleeping pills increases the frequency and duration of breathing pauses in people with sleep apnea.

How Is Normal Breathing Restored During Sleep?

During the apneic event, the person is unable to breathe in oxygen and to exhale carbon dioxide, resulting in low levels of oxygen and increased levels of carbon dioxide in the blood. The reduction in oxygen and increase in carbon dioxide alert the brain to resume breathing and cause an arousal. With each arousal, a signal is sent from the brain to the upper airway muscles to open the airway; breathing is resumed, often with a loud snort or gasp. Frequent arousals, although necessary for breathing to restart, prevent the patient from getting enough restorative, deep sleep.

What Are the Effects of Sleep Apnea?

Because of the serious disturbances in their normal sleep patterns, people with sleep apnea often feel very sleepy during the day and their concentration and daytime performance suffer. The consequences of sleep apnea range from annoying to life-threatening. They include depression, irritability, sexual dysfunction, learning and memory difficulties, and falling asleep while at work, on the phone, or driving. It has been estimated that up to 50 percent of sleep apnea patients have high blood pressure. Although it is not known with certainty if there is a cause and effect relationship, it appears that sleep apnea contributes to high blood pressure. Risk for heart attack and stroke may also increase in those with sleep apnea. In addition, sleep apnea is sometimes implicated in sudden infant death syndrome.

When Should Sleep Apnea Be Suspected?

For many sleep apnea patients, their spouses are the first ones to suspect that something is wrong, usually from their heavy snoring and apparent struggle to breathe. Co-workers or friends of the sleep apnea victim may notice that the individual falls asleep during the day at inappropriate times (such as while driving a car, working, or talking). The patient often does not know he or she has a problem and may not believe it when told. It is important that the person see a doctor for evaluation of the sleep problem.

How Is Sleep Apnea Diagnosed?

In addition to the primary care physician, pulmonologists, neurologists, or other physicians with specialty training in sleep disorders may be involved in making a definitive diagnosis and initiating treatment. Diagnosis of sleep apnea is not simple because there can be many different reasons for disturbed sleep. Several tests are available for evaluating a person for sleep apnea.

Polysomnography is a test that records a variety of body functions during sleep, such as the electrical activity of the brain, eye movement, muscle activity, heart rate, respiratory effort, air flow, and blood oxygen levels. These tests are used both to diagnose sleep apnea and to determine its severity.

The ***Multiple Sleep Latency Test*** (MSLT) measures the speed of falling asleep. In this test, patients are given several opportunities to fall asleep during the course of a day when they would normally be awake. For each opportunity, time to fall asleep is measured. People without sleep problems usually take an average of 10 to 20 minutes to fall asleep. Individuals who fall asleep in less than 5 minutes are likely to require some treatment for sleep disorders. The MSLT may be useful to measure the degree of excessive daytime sleepiness and to rule out other types of sleep disorders.

Diagnostic tests usually are performed in a sleep center, but new technology may allow some sleep studies to be conducted in the patient's home.

How Is Sleep Apnea Treated?

The specific therapy for sleep apnea is tailored to the individual patient based on medical history, physical examination, and the results of polysomnography. Medications are generally not effective in the treatment of sleep apnea. Oxygen administration may safely benefit certain patients but does not eliminate sleep apnea or prevent daytime sleepiness. Thus, the role of oxygen in the treatment of sleep apnea is controversial, and it is difficult to predict which patients will respond well. It is important that the effectiveness of the selected treatment be verified; this is usually accomplished by polysomnography.

Behavioral Therapy

Behavioral changes are an important part of the treatment program, and in mild cases behavioral therapy may be all that is needed. The individual should avoid the use of alcohol, tobacco, and sleeping pills, which make the airway more likely to collapse during sleep and prolong the apneic periods. Overweight persons can benefit from losing weight. Even a 10 percent weight loss can reduce the number of apneic events for most patients. In some patients with mild sleep apnea, breathing pauses occur only when they sleep on their backs. In such cases, using pillows and other devices that help them sleep in a side position is often helpful.

Physical or Mechanical Therapy

Nasal *continuous positive airway pressure* (CPAP) is the most common effective treatment for sleep apnea. In this procedure, the patient wears a mask over the nose during sleep, and pressure from an air blower forces air through the nasal passages. The air pressure is adjusted so that it is just enough to prevent the throat from collapsing during sleep. The pressure is constant and continuous. Nasal CPAP prevents airway closure while in use, but apnea episodes return when CPAP is stopped or used improperly.

Variations of the CPAP device attempt to minimize side effects that sometimes occur, such as nasal irritation and drying, facial skin irritation, abdominal bloating, mask leaks, sore eyes, and headaches. Some versions of CPAP vary the pressure to coincide with the person's breathing pattern, and others start with low pressure, slowly increasing it to allow the person to fall asleep before the full prescribed pressure is applied.

Dental appliances that reposition the lower jaw and the tongue have been helpful to some patients with mild sleep apnea or who snore but do not have apnea. Possible side effects include damage to teeth, soft tissues, and the jaw joint. A dentist or orthodontist is often the one to fit the patient with such a device.

Surgery

Some patients with sleep apnea may need surgery. Although several surgical procedures are used to increase the size of the airway, none of them is completely successful or without risks. More than one procedure may need to be tried before the patient realizes any benefits.

Some of the more common procedures include removal of adenoids and tonsils (especially in children), nasal polyps or other growths, or other tissue in the airway and correction of structural deformities. Younger patients seem to benefit from these surgical procedures more than older patients.

Uvulopalatopharyngoplasty (UPPP) is a procedure used to remove excess tissue at the back of the throat (tonsils, uvula, and part of the soft palate). The success of this technique may range from 30 to 50 percent. The long-term side effects and benefits are not known, and it is difficult to predict which patients will do well with this procedure.

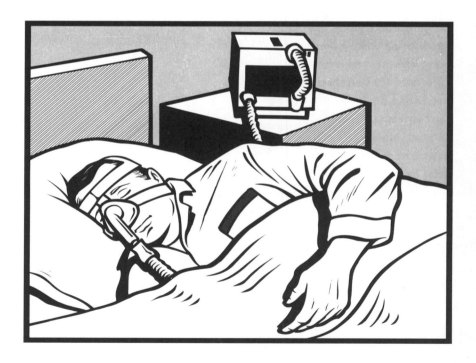

Figure 52.2. A patient using CPAP (continuous positive airway pressure).

Laser-assisted uvulopalatoplasty (LAUP) is done to eliminate snoring but has not been shown to be effective in treating sleep apnea. This procedure involves using a laser device to eliminate tissue in the back of the throat. Like UPPP, LAUP may decrease or eliminate snoring but not sleep apnea itself. Elimination of snoring, the primary symptom of sleep apnea, without influencing the condition may carry the risk of delaying the diagnosis and possible treatment of sleep apnea in patients who elect LAUP. To identify possible underlying sleep apnea, sleep studies are usually required before LAUP is performed.

Tracheostomy is used in persons with severe, life-threatening sleep apnea. In this procedure, a small hole is made in the windpipe and a tube is inserted into the opening. This tube stays closed during waking hours, and the person breathes and speaks normally. It is opened for sleep so that air flows directly into the lungs, bypassing any upper airway obstruction. Although this procedure is highly effective, it is an extreme measure that is poorly tolerated by patients and rarely used.

Other procedures. Patients in whom sleep apnea is due to deformities of the lower jaw may benefit from surgical reconstruction. Finally, surgical procedures to treat obesity are sometimes recommended for sleep apnea patients who are morbidly obese.

Chapter 53

Spasmodic Dysphonia

What Is Spasmodic Dysphonia?

Spasmodic dysphonia (or laryngeal dystonia) is a voice disorder caused by involuntary movements of one or more muscles of the larynx or voice box. Individuals who have spasmodic dysphonia may have occasional difficulty saying a word or two or they may experience sufficient difficulty to interfere with communication. Spasmodic dysphonia causes the voice to break or to have a tight, strained or strangled quality. There are three different types of spasmodic dysphonia.

What Are the Types of Spasmodic Dysphonia?

The three types of spasmodic dysphonia are adductor spasmodic dysphonia, abductor spasmodic dysphonia and mixed spasmodic dysphonia.

What Are the Features of Spasmodic Dysphonia?

In adductor spasmodic dysphonia, sudden involuntary muscle movements or spasms cause the vocal folds (or vocal cords) to slam together and stiffen. These spasms make it difficult for the vocal folds to vibrate and produce voice. Words are often cut off or difficult to start because of the muscle spasms. Therefore, speech may be choppy and sound similar to stuttering. The voice of an individual with adductor

National Institute on Deafness and Other Communication Disorders, July 1996.

413

spasmodic dysphonia is commonly described as strained or strangled and full of effort. Surprisingly, the spasms are usually absent while whispering, laughing, singing, speaking at a high pitch or speaking while breathing in. Stress, however, often makes the muscle spasms more severe.

In abductor spasmodic dysphonia, sudden involuntary muscle movements or spasms cause the vocal folds to open. The vocal folds can not vibrate when they are open. The open position of the vocal folds also allows air to escape from the lungs during speech. As a result, the voices of these individuals often sound weak, quiet and breathy or whispery. As with adductor spasmodic dysphonia, the spasms are often absent during activities such as laughing or singing.

Mixed spasmodic dysphonia involves muscles that open the vocal folds as well as muscles that close the vocal folds and therefore has features of both adductor and abductor spasmodic dysphonia.

What Causes Spasmodic Dysphonia?

The cause of spasmodic dysphonia is unknown. Because the voice can sound normal or near normal at times, spasmodic dysphonia was once thought to be psychogenic, that is, originating in the affected person's mind rather than from a physical cause. While psychogenic forms of spasmodic dysphonia exist, research has revealed increasing evidence that most cases of spasmodic dysphonia are in fact neurogenic or having to do with the nervous system (brain and nerves). Spasmodic dysphonia may co-occur with other movement disorders such as blepharospasm (excessive eye blinking and involuntary forced eye closure), tardive dyskinesia (involuntary and repetitious movement of muscles of the face, body, arms and legs), oromandibular dystonia (involuntary movements of the jaw muscles, lips and tongue), torticollis (involuntary movements of the neck muscles), or tremor (rhythmic, quivering muscle movements).

In some cases, spasmodic dysphonia may run in families and is thought to be inherited. Research has identified a possible gene on chromosome 9 that may contribute to the spasmodic dysphonia that is common to certain families. In some individuals the voice symptoms begin following an upper respiratory infection, injury to the larynx, a long period of voice use, or stress.

How Is Spasmodic Dysphonia Diagnosed?

The diagnosis of spasmodic dysphonia is usually made based on identifying the way the symptoms developed as well as by careful

414

examination of the individual. Most people are evaluated by a team that usually includes an otolaryngologist (a physician who specializes in ear, nose and throat disorders), a speech-language pathologist (a professional trained to diagnose and treat speech, language and voice disorders) and a neurologist (a physician who specializes in nervous system disorders). The otolaryngologist examines the vocal folds to look for other possible causes for the voice disorder. Fiberoptic nasolaryngoscopy, a method whereby a small lighted tube is passed through the nose and into the throat, is a helpful tool that allows the otolaryngologist to evaluate vocal cord movement during speech. The speech-language pathologist evaluates the patient's voice and voice quality. The neurologist evaluates the patient for signs of other muscle movement disorders.

What Treatment Is Available for Spasmodic Dysphonia?

There is presently no cure for spasmodic dysphonia. Current treatments only help reduce the symptoms of this voice disorder. No medication can rid individuals of the vocal symptoms. Voice therapy may reduce some symptoms, especially in mild cases. An operation that cuts one of the nerves of the vocal folds (the recurrent laryngeal nerve) has improved the voice of many for several months to several years but the improvement is often temporary. Others may benefit from psychological counseling to help them to accept and live with their voice problem. Still others may benefit from job counseling that will help them select a line of work more compatible with their speaking limitations.

Currently the most promising treatment for reducing the symptoms of spasmodic dysphonia is injections of very small amounts of botulinum toxin (botox) directly into the affected muscles of the larynx. Botulinum toxin is produced by the Clostridium botulinum bacteria. This is the bacterium that occurs in improperly canned foods and honey. The toxin weakens muscles by blocking the nerve impulse to the muscle. The botox injections generally improve the voice for a period of three to four months after which the voice symptoms gradually return. Reinjections are necessary to maintain a good speaking voice. Initial side effects that usually subside after a few days to a few weeks may include a temporary weak, breathy voice or occasional swallowing difficulties. Botox may relieve the symptoms of both adductor and abductor spasmodic dysphonia.

Botox has not yet been approved by the Food and Drug Administration (FDA) for spasmodic dysphonia and is therefore considered experimental. It has been approved, however, for other muscle movement disorders such as blepharospasm and strabismus (misalignment of the eyes). Botulinum toxin has been found to be a safe form of treatment for these disorders when given in correct doses by experienced physicians. Since this is a relatively new form of treatment, the long-term effects of repeated injections are unknown. Because the effects of botox on fetal and neonatal development has not been fully examined, women of childbearing age or who are breastfeeding are cautioned to avoid the injections.

Where Can I Get Additional Information?

American Academy of Neurology
2221 University Avenue SE, Suite 335
Minneapolis, MN 55414
(612) 623-8115 (voice); (612) 623-3504 (fax)

American Academy of Otolaryngology–Head and Neck Surgery
One Prince Street
Alexandria, VA 22314
(703) 836-4444 (voice); (703) 519-1585 (TTY)
(703) 683-5100 (fax)

American Speech-Language-Hearing Association
10801 Rockville Pike
Rockville, MD 20852
(301) 897-5700 (voice/TTY); (800) 638-8255 (toll free);
(301) 571-0457 (fax)

Dystonia Medical Research Foundation
One East Wacker Drive, Suite 2430
Chicago, IL 60601-1905
(312) 755-0198 (voice); (312) 803-0138 (fax)

National Spasmodic Dysphonia Association
P.O. Box 203
Atwood, California 92601-0203
(800) 795-6732 (voice); (714) 961-0945 (fax)

Our Voice
365 West 25th Street, Suite 13E
New York, NY 10001
(212) 929-4299 (voice); (212) 929-4099 (fax)

Chapter 54

Laryngeal Diseases and Disorders

Overview

Normal Structure and Function

The voice supports spoken communication and the acoustic representation of language. Speech is the product of adjustments of the larynx and upper aerodigestive tract that act upon and interact with the respiratory airstream to create the physical disturbances that are perceived as speech sounds. Although most people take voice production for granted, reduction or loss of the ability to produce the voice can disrupt or preclude spoken communication, and thus can have far-reaching personal, professional and social consequences. A good voice is important in modern society because there is great demand for effective spoken communication.

The normal voice is produced by using structures in the larynx to rapidly modulate air that is exhaled from the lungs. The larynx acts as a valve between the pharynx (throat) and trachea (windpipe) and, along with other structures in the region, also forms a crossroads between the respiratory and digestive systems. The laryngeal skeleton consists of several cartilages and is suspended in the neck through attachments to the hyoid bone above and trachea below.

The primary laryngeal structures for voice production are the vocal folds (cords). The vocal folds are formed by muscles that are covered with

Excerpted from *National Strategic Research Plan*, National Institute on Deafness and Other Communication Disorders, 1994-1995; NIH Pub. No. 97-3217.

417

mucous membrane and are moved apart to open the larynx or brought together for closure. The voice is produced by bringing the vocal folds close together and exhaling. When air pressure in the lungs reaches a sufficient level, the vocal folds are blown into vibration, causing the airflow from the lungs to become pulsed. The pulsed airflow is further modified by vocal tract shaping which occurs above the larynx in the hypopharynx, pharynx, nasopharynx, oral cavity and nasal cavities and that affects the quality of the voice during the production of speech. The respiratory system, which is an integral part of the voice production system, provides the energy source and must be coordinated with laryngeal valving and upper aerodigestive tract modulation of the respiratory airflow. Normal voice production is not possible without normal vibration of the vocal folds.

Another important role of the larynx is protection and regulation of the airway. During inspiration, the vocal folds are separated and air passes through the trachea to the lungs. During expiration, movements of the vocal folds participate in the control of the rate of airflow out of the lungs. During swallowing, the larynx is elevated, moved forward and closed tightly, while the tongue and pharyngeal muscles move food or fluid through the oral cavity and pharynx into the esophagus. During a cough, the vocal folds close while expiratory muscles contract to increase pressure in the lungs. The larynx opens abruptly, air rushes out and mucus or foreign material is ejected from the tracheobronchial tree. If the larynx is irritated by particulate matter, reflex closure of the vocal folds and coughing occur. These actions prevent life-threatening aspiration pneumonia.

The same upper aerodigestive tract structures involved in voice and speech production are also required to coordinate the activity of swallowing. Although normal structure and function of the larynx and diseases and disorders of the voice can be studied independently, their interrelations should also be studied. Such integrated studies are critical to improving methods for diagnosis and treatment.

However, there is still a lack of basic information on the structure and function of the laryngopharynx. For example, even now scientists remain unsure of the embryonic origins of parts of the laryngopharynx. As a result, large gaps in knowledge persist regarding innervation of the laryngopharynx, especially sensory innervation.

Information from several domains, such as the neural, muscular, structural, aeromechanical, acoustical and perceptual, will be required to improve the understanding of the complex nature of voice production. This effort will necessitate the involvement of scientists and practitioners from a multitude of disciplines, including basic biological sciences, medicine, physics, engineering, behavioral sciences, communication sciences and the arts. It will also be important to relate such knowledge to specific functions and forms of expression, including those that are psycholinguistic and artistic.

Examples of such disciplines that are of primary importance are molecular biology and genetics. Hundreds of genes have been identified as having a role in normal and abnormal development. Yet, there remains a paucity of information regarding the molecular basis of laryngeal structure and function. Elucidation of the normal development and function of the vocal system at the molecular level is a critical area of research. The application of molecular technology to such studies is essential, and their results will serve as a basis for further studies of the complex cellular and physiologic processes of the vocal system. In particular, these studies will identify genetic factors and distinguish them from environmental effects.

There is also a great need to expand normative database studies to include modifying factors of gender, age and ethnicity.

Diseases and Disorders of the Larynx

Diseases and disorders of the larynx are common, affecting nearly everyone at some time in life. They range in severity from acute laryngitis to airway obstruction and loss of airway protection.

Much of the American workforce depends on good vocal quality to do their work. Consequently, voice disorders can have a substantial negative impact on an individual's productivity and the nation's economy. That impact becomes evident when, for example, a lawyer cannot be heard in court and fails to communicate with the jury, a teacher cannot be heard in the classroom and must cease teaching or a supervisor cannot direct workers at a construction site. Furthermore, for the individual with such a disorder, the social and psychologic effects stemming from inability to be understood are great as is the economic impact.

Most of the activities of the larynx are automatic, and therefore they tend to be taken for granted until there is a disorder that disturbs the normal function. When disease disrupts an individual's vocal or swallowing mechanisms, the consequences can be devastating to the health, well-being and livelihood of the person.

Because of their anatomic location and high-frequency vibration, the vocal folds and larynx have been difficult to examine and study, a fact that delayed research on these important structures in the past. Increased knowledge of the normal functions of the larynx and the availability of new diagnostic tools and new means of analyzing laryngeal function have greatly enhanced scientists' ability to understand the disorders that affect the vocal and swallowing mechanisms. Important progress has been made in diagnosing and treating neoplasms and other lesions of the larynx while preserving function. Less progress has been made toward understanding the molecular basis of laryngeal disorders, especially trauma and scarring. Molecular biological studies of the processes that control wound healing, scar contraction, inflammation and neurogenic abnormalities offer important opportunities for dealing with these problems.

The most prevalent voice disorders result from the way in which the voice is produced. Research is providing new insights into how damage occurs to the vocal mechanism in misuse and abuse of the voice. With that information, early identification and prevention of these voice disorders can be improved. Significant progress has been made in identifying causes of chronic recurring inflammation of the larynx. Important information is being obtained about viral and other infections that cause life-threatening diseases. This work has pointed out important opportunities for further research.

Significant progress has been made in understanding the neural control of the larynx and how it is disturbed by disease. These insights have been translated into more effective treatment for several disorders, such as Parkinson's disease and dystonia. These findings have pointed out important opportunities for research that could lead to great improvements in the treatment of neural abnormalities of phonation and swallowing. Understanding of the growth and control factors that influence the reinnervation of muscles could eventually result in relief for a large number of individuals who suffer from injuries to the laryngeal nerves.

Although progress made so far has been promising, the opportunities for better understanding of the disorders of the vocal system have barely been explored. These opportunities constitute a vital area of research that could lead to improved lives for many individuals.

Application of Technology to Prevention, Diagnosis and Treatment

Advances in technology have led to improvement in the prevention, diagnosis and treatment of disorders of the vocal tract. There has been a steady improvement in technology applicable to molecular and clinical research on disorders that affect voice, swallowing and respiration. Clinicians treating swallowing and voice disorders now have easier access to technologically advanced measurement and analytic computing tools that are useful in the diagnosis and treatment of voice and swallowing disorders. The use of new imaging modalities such as synchronized videostroboscopy, high-speed digital imaging of vocal fold vibration and dynamic magnetic resonance imaging is making it easier to evaluate vocal tract disorders. The widespread use of laryngeal electromyography has led to improved electrodiagnosis of vocal tract abnormalities. Multimodality applications of electrodiagnostic, physiologic and acoustic measurements are now available for the investigation of the normal and abnormal states of voicing and swallowing.

New surgical techniques have been developed to improve the voice and alter voice quality. Restoration of voice after complete loss of voice as a result of cancer or trauma may now be achieved with operations based on the innovative application of technology, including lasers, intralaryngeal framework surgery and new biocompatible implants. The implantation of nerve stimulators and artificial voice devices holds promise as methods for restoring the voice. Work continues on testing the feasibility of laryngeal transplantation in animal models. New voice therapy techniques have been developed to improve rehabilitation of the voice in a variety of disorders, including Parkinson's disease, postsurgical scarring and spasmodic dysphonia.

Augmentative communication and multimedia communication have been improved and offer a better quality of life to individuals with communication impairments. Improvements in speech analysis, synthesis and recognition should further improve technology transfer to industry and lead to clinical applications for people with voice disorders.

There have been advancements in the pharmacotherapeutic and behavioral control regimens for treatment of gastroesophageal reflux laryngitis, a common affliction in professional voice users. The efficacy of systemic and locally injected therapeutic agents has been demonstrated in ameliorating a variety of neurogenic, inflammatory, infectious and aging processes that have a negative impact on the voice. The side effects of common medications on the voice also are being recognized more frequently. In individuals with voice disorders, multidisciplinary evaluation and treatment are usually a more effective approach to delivering voice care.

Recognition of the effects of systemic disease, medication, smoking and environmental toxins on vocal and swallowing function has led to improved efforts at prevention.

The harmful effects of pollution and environmental toxins on vocal health are increasingly being recognized in industrialized urban

421

centers. Similarly, the deleterious effect of smoking on the larynx is well recognized.

Recent Accomplishments

Normal Structure and Function

Anatomy, Cellular and Molecular Biology, and Genetics

Progress is being made in understanding brain function in vocal control through the use of noninvasive techniques such as positron emission tomography and transcranial magnetic stimulation of the cerebral cortex. Both techniques are demonstrating that cortical control over laryngeal muscles is predominantly located in the left hemisphere. In addition, there has been direct electrical stimulation of the cerebral cortex in individuals undergoing neurologic surgery.

Progress has also been made in understanding the innervation of the larynx. One advance has resulted from the introduction of a nerve-tracing technique using Sihler's stain, which renders specimens of non-neural laryngeal tissue transparent while staining the nerve supply. Several novel observations have been made through the use of this technique.

Progress has been made in understanding the structure of human laryngeal muscles. Certain muscles have been found to be composed of several compartments that may have different functions. An important example is the thyroarytenoid muscle. This muscle, in the vocal fold, can be differentiated into two compartments, the muscularis and the vocalic, that may have different functions.

Organotypic cell cultures, composed of both epithelial and mesenchymal cells in a three-dimensional structure, permit near-normal epithelial differentiation. Application of this technique to primary laryngeal epithelial cells has provided insight into the plasticity of the adult human laryngeal epithelium. A single culture of cells can be induced to differentiate along two different pathways, forming either a ciliated columnar or stratified squamous epithelium, as a function of concentrations of retinoic acid in the medium.

The molecular basis for structure and function of cells and tissues is rapidly being defined. Advances in this area include the identification of the role of cell-surface receptors, their ligands, and the subsequent activation of multiple complex signal transduction pathways. The advent of molecular biologic technology has made it possible to study genetic material and identify genetic factors involved in normal development. The Human Genome Project, with its exponential increases in the information in sequence databases, continues to enhance rapidly scientists' ability to identify and clone genes of interest for any tissue. These advances can provide the framework for the definition of the molecular basis of the development and function of the respiratory tract.

Development and Lifespan Alterations

Current knowledge of embryology consists of well-defined descriptions of the stages of laryngeal development in several species, including humans.

Detailed anatomic measurements of the normal larynx have been performed. These studies have shown that the internal structure of the vocal folds is not the same in young children as it is in adults. For example, young children lack a fully developed vocal ligament and have different elastin content in the vocal fold muscle. Current acoustic, aerodynamic and kinematic research is examining the functional consequences of different anatomic structures. Children's physiologic mechanisms for controlling pitch, loudness and vocal quality are different from those of adults. Comparative descriptions have contributed to the study of the structure and function of the human larynx. In particular, ongoing investigations are addressing the neuro-development of the larynx.

Critical periods for optimum development of vocal control, as well as periods when a speaker may be at risk for developing dysphonia, have been recognized, but they have not been completely studied. The critical periods that are particularly important for the prevention and treatment of voice disorders include infancy, childhood, puberty and other life-cycle stages characterized by hormonal changes. The onset of a hearing impairment or work in a noisy environment may produce critical periods for the development of voice disorders.

Hormones (growth hormone, androgens and estrogens) affect voice development. Studies have shown that they alter adult pitch; for example, androgen therapy in postmenopausal women lowers the fundamental frequency. Masculinizing neoplasms, male hormone therapy, pregnancy and menopause result in edematous changes in the larynx. Animal studies have shown that androgens alter laryngeal muscle-fiber properties. Molecular biology studies of androgen-regulated laryngeal muscle and cartilage differentiation have shown that two androgen mRNA receptor isoforms are expressed at various stages of the masculine development program in the *Xenopus laevis* model system. These receptors may play a regulatory role in the onset of androgen-mediated myosin expression and cell addition during laryngeal maturation. The effect of androgens on proliferation, survival, synaptic connectivity and function of laryngeal motor neurons is also being studied.

Recent studies have shown that endocrine-type cells in the larynx and trachea express a variety of peptides. Serotonin, calcitonin gene-related peptide and calcitonin appear during development. The significance of these cells is not understood.

Gender Differences. Gender differences in vocal production are currently under investigation. Research has shown that alterations in estrogen and progesterone levels cause cytologic and physiologic changes in the vocal folds. Reinke's edema has been shown to have an increased incidence in postmenopausal women. There is an increased incidence of vocal fold nodules in women. Differences in glottal configuration have been noted between women and men and deserve further investigation. Preliminary work on breathing during speech has resulted in controversy about functional differences between women and men.

Lifestyle and Cultural Influences. Although studies have demonstrated the association of alcohol and tobacco use with cancers of the oropharynx and larynx, relatively little is known about other lifestyle or cultural influences (diet, drug use and exercise) on the function of the laryngeal, respiratory and upper aerodigestive systems. In general, the degree to which these factors lead to deterioration of the structure and function of the pharynx and larynx and vocal quality has not been clearly determined.

Role of Auditory Feedback in the Development and Maintenance of Vocal Control. Individuals with congenital and late-onset hearing impairment display phonation-induced disorders that include voicing errors for consonants, poor voice quality and suprasegmental anomalies of pitch and loudness. Such phonation-related abnormalities have been linked to deficits in the control and coordination of both the laryngeal and respiratory systems. For example, voice-quality aberrations (such as excessive breathiness) in individuals with hearing impairment have been linked to underadduction of the vocal folds, and deviant phrasing has been attributed to air wastage owing to incoordination between the laryngeal and respiratory systems.

Results from recent studies of vocal function in adults and children who are deaf and have received cochlear implants have served to reinforce the importance of auditory feedback in the development and maintenance of vocal control; that is, the acquisition and recovery of vocal control seem to be aided by the auditory feedback provided by cochlear implantation.

Aging

Research has revealed specific anatomical, physiological and biochemical alterations that occur with maturation of the upper aerodigestive system. Laryngeal position and configuration change during development and with aging. Swallowing is also affected by aging. Prolongation of oral transit times and delay in initiating the pharyngeal phase of swallowing have been defined in the elderly. Changes in laryngeal muscle contraction behaviors with maturation also have been reported.

Neurophysiologic studies to examine laryngeal mechanoreceptor (sensory) activity are in progress and will provide better understanding of the neural changes that occur as the larynx ages. In addition, studies of the human superior laryngeal nerves have revealed a large, selective loss of the smallest nerve fibers. This finding may help to explain the age-related dysfunction of laryngeal protection of the airway against aspiration.

A series of histochemical, ultrastructural and stereological studies have been initiated to investigate the aging human larynx and its innervation. Studies of comparative models have demonstrated a number of changes in morphologic parameters that are likely to play key roles in the mechanisms underlying age-related laryngeal dysfunction. Prenatal development of the mouse larynx has been shown to pass through critical stages similar to those in human laryngeal development. Investigations using the murine model make it possible to manipulate the factors thought to have a role in regulating development and aging. In addition, the increasing number of transgenic and knockout mouse lines provides a wealth of possibilities for investigations of the anatomical, cellular and biochemical changes that accompany lifespan changes.

The cellular biology of the upper aerodigestive system also has been found to change with age. Morphological, biochemical and immunohistochemical techniques are being used to examine the distribution of the various types of collagens, other extracellular matrix proteins and basement membrane zone components in the developing and adult larynx.

Muscle Atrophy. It is known that muscle tissue gradually degenerates with age. The main reasons for the degeneration include (1) paralysis of the vasomotor fibers of the sympathetic nerves supplying the muscles, (2) decreased blood supply, (3) decreased levels of mitochondrial enzymes and glycogen and (4) overall reduced metabolic capabilities. This degenerative process involves the age-related death of motoneurons with subsequent reinnervation of denervated muscle fibers by the surviving motoneurons. Since this remodeling can alter the number of muscle fibers innervated by each of the surviving motoneurons, it can contribute to changes in motor control. In addition, the muscle fibers may undergo age-related atrophy, hypertrophy or cell death, which may be specific to the muscle-fiber type.

Deterioration of Joints, Ligaments, Membranes and Other Tissues of the Laryngeal, Pulmonary and Secretory Systems. Vocal deterioration or swallowing disorders may result from restrictions in the movement of the glottal structures, as well as from reductions in lubrication. Specifically, the cricoarytenoid joint, which subserves vocal fold abduction and adduction, can lose its freedom of movement if the capsule of the joint deteriorates. Changes in articular cartilage with thinning and irregularities of the articular surface have been noted with age. Further arthritic changes can result in a joint that is fixed.

Stiffness and lack of elasticity limit the pliability of the aging larynx. This state affects the membranous cover of the vocal fold which results in less motion of the mucosal wave. With vocal stress, the vocal mechanism is less resilient.

Atrophy of mucus-producing glands with aging can lead to changes in the fluid layer of the vocal folds, making normal-quality phonation more difficult.

Biomechanics of the Larynx and Upper Aerodigestive Tract During Vocalization, Respiration and Swallowing

Biomechanics of the Larynx. Biomechanics is concerned with the passive and dynamic characteristics of laryngeal tissues and how these tissues interact to cause motion. The biomechanical problems of the larynx are unique since the vocal folds vibrate. A wide variety of experimental techniques have been applied to the study of vocal fold vibration. Ongoing research is directly or indirectly examining vocal fold vibration in human subjects. Another series of experiments is examining comparative models of vocal fold vibration. Research also is being carried out on excised larynges and on mechanical and theoretical models of vocal fold vibration. All of these studies seek to understand the complex aerodynamics and tissue interactions that produce vocal fold vibration.

Control of Pitch, Loudness and Vocal Quality. Recent investigations have used aerodynamic, acoustic, kinematic, electromyographic, analog and mathematical models to study the control of pitch, loudness and vocal quality. Primary mechanisms for controlling pitch include activity of the intrinsic and extrinsic laryngeal muscles, as well as subglottal pressure. Factors that affect fundamental frequency include vocal fold stiffness (vocal fold tension) and mass. Recently, other factors have been identified that can affect the elastic and stiffness components of the vocal folds: metabolic factors such as nutrients, hydration and temperature, and population factors such as gender and age.

The active and passive forces that contribute to the control of fundamental frequency are also those that serve to alter vocal intensity. In this case, a major force responsible for intensity control is subglottal pressure or the aerodynamic power used to drive the larynx. The control of the aerodynamic power also is regulated by glottal configuration. For example, current research using functional and comparative models has indicated that glottal width is an important variable. Loudness also can be varied by adjusting the supraglottal cavity (pharynx, oral and nasal cavities). Recent research in these areas has focused on the interaction of respiratory, laryngeal and supralaryngeal components for controlling pitch and loudness.

Control of vocal quality is not as clearly defined but is typically described as consisting of various mixes of frequency and intensity components. Examples of terms used to describe vocal quality are "hoarse," "harsh," "breathy," and "register." "Register" has been used to describe different vocal qualities over similar pitch ranges. Terms associated with registers are "pulse" (fry), "modal" (chest) and "loft" (falsetto).

Vocal-Tract Component Interactions. The traditional view of the speech mechanism is that it consists of three systems: the respiratory system, the laryngeal system and the supralaryngeal system. Because of this approach to describing the speech mechanism, investigators historically have tended to treat the three systems as independent functioning mechanisms. More recently though, an emphasis has been placed on studying the interaction of these three systems. The pulmonary and laryngeal components of respiration have a common neural control mechanism so that the vagal-volume response simultaneously regulates thoraco-abdominal and laryngeal muscle functions. Recent aerodynamic studies using both comparative and human models have investigated the simultaneous function of passive forces (subglottal and supraglottal pressures) and active muscular forces (laryngeal muscles) affecting glottal resistance during speech, singing and swallowing.

Swallowing. Swallowing consists of a set of complex muscular actions in the oral, pharyngeal, laryngeal and esophageal regions that are integrated into a functional pattern to prepare and transport food while simultaneously protecting the airway. As such, swallowing is viewed not as one behavior but as a set of coordinated behaviors that vary in their temporal and kinematic characteristics.

The application of electromyography, endoscopy, manometry and combined techniques (such as videofluoroscopy and manometry with computer image analysis) continue to offer new insights and provide more accurate details concerning normal swallowing mechanisms. The physiology of the upper esophageal sphincter has received special attention relative to the mechanisms of opening. The major elements responsible for opening the upper esophageal sphincter have been defined as (1) relaxation of the cricopharyngeal muscle; (2) anterior and vertical laryngeal movement, which opens the sphincter and (3) bolus pressure, which modulates the width of the opening. Recent work has also further specified the influence of bolus variables (for example, volume, viscosity and temperature) on swallowing function. In addition, there have been ongoing efforts to document more fully the nature and extent of normal volitional control over important components of swallowing function, including laryngeal movement, cricopharyngeal opening and airway closure.

Results from recent simultaneous studies of swallowing and respiration have further served to delineate the well-timed pattern between respiratory and swallowing events, including the timing of swallows relative to the respiratory cycle and apneic (breath-holding) interval durations.

Progress continues to be made in efforts to understand the central and peripheral neural control of swallowing. Studies of peripheral control have involved humans and other mammals. Most of the work on central control has been carried out in nonhuman mammals. Recordings from peripheral nerves and muscles and stimulation of peripheral nerves and their receptive fields have provided new information on the sensory receptive fields that evoke or facilitate swallowing. Studies of central control have involved ablation studies, electrical stimulation of and recordings from central neural tissue and the application of pharmacologic agents and immunochemical techniques. These various techniques are serving to provide insights into the general organization of the central swallowing pathway.

Recent studies have begun to examine potential changes that may occur in swallowing function with normal aging. From this work, evidence is emerging that normal aging alters some aspects of swallowing function, including increased oral and pharyngeal transit times, increased magnitudes and durations of pharyngeal pressures and a higher incidence of pharyngeal residue after swallowing.

Comparative and Theoretical Models of Voicing

Comparative Models. Comparative models are an irreplaceable resource for studying the basic processes of voicing. Research is examining the ways in which some species use their vocalizations for social purposes, the basic "grammar" of these vocalizations and how the vocalizations change throughout development. Other investigations seek to understand what aspects of vocalization are lateralized to the left cerebral hemisphere and how they are disrupted by lesions similar to human strokes. Research also is examining how some species learn certain vocalizations. This research is examining what is genetic and what is learned in these vocalizations and how they may reflect a primitive version of human language. Related research is being done on how the brain areas subserving emotion are related to vocalization areas. Ongoing research is investigating the interaction of subcortical structures (periaqueductal gray area) with the nucleus ambiguous in voicing control. This research integrates many different experimental levels: recording, stimulation, neural tracing and ablation of identified cells, and the correlation of these manipulations with vocalization. Other research is studying the mechanism by which subcortical structures (medial geniculate nucleus) distinguish vocalization from other, albeit similar, sounds.

Progress has been made in understanding the sensory physiology of the larynx and pharynx. Recordings have been made from single neurons in the superior laryngeal nerve while changes in pressure and temperature and other variables are applied to isolated regions of the laryngopharynx. Similar research is characterizing the proprioceptive feedback to the brain during phonation.

The structure and biomechanics of the larynx are being studied in a variety of research projects. The intramuscular fluid pressure for different laryngeal muscles is being examined as an indicator of

429

muscle function. This technique may allow small regions of contraction to be measured more accurately and may have advantages over electromyography, in which localization and quantification of muscle contraction can be difficult. Various projects are examining the aerodynamic and mechanical forces in larynges *in vitro* and *in vivo*. This line of research seeks to understand the basic mechanisms of vocal fold vibration. Finally, experiments in lower vertebrates are using the vocalization system as a tool for studying basic brain mechanisms such as learning, memory, motor control, and lateralization and genetic, hormonal, and environmental influences on brain structure and function.

Computational Analysis, Modeling and Speech Synthesis. Methods of computer simulation of vocal fold vibration have been effectively used to compare physiologic mechanisms and their control of acoustic signal characteristics. Modern computers make possible the three-dimensional, realistic simulation of vocal activities in real time. A parametric model that characterizes normal voice source signals has been developed and used as a mathematical framework for voice analysis and synthesis.

Exceptional Vocal Behavior

A majority of research on the exceptional voice has dealt with trained singers. There has been an increased use of quantitative methods (that is, objective measures of vocal function, the application of vocal fold and tract modeling and use of voice synthesis) to provide insights into the physical mechanisms that underlie the perception of singing-voice quality, as well as such singing phenomena as the singer's formant and vibrato.

Other studies have sought to compare the vocal capabilities of trained singers with those of nonsingers. Results of this work indicate that trained singers tend to have greater vocal capabilities in the form of larger frequency (pitch) and intensity ranges than nonsingers. In addition, trained singers display higher vocal efficiency than nonsingers, as evidenced by studies showing that singers can produce higher levels of vocal intensity than nonsingers while expending equivalent amounts of aerodynamic energy.

A growing awareness of the special vocal capabilities and behaviors of trained singers has led to recent efforts to include trained singers as special groups in research studies and descriptive databases; that is, to generate separate normative group data for trained singers that can be used in evaluating the voices of individuals who have had singing training.

Advances in the Diagnosis and Treatment of Voice Disorders

Population- and Outcome-Based Research

Existing data indicate that voice disorders affect three to 10 percent of the population in the United States, and an even greater percentage of school-age children and senior citizens. Use of the voice is one of the forms of human communication that is vital for quality of life; loss of the voice is devastating and may be associated with severe depression, stress and withdrawal. The voice also is essential to the functioning of the national economy. Within the working population of the United States, 28 million workers have jobs that require voice use, and 3.8 million have occupations in which voice use is essential for public safety (for example, air traffic controllers, pilots and police).

Data on the incidence of various types of voice and swallowing disorders currently are available primarily from retrospective reviews of selected populations of individuals who have been treated. Extensive data on neoplasms of the vocal tract are available from tumor registries and population databases. Misuse, abuse and overuse (hyperfunction) disorders causing vocal fold nodules, polyps, edema, and dysphonia are prevalent, and they have been cited in numerous studies. Voice and swallowing disorders in association with neurogenic diseases are common; they include Parkinson's disease, amyotrophic lateral sclerosis, multiple sclerosis, stroke and closed head injury. Neoplasms of the vocal tract affect 1,500 children and 50,000 adults annually and result in 5,000 deaths, accounting for two percent of all cancer deaths. Vocal tract neoplasms are associated with tobacco and alcohol use, but the recent identification of potential viral and genetic variables provides new opportunities to explore the interaction of these factors within the population. An apparent increase in death rates among women, African-American and Hispanic-American subpopulations is of concern. Population-based studies that analyze contributing variables remain to be carried out.

Congenital and Acquired Structural Lesions

Congenital and acquired lesions result in serious dysfunction of the vocal, swallowing and breathing mechanisms in thousands of infants, children and adults each year. Such life-threatening disorders include cysts, webs, scarring, lack of normal development and tumors. As the treatment of life-threatening disorders improves, the consequences of interventions (for example, scarring or subglottic stenosis from prolonged intubation) become evident. Important advances have been made in the early detection and diagnosis of congenital and acquired structural lesions of the larynx and pharynx; they include the use of telescopes and fiberoptic technology. The early diagnosis of laryngeal and pharyngeal cancers and other neoplasms is possible in almost all cases if the individual can be evaluated when first experiencing symptoms. Office endoscopy with documentation of the examination has improved the accuracy of diagnosis and follow-up of individuals with neoplasms and other lesions of the larynx without the need for endoscopy under general anesthesia. This improvement has reduced the cost and morbidity of caring for individuals with these disorders. Important progress has been made in developing an understanding of how vocal nodules and polyps develop, and early diagnosis of abnormal phonation patterns offers the possibility of prevention of vocal nodules and polyps.

Major advances have been made in the treatment of non-neoplastic congenital and acquired structural lesions such as subglottic stenosis. New approaches to laryngotracheal reconstruction have greatly improved the mortality rate in children affected with this disorder. New laser technology is available for treating subglottic hemangiomas in infants and papillomas in children and adults.

Laryngeal and respiratory tract papillomas are benign neoplasms in children and adults that are caused by human papilloma virus infection. These neoplasms may rapidly obstruct the airway. Prevention of death from suffocation often requires repeated surgical removal of the papillomas, sometimes every few weeks. The scarring from repeated surgical procedures frequently results in permanent voice damage, even though the neoplasms are controlled. Recent advances in the understanding of recurrent respiratory papillomatosis should eventually improve management of this disease. Abnormal response to growth factors appears to be important in papilloma proliferation and contributes to the failure to differentiate into normal tissue. Genetic susceptibility to development of neoplasms after papillomavirus infection also has been identified. Several clinical trials are currently under way to evaluate alternative or adjunctive therapies for respiratory papillomatosis. These experimental approaches include the use of interferon, ribavirin and photodynamic therapy with new photosensitizers.

Numerous recent studies have explored the possible role of human viruses in the development of head and neck cancers. Epstein-Barr virus is associated with nasopharyngeal cancers. It appears that the human papillomaviruses are present in perhaps 30 percent of neoplasms of the vocal tract, and that these viruses may play a significant role in cancers of the tonsils, base of the tongue and adenoids. In contrast, human papillomaviruses appear to be present in only two to five percent of other head and neck cancers. Therefore, even among mucosal squamous cell carcinomas there are probably differences in the specific mechanisms of malignant transformation. Important questions about the mechanisms of specific tissue susceptibility to viruses and other carcinogens demonstrate the need to study the role of environmental and genetic cofactors in the etiology of specific types of head and neck cancers.

Important and constant progress has been made in the early detection of cancers of the larynx and pharynx. Genetic markers for several different types of malignancies have been identified, and these markers can now be detected in cells from the respiratory tract by using molecular biology methods. This new finding provides the potential for very early detection of preneoplastic and neoplastic lesions and potentially can be used to monitor the progression and recurrence of cancer. Progress has been made in the identification of specific proteins that are expressed in cancers, and may provide opportunities for screening tests for early identification and new targets for therapy.

There have been important advances in treatment for individuals with precancers and early cancers. The efficacy of conservation surgery has been demonstrated, and reconstruction has been refined to improve the options available in individuals with cancer of the vocal tract. Treatment of laryngeal cancers with combination chemotherapy and radiation therapy has shown promising results in sparing the functions of the larynx without compromising survival. Retinoids may have promise in the chemoprevention of cancers in individuals at increased risk for vocal tract cancers. Photodynamic therapy is being tested as a treatment for superficial malignancies of the pharynx and larynx. Important progress has been made in the ability to diagnose and treat swallowing dysfunction after treatment of vocal tract cancers, and research on evaluation of the swallowing function has been translated into the training of therapists who can be effective in the rehabilitation of individuals with swallowing dysfunction. Important progress has also been achieved in the development of prostheses for the production of speech in individuals who have undergone laryngectomy.

Some scientists believe there is a relationship between chronic or recurrent irritation and development of epithelial tumors. Gastroesophageal reflux—or more accurately, gastropharyngeal reflux—is now recognized as commonly associated with chronic laryngeal problems and recurring inflammation. Signs of gastropharyngeal reflux include chronic sore throat and dryness, hoarseness, chronic cough, chronic throat clearing, and contact ulcers. An entirely new understanding has emerged of the role of gastropharyngeal reflux of stomach acid in causing inflammatory disease of the larynx. This finding has resulted from investigators having a greatly enhanced ability to view the posterior larynx and glottic wall and to appreciate color differences. The use of magnifying telescopes with superior light-carrying fiber optics has led to greatly improved recognition of posterior chronic laryngitis as a very common disorder. This has enhanced the 'ability of clinicians to prevent inflammation in individuals who are at higher risk of complications during and after surgical procedures.

New phonosurgical procedures have been developed to treat voice disorders caused by paralysis, aging and scarring. Phonosurgery is a new surgical discipline specifically designed to improve the voice. Helped by better assessment techniques and better understanding of pathophysiology of voice production, new phonosurgery may be anticipated.

One of the major problems in treating individuals who have had laryngeal disease is dealing with glottic insufficiency. There are now a number of new phonosurgical procedures available to augment the position and shape of the vocal folds to improve the control of airflow and quality of voice in individuals who have experienced damage to the larynx or its nerve supply. Advances have been made in the application of objective measurements developed through basic voice research to the evaluation of the efficacy of these techniques. There has been important growth in the amount of research on the ways in which diseases and disorders of the larynx affect voice and other important functions of the larynx.

Trauma

Progress has been achieved in the reconstruction of tracheal defects, but there remains a need for more research on better treatment of the life-threatening problems in the airway that can result from trauma.

Although important research has been undertaken to improve methods of dealing with scarring of the larynx after injury or surgical treatment, more work needs to be done. There have not been major changes in clinicians' ability to treat trauma of the vocal tract, and there are great opportunities for research in this key area.

Neural Lesions and Disorders

Neural-based laryngeal problems account for a substantial portion of all voice and swallowing disorders. Voice and swallowing disorders may be the first sign of a neurogenic disease, including peripheral disorders such as laryngeal paralysis or central disorders such as Parkinson's disease, amyotrophic lateral sclerosis, multiple sclerosis, dystonia, closed head injury and stroke. Symptoms of neural voice disorders may range from a mild reduction in vocal quality to a severe reduction in speech intelligibility.

Major improvements have been achieved in ways to evaluate and diagnose neural disorders of the larynx. Being able to view and record the movements of the larynx has improved investigators' understanding of how particular neural disorders affect laryngeal functions. Acoustic, glottographic, aerodynamic and electromyographic techniques have emerging roles in the documentation and diagnosis of neural laryngeal disorders. Progress has been made in the treatment of some neural disorders of the larynx, such as Parkinson's disease and focal laryngeal dystonia.

Peripheral Disorders. Injuries to the laryngeal nerves affect the larynx and upper aerodigestive tract. Injuries to the recurrent laryngeal nerve results in paralysis of the vocal fold. The most frequent causes of the injury are operations of the skull base, neck and chest. Tumors, radiation treatment or infections along the path of the vagus nerve also can affect laryngeal function, producing alterations of phonation, airway protection and respiration. Unilateral laryngeal paralysis can result in hoarseness and aspiration owing to incomplete closure of the vocal folds. Compensatory behavior may include hyperadduction of the mobile vocal fold and associated structures. Bilateral paralysis is potentially life threatening because the airway may be compromised. Vocal fold paresis or paralysis also may accompany peripheral neuromuscular disorders such as myotonic muscular dystrophy and myasthenia gravis.

Central Disorders. Laryngeal dysfunction accompanying disorders of the central nervous system is now being studied in relation to problems with vocal fold closure and steadiness. Parkinson's disease, closed head injury and multiple sclerosis are examples of neurologic disorders that may result in limited vocal fold closure (hypoadduction) and reduced vocal loudness. Dystonia and Huntington's disease are examples of neurologic disorders that may result in increased vocal fold closure (hyperadduction) and tight "pressed" voice. Vocal unsteadiness includes tremor, voice breaks or hoarseness. Vocal tremor accompanies a number of neural disorders including essential tremor, Parkinson's disease and cerebellar disorders. The voice disorders accompanying these diseases may severely reduce the individual's ability to communicate. The swallowing disorders associated with these diseases may significantly limit the individual's oral intake of nutrients.

Systemic Disorders Affecting the Larynx and Upper Aerodigestive Tract

Systemic disorders can alter the function of the vocal system. They include effects of pharmacotherapeutic agents for unrelated diseases, hormone fluctuations and imbalances, connective tissue diseases and genetically determined keratin disorders. A key advance has been the growing awareness that these factors have a profound effect on voice production and swallowing. Hormone receptors have been identified on laryngeal epithelium, and the tissues clearly respond to hormone changes associated with endocrine disorders, hormonal therapy for diseases and age-related changes. The impact of connective tissue disorders, including arthritis, lupus and sarcoidosis, has been recognized, but more research is needed to define mechanisms and management of these diseases. The continuously increasing use of drugs for nonvoice disorders will have increasing effects on the vocal system. These effects need to be considered in drug evaluations and usage. Diseases of keratin structure and function, generally considered as skin diseases, also impact the epithelium of the larynx. Transgenic mice that mimic these keratin disorders have recently been developed. They will be useful in studying the effects of expression of specific keratin gene mutations on vocal tract epithelia.

Psychogenic Disorders of the Larynx and Upper Aerodigestive Tract

Psychogenic disorders of the larynx and upper aerodigestive tract are encountered occasionally in the clinical setting. However, because they are often not well understood etiologically, accurate incidence data are not available. It is estimated that the incidence may be from 4.4 percent to more than 30 percent, depending upon ages included in a given survey and definitions utilized. For example, hyperfunctional vocal fold behaviors and laryngeal disorders resulting from vocal abuse may be clustered with a psychologic disorder such as a conversion reaction. It should be noted that data on the incidence of various psychogenic voice disorders are primarily available from retrospective reviews of clinical cases.

Psychogenic disorders may be primary disorders or may be secondary to a loss of communication skills. Disorders of a psychogenic nature include aberrant breath control, pitch, loudness and quality of the voice, as well as muscle tension dysfunction, vocal fold hypofunction and paradoxical vocal fold adduction. It is often difficult to distinguish voice symptoms caused by a psychogenic problem from those evidenced by an idiopathic organic disorder. For example, a conversion aphonia is the manipulation of psychologic stress into a physical manifestation—in this case, no voice.

Misuse and Abuse Disorders

Disorders of misuse, abuse and overuse are the most prevalent and preventable of the voice disorders. They represent a reported 25 percent of adult disorders in otolaryngology practice and 36 percent of children treated for speech disorders. Vocal misuse or abuse implies a mode of vocal production that places undue strain or stress on the structures participating in the production of the voice. The result may be frank changes or damage to the tissues of the vocal folds and related structures, resulting in dysphonia.

Vocal misuse implies inappropriate breath-control pattern, pitch, loudness or quality inappropriate for the individual's laryngeal mechanism, placing strain on the system. Vocal abuse is typified by loud vocalization, throat clearing, chronic coughing or excessive vocalization without periods of vocal rest. Overuse is the ongoing use of the voice for long periods of time with insufficient rest or the use of the voice over a shorter time in abusive ways. Risk factors include loud talking in a noisy, smoke-filled or dry atmosphere, chronic coughing, throat clearing and use of an inappropriate habitual speaking posture. Many forms of vocal abuse are associated with disease processes such as upper respiratory infection, asthma and gastroesophageal reflux that may increase the tendency to cough. Some medications prescribed for asthma, for example, may actually contribute to reduced efficiency of the vibrating structure. This condition may lead to chronic abuse or increased tension in vocalization and subsequent vocal fold irritation or swelling. These vocal behaviors cause a variety of lesions, including vocal nodules, polyps, hemorrhage, polypoid degeneration, chronic edema and vocal fatigue. Further, toxic environmental elements in the workplace have been shown to contribute to allergy and upper respiratory disease that, in turn, may lead to chronic cough and vocal fold irritation. Studies that lead to a better understanding of the anatomy and physiology of the vocal mechanism have been useful in furthering knowledge of this category of voice disorders. For example, histologic studies of the larynx, defining the ultrastructure of the vocal fold in injury, suggest that vocal nodules are the result of damage to basement membrane zone structures.

Influencing Variables

Multicultural Issues. Much of what is known about vocal diversity and pathology across races or cultures is based upon clinical observations, anecdotal evidence and doctoral dissertations. Therefore, our current responses to even the most basic queries in this area of communication disorders are limited to pitch and its physical correlate, fundamental frequency, which appears to have garnered most of the research focus, and to clinical data on disorders associated with specific lesions. It is likely that non-Caucasian and non-European individuals participated in surveys and large-scale studies of voice disorders. However, the pertinence of cultural identity and ethnicity, including religious values and observances, nutrition, attitude toward medicine and illness was not noted or reported.

Hoarseness continues to be the predominant dysphonia in children up to age 18, with vocal nodules being the most frequent cause of hoarseness. Evidence suggests that African-American youngsters from economically depressed inner cities exhibit more than twice the incidence of hoarseness than do Caucasian children in other communities, and Hispanic-American teenagers from southern California have more than twice the incidence of dysphonia as Caucasian adolescents in the same or similar communities. The oncology literature offers an uneven distribution of laryngeal carcinoma across race.

The Surveillance, Epidemiology, and End Results (SEER) Program of the National Cancer Institute (NCI) has gathered current and comprehensive data on United States incidence and survival statistics since 1973 in nine regions or registries (Atlanta, Connecticut, Detroit, Hawaii, Iowa, New Mexico, San Francisco, Seattle and Utah). It contains an analysis of Caucasian, African-American, Native-American and Asian/Pacific Islander-American populations for a multitude of cancer sites. SEER findings indicate that the African-American population has an incidence rate for laryngeal cancer 50 percent higher than the Caucasian population, with the higher incidence spanning all age categories above 25 years. There is an even higher incidence for Hispanic Americans over age 65, and a relatively low incidence of laryngeal cancer in Native Americans.

These SEER findings may have cultural implications as well. Choices of diet and lifestyle factors, attitude toward illness, and the use of medical practitioners and medicines are culturally based, and adequate medical services may be limited in large portions of non-Caucasian and non-European ethnic populations of American society. Ethnic rather than racial analysis might provide more valuable insight into risk factors in culturally diverse populations in the United States.

Gender. Male and female voices differ acoustically and perceptually, and there are clear gender differences in laryngeal and respiratory anatomy and physiology. Hormonal, metabolic and genetic factors differ by gender. Menstruation and pregnancy cause changes in fluid retention in the vocal folds and in the degree of dryness of the mucosal lining of the respiratory tract. Vocal fold edema and increased risk of hemorrhage have also been observed during menses. Women seek treatment with greater frequency than men for many voice disorders, including vocal nodules, spasmodic dysphonia, Reinke's edema and changes in pitch range and quality. On the other hand, contact granuloma and contact ulcers are more often observed in men.

Psychosocial and cultural factors that affect men and women differently also affect vocal health. They include diet and other aspects of lifestyle, use of medication, willingness to seek treatment and choice of occupation. Bulimia, which is predominantly a disease of young women, may damage the mucosal lining of the larynx. Occupations typically associated with women, such as teaching and aerobics instruction, appear to involve increased vocal stress, and men in sales tend to exhibit a higher incidence of benign vocal fold lesions than men in other careers. Society places vocal role expectations on both genders that can result in inappropriate pitch, loudness, vocal quality and breathing patterns.

Aging. People over the age of 65 years represent a growing and changing segment of American society. Increased longevity and activity increase the demand for an enduring voice. Age-related changes in the larynx include loss of elasticity and muscle tone, calcification of laryngeal cartilages and increased dryness of the mucosal lining. The most frequently observed vocal pathophysiology during these years is bowing of the vocal folds, although several neurogenically based conditions, including secondary voice problems, may also occur at this time. In addition, senior citizens may exhibit benign mucosal lesions of the vocal folds, as well as vocal fold swelling and hyperfunctional vocal fold activity owing to occupation and personality. Studies have shown that the voice of the elderly is characterized by a decrease in pitch in women and a slight increase in men. Reduction in loudness and altered vocal quality often occur. Although these changes may not be abnormal, voice therapy is sometimes sought to minimalize them.

Environment. Environmental factors are thought to cause or perpetuate voice disorders. Noise, air pollution (including gases, fumes and smoke) and relative humidity are factors that singularly or in combination may cause or maintain a particular disorder. Allergic reactions causing vocal disorders, which may be aggravated by ongoing environmental changes, are being reported with greater frequency.

Lifestyle. There is growing awareness of the effects of lifestyle including diet, smoking, rest and sleep, drug use, exercise and alcohol consumption on the functions of the larynx and upper aerodigestive tract. Gastroesophageal reflux causing throat and voice complaints can be controlled by changes in lifestyle and eating habits. This correlation implies a critical need for outcome research in voice disorder prevention, diagnosis and treatment.

Application of Technology to Prevention, Diagnosis and Treatment

Recent Advances in Electromyography

Electromyography of intrinsic and extrinsic laryngeal muscle activity has been used to investigate peripheral vocal fold paralysis, to diagnose spasmodic dysphonia and to differentiate myopathic from neuropathic disorders. The results have been used to understand the basis of both normal and pathologic speech processes. Bipolar hooked-wire electrodes have been used to investigate laryngeal kinesiology and are increasingly being applied in voice and swallowing investigations. In selected centers, multimodality recordings of simultaneous acoustic, electrophysiologic, aerodynamic and stroboscopic data are being applied to the study of normal and abnormal voicing gestures in individuals with and without dysphonia.

The fabrication and manufacture of implantable devices for pacing the nerves and muscles of the larynx have been accomplished. These devices are transfers of technology already in use in other implantable devices in the body, and they offer new areas for rehabilitation of the paralyzed larynx.

Intraoperative monitoring of laryngeal nerves during thyroid, neck and skull base surgery is being applied to attempt to decrease the risk of injury. Monitoring of the laryngeal and pharyngeal muscles for biofeedback is being done in dysphagia therapy and has important rehabilitation implications for individuals with head injury, neural injury and neuromotor system degeneration associated with the aging process.

Laryngeal and pharyngeal electromyography has had wide clinical application in the diagnosis of and botulism toxin treatment for movement disorders of the larynx and pharynx. For individuals with spasmodic dysphonia, tremor and stuttering, intralaryngeal injection of botulinum type A using electromyography monitoring now offers a new, less invasive treatment.

Chemodenervation with botulism toxin has also been used to treat disorders of the upper esophageal sphincter in selected individuals with dysphagia after stroke and head injury. These ongoing studies offer promise of new treatment for dysphagia.

Acoustic Signal Analysis

The acoustic signal is the most readily available, physical representation of voice and carries all perceptually significant information. Recent developments in technology permit fast and accurate analysis of acoustic signals. Effective acoustic signal analysis continues to be a useful quantitative tool for the evaluation and treatment of voice disorders. Acoustic recording and analysis are now routinely used in voice clinics. New signal processing chips and computer engines now provide clinicians with mainframe computing capabilities, thereby making it easier to quantify the voice. Low-cost digital audio tape technology and digital sound boards enable retrieval of voice samples quickly and accurately for analysis and research.

Imaging

Technologic advances have been achieved in the imaging of the larynx and pharynx. Imaging using real-time magnetic resonance imaging (MRI) has been improved in the last three years. Echo-planar MRI now allows viewing of the laryngeal and pharyngeal structures

441

in the coronal, axial and saggital planes with a sampling time of less than 100 milliseconds. Such applications in the evaluation of pharyngolaryngeal gestures, swallowing dysfunction and voice production problems hold great promise. Ultrasound has been used with increasing success for the evaluation of laryngeal anatomy and function. Scientists have used ultrasound successfully to demonstrate impairment in vocal fold function in the adult and pediatric population.

Imaging of the upper aerodigestive tract is currently most often performed with videofluoroscopic techniques. Combining videofluoroscopic imaging with various physiologic and electrophysiologic measures is now easily performed. These measures include videofluoroscopy and multichannel manometry in the study of swallowing and voice production. Laryngeal electromyography, airflow and videostroboscopy can now be combined with videofluoroscopy. Advances in signal acquisition and computer enhancement will likely reduce radiation dosage. Research should continue in all of these technologies to promote a greater understanding of the complex interactions of the upper aerodigestive tract.

Direct visualization of the laryngopharyngeal region continues to improve with advances in fiber-optic endoscopes and rigid telescopes. The widespread application of this technology has improved patient care and provided the means for direct observation of the larynx and pharynx. Further improvements should be pursued in this technology in the areas of image quality and analysis. Better techniques to quantitate three-dimensional laryngeal images and their changes through the glottal cycle must be developed, and meaningful applications of these images should be used in research and clinical settings.

Visualization of the larynx and its vibratory characteristics using videostroboscopy remains the most valuable tool for the assessment of vocal production and dysfunction. Quantification of the laryngeal image to correlate with other physiologic modalities should remain a high priority.

High-speed photography of the larynx with digital storage has been used to study problems such as voice break, diplophonia and those during voice onset gestures. These findings are being correlated with other physiologic data and hold promise for expanded clinical applications.

Various projects are exploring the use of laser light properties to track mucosal wave characteristics and to estimate absolute laryngeal image size. With lowering costs of computing, digital image analysis of laryngeal motion and vibratory function is now commercially available. The validity of these approaches should be verified. Advances also have been made in the use of radionuclear imaging for evaluating aspiration and swallowing function; such applications hold promise for better evaluation of aspiration and dysphagia.

Dynamic imaging during the formulation and production of language, voice and speech, which is based on increased blood flow during activation of areas of the brain involved in these functions, is under investigation through the use of positron emission tomography (PET). Functional imaging of the brain with MRI techniques also holds promise for such investigations. Differences in flow in certain regions of the two hemispheres of the brain have been identified in the development of sign language, in people who stutter, and following stroke. MRI angiography offers another potential tool for these studies. Fast spin echo MRI techniques have been used to reconstruct the vocal tract to study the effect of alterations in the supraglottic larynx on voice production and swallowing. These methods should be used to study other conditions, and new methods should be developed for imaging of the central nervous system in the study of voice, speech and language.

Improvements in the resolution of static computerized tomography (CT) and MRI have facilitated detection of the presence and extent of congenital and acquired lesions of the larynx, including neoplasms, inflammation and trauma. Two- and three-dimensional imaging have improved modeling for reconstruction of laryngeal trauma and planning of radiotherapy fields. Parameters have been defined for early diagnoses of nonpalpable regional lymph node metastases and correlation with clinical and pathologic findings. The clinical indications for these procedures and the utility of these results require further study.

PET and scintigraphy with radiolabeled monoclonal antibodies specific for tumor-associated antigens have been used to image malignant neoplasms of the upper aerodigestive tract, including the larynx and regional metastases. Improvement is needed in the sensitivity and specificity of these methods, and their potential role in diagnosis, staging and therapy should be determined.

Observations obtained by using a combination of these technologies should be correlated with each other and with measures from nonimaging techniques to develop appropriate models for understanding voice production.

Augumentative and Alternative Voice Sources

Augmentative or alternative communication can replace the speaking mechanism in congenital and acquired disorders of the larynx.

443

Advances have been made in the development of electronic communication aids, artificial larynges (external, internal and implantable) and in tracheoesophageal shunts (with and without alloplastic voice prostheses). Further study in this area is required. Also needed are efficacy studies to evaluate the relative benefits of these prostheses and to predict which prostheses are appropriate for various populations.

There has been increased recognition of the need for better augmentative communication devices in communicatively disadvantaged populations (low birth weight infants, individuals in the aging population and stroke victims). Advances have been made in augmentative communication devices for the postlaryngectomy population.

One of the major purposes of communication is to express affect or emotion. In the development of augmentative and alternative communication devices and aids, research is needed to develop more normal vocal quality so that the full meaning of vocal communication can be expressed.

There are now augmentative communication systems that have the ability to produce varied voices with multiple pitch ranges. New software has given augmentative communication users the ability to produce speech at a rate similar to that heard in normal conversation; the software incorporates a word prediction program that helps to speed the production of artificial speech. Improvement in the portability of augmentative communication devices provides users with a greater freedom of movement.

There has been increasing interest in forms of augmentative communication for individuals with autism. Further research into the effectiveness and validity of facilitated communication must be undertaken. Studies should be performed to evaluate ways of improving communication in the autistic adult and child.

As the mortality rate in low birth weight infants decreases, the consequences of aggressive intervention becomes apparent. Additional research is needed in ways to improve communication in certain populations, such as low birth weight infants, individuals with tracheostomies and the aged, who are at risk for significant alterations of voice production. Further research is needed to improve the use of augmentative communication in the pediatric population.

Surgical Technology

Recent methodologic developments have given surgeons the potential to alter the structure and improve the function of the larynx reliably. Investigation into the individual controlling variables of voice production has led to a better understanding of disorders of voice production and their treatment.

Phonosurgery enables surgeons to alter the laryngeal framework and its muscular function to improve vocal function. Laryngoplastic phonosurgery is designed to change the laryngeal framework to improve vocal function, and endoscopic phonosurgery of the vocal folds is designed to improve the voice. There have been advances in improving surgical technique in both areas. Research is needed to address the role of these technical advances and the outcome of laryngeal phonosurgery.

Improvement continues to be achieved in the use of laryngotracheal reconstruction, as measured by successful decannulation, to treat congenital and acquired laryngotracheal stenosis. However the effect of laryngotracheal reconstruction on vocal quality deserves further investigation. Research must address uniform methods for reporting voice and speech results in the pediatric population.

Surgical technology continues to advance with the refinement of instruments available for surgery of the vocal fold and the expanded use of lasers for treatment of vocal tract disorders. Newer laser wavelengths and the expanded use of existing lasers have led to improvement of surgical technique and reduction of complications such as scarring and abnormalities of vibratory function. Advances in the anesthetic management of patients have produced a variety of laser-safe endotracheal tubes, as well as improvements in anesthetic techniques that make possible more precise surgical control.

Intraoperative monitoring of the recurrent and superior laryngeal nerves as well as intraoperative monitoring of the voice during phonosurgery have helped to improve surgical outcomes.

There have been new developments in the fabrication of implantable electrode arrays for stimulation of the posterior cricoarytenoid muscle. These new devices offer promise as a tool for adjusting the servomechanism of the larynx. This technology has important potential applications. Implantable devices also are being developed in several major centers for rehabilitation of the paralyzed larynx. These devices with nerve-stimulating cuff electrodes have been implanted with success in animal models, and ongoing study is being carried out with the future goal of implantation in humans.

Aeromechanical and Respiratory Measures

Laryngeal disorders can disrupt the normal pattern of vocal fold valving during speech and affect respiratory patterns and aerodynamic events. For example, vocal nodules, polyps or vocal fold paralysis may

445

change the amplitude and shape of the glottal airflow waveform. These changes in the structure or function of the vocal folds also may change the respiratory and supraglottal aeromechanical activity. Recent studies support consideration of this interaction in the description, diagnosis and treatment of phonatory disorders. To date, few investigators have simultaneously observed speech and abnormal aeromechanical function of the respiratory and laryngeal components. Inverse filtering has made it possible to study the alternating and direct current components of the airflow signal, and this method is being evaluated for its usefulness in differential diagnosis and quantification of the effects of various phonatory treatments.

Behavioral Treatment

The goal of behavioral voice treatment is to maximize vocal effectiveness relative to an existing laryngeal disorder. Behavioral voice treatment may be undertaken (1) as the preferred treatment to resolve a voice disorder when surgery or pharmacotherapy is not indicated, (2) when recommended as the initial treatment in patients in whom medical treatment appears indicated and may obviate the need for surgery or (3) when recommended before and after laryngeal surgery to maximize the postsurgical voice.

Data exist to support the efficacy of techniques of behavioral voice treatment for disorders related to misuse and hyperfunction, medical or physical conditions and psychologic disorders. For example, there are data to support the efficacy of techniques designed to reduce vocal abuse to improve characteristics of the voice and to reduce the recurrence of laryngeal lesions. There are data to support the efficacy of techniques such as musculoskeletal tension reduction to elicit phonation in disorders associated with psychologic stress. Recently, the efficacy of techniques focusing on increased vocal fold adduction and respiratory support has been established in the treatment of the voice disorder accompanying Parkinson's disease. Although data on the efficacy of behavioral treatment have been obtained from group designs, case studies and retrospective analyses, there is still a need for additional comprehensive studies.

Molecular Biology

Recent advances in molecular biology have revolutionized the approach to many diseases and disorders. It is now possible to identify the regulatory factors that contribute to the causation of many diseases at a subcellular level, thereby facilitating precise diagnosis. For example, many steps in the progression of premalignant lesions can now be distinguished. Defects in development can now be studied at a level never before possible. Gene sequences in the Human Genome Project Database facilitate identifying the genetic basis of hereditary disorders. Knowledge of molecular pathology also opens the possibility of completely new approaches to treatment, such as gene therapy or the modulation of cell-surface receptors to alter cell function.

Psychophysical and Perceptual Measures

A great deal of work in the past has attempted to equate descriptive terms, such as "roughness" and "hoarseness," in the perceptual domain with recorded voice signals in the acoustic domain. Such efforts have been disappointing and appear not to have led to a productive endpoint. There are key parameters that must be taken into account in attempting to relate the acoustic voice signal to the listener's voice-quality ratings. For examples, whether a listener is experienced or naive, and the person's internal standards, for what constitute degrees of abnormal voice quality, will vary. In recent years, there has been renewed interest in assessing the reliability and validity of procedures involved in the use of abnormal speech samples and increased attention has been devoted to the use of synthetic speech stimuli. In addition, psychoacoustic experiments have incorporated complex speechlike stimuli in an attempt to simulate the speech signal more closely while maintaining a high level of control of important acoustic stimuli. The role of phonation in speech intelligibility is now being constructed. The importance of laryngeal participation in articulation of the produced sound is now being recognized more and more.

Measurement of Laryngopharyngeal Gestures

Voice quality is controlled by subtle alterations in the setting or resetting of laryngeal and pharyngeal postures, such as laryngeal height, supraglottic constrictions and agonistic or antagonistic interaction of the intrinsic and extrinsic musculature. In recent years, a variety of techniques have been employed to measure these gestures directly or indirectly using electromyography, electroglottography, photoglottography, high-resolution MRI, inverse filtering, stroboscopic imaging, direct fibroscopic imaging and digital storage.

There has been increased understanding of the range of normal laryngopharyngeal activity because of more prevalent and concurrent use of various types of instrumentation, such as videofluoroscopy and pressure-sensing devices. The understanding of the biomechanics of propulsion of the bolus of food during swallowing has been improved. Also, the use of improved imaging procedures has led to a greater understanding of the various forms of upper airway obstruction.

Chapter 55

Recovering Speech after a Laryngectomy

Laryngectomy: The Operation

The Important Anatomy

A laryngectomy is surgical removal of the larynx, also called the voice box. The larynx is located at the point where a division occurs from the single tube that makes up the throat (also called the pharynx) into a separate tube for food going to the stomach (the esophagus) and air going to the lungs (trachea, or windpipe). One important function of the larynx is to protect the airway by ensuring that swallowed foods and liquids pass down the esophagus instead of going into the lungs.

The vocal folds, responsible for sound generation in speech and singing, are also located in the larynx. As air is exhaled past the vocal cords, it can be made to produce the sounds necessary for speech.

If the larynx is removed, air can no longer pass from the lungs into the mouth. The connection between the mouth and the windpipe no longer exists. In order to allow air to get into the lungs, an new opening must be made in the front of the neck. The upper portion of the trachea (windpipe) is brought out to the front of the neck to create a permanent opening called a stoma. When a laryngectomy patient inhales, air passes directly through the stoma into the trachea and then

Information in this chapter was produced by The Voice Center at Eastern Virginia Medical School, Norfolk, VA 23507. URL: http://www.voice-center.com/index.html, last updated September 20, 1997; reprinted with permission.

449

into the lungs. The connection between the mouth and the esophagus is usually not affected, so food and liquid can be swallowed just as they were before the operation. Removal of the vocal cords means that a laryngectomy patient will no longer have laryngeal speech. This does not mean that speech is lost, as there are ways to talk without a larynx. These are described [in separate sections below].

The operation itself is done through an incision in the neck. Many times a operation called a neck dissection is done at the same time to remove lymph nodes in the neck that may be involved with cancer.

What to Expect Immediately after a Laryngectomy

The first night after a laryngectomy is usually spent in the intensive care unit (ICU). As with most other operations for head and neck cancer, the patient will have one or more suction drains under the skin to collect any small amount of fluid collection in the neck. The drains are removed after several days. There also will be intravenous lines (IVs) in order to give fluids and medicine.

While the lower portion of the throat is healing after a laryngectomy, the patient will not be able to swallow food or liquids. In order to supply nutrition, a small flexible plastic feeding tube will be placed into the stomach. The tube is placed either through the nose or the neck. If all goes well, the patient will be able to start swallowing about one week after the operation, and the feeding tube can be removed at that time. If there is concern that the tube may be needed for a much longer time, a tube can be placed through the skin of the abdomen directly into the stomach. Placement of this tube, called a PEG, is more involved, but once in it is easier to take care of and less conspicuous.

In some cases a tracheotomy tube is placed into the stoma after the operation. However, this is usually done on a temporary basis until the stoma will stay open on its own.

Total hospital stay after a laryngectomy is usually about 5-7 days. Some patients may not be quite ready to go home after they leave the hospital and will, therefore, first spend a few days at a Nursing Care Center.

What to Expect on a Long-Term Basis after a Laryngectomy

When we breathe, air normally passes through our nose or mouth and is both warmed and humidified before reaching the windpipe, or trachea. After a laryngectomy the air will instead pass directly into the windpipe through the stoma. As a result, the lining of the windpipe will be exposed to air that is much drier and cooler than usual. The mucous that normally lines the trachea will become thicker and crusting can develop. The crusts that form can actually block the airway and can also lead to infection.

In order to prevent this, after a laryngectomy a small mask with humidified air will be placed over the stoma. The patient will need to use this mask as much as possible until the lining of the windpipe "matures" and can tolerate the drier air.

The stoma is the only airway for a laryngectomy patient and its care is important. The misted air mentioned above is obviously important. Also important is cleaning and suctioning of the stoma. Certain individuals will develop crusting around the stoma, and these crusts will need to be cleaned. The trachea itself may need suctioning. It is important that the patient as well as his family and friends become familiar with stomal care. The stoma is the patient's only airway, and any blockage of the stoma can therefore be very serious. With proper care, these blockages are very rare.

Electrolaryngeal Speech

An electrolarynx is a mechanical device that is used to help produce speech in individuals who have had a laryngectomy, or for some other reason cannot use their larynx.

The electrolarynx is a hand-held device about the size of a small electric shaver that has a vibrating plastic diaphragm. In order to speak, the end of the electrolarynx is placed against the neck and a small button in pushed. This causes the diaphragm to vibrate and produces a vibration in the throat that duplicates the vibration of the vocal cords. The speaker then articulates with the tongue, palate, throat, and lips as usual.

Some people require practice in placing the electrolarynx in just the right spot on the neck in order to produce good speech. Practice is also needed in articulation. The speech from an electrolarynx has a mechanical sound but is very clear and easily understood. The speech, when done properly, is also easily understandable over a telephone.

Advantages and Disadvantages of Electrolaryngeal Speech

Advantages

1. One can speak in long sentences that are easily understood.

2. No special care requirements are needed; the electrolarynx only has to be placed up against the neck and turned on.

3. The electrolarynx can be used by almost everybody, regardless of the post-operative changes in the neck. In those few cases where scarring prevents proper placement of the electrolarynx, an intraoral version can be used.

Disadvantages

1. The electrolarynx has a very mechanical sound that does not sound natural. There usually is little change in pitch or modulation.

2. One must have good hand control to use an electrolarynx.

Esophageal Speech

This section describes esophageal speech, which is one of the techniques that can be used to speak after a laryngectomy has been performed. Other sections describe what a laryngectomy is, and the other types of speech after a laryngectomy, including electrolaryngeal speech and tracheo-esophageal speech.

After a laryngectomy, air flow enters and leaves the lungs through a permanent opening in the neck called a stoma. Since the larynx and its vocal folds are no longer present, there is nothing that vibrates as the air moves in and out of the lungs. As a result, no sound is produced and speech is not possible.

In esophageal speech, the sound is not produced by the vocal folds but rather by vibrations in the esophagus. The principle is that the individual swallows air and then allows it to escape in a controlled fashion.

As the air escapes it causes the walls of the esophagus to vibrate. This produces a sound, which can then be articulated by the mouth an lips to produce speech.

Advantages of esophageal speech are that it requires no additional operations or any special prosthesis. It is relatively easy to learn.

The major drawback with esophageal speech is that the sounds have a rough, almost burp-like sound, and one is usually limited to relatively short segments of speech between interruptions to take in more air.

Tracheo-Esophageal Speech Following Laryngectomy

One of the most effective techniques for speaking following a laryngectomy is tracheo-esophageal speech (TE speech).

To understand how TE speech works, you have to be familiar with the anatomy of the neck after laryngectomy. That is described above, but briefly after a laryngectomy the end of the trachea (windpipe) is brought out to the front of the neck. This opening is called the stoma, and one breathes in and out of the stoma. No speech is possible as one exhales through the stoma, since air just travels out without causing any vibration or sound. Just behind the trachea is the esophagus, which is the tube through which food travels from the mouth to the stomach.

The principle in TE speech is that during exhalation, air is diverted into the esophagus. The air eventually flows out the mouth. That air flow causes the esophagus to vibrate, which produces a sound. By moving the lips, tongue, etc, the sound is articulated into speech.

In order to divert air to the esophagus during exhalation, a small opening called a fistula is created between the trachea and the esophagus. A small valved tube is placed into the opening or fistula to keep it open and to prevent swallowed food and liquid from getting down the trachea. This tube is usually called a voice prosthesis.

The fistula can be created at the time of the original laryngectomy, or at a later time. It is a relatively minor operation.

The voice prosthesis connects the trachea (windpipe) and the esophagus. The prosthesis is constructed with a small valve on the end that goes into the esophagus. This is done to prevent swallowed food from going into the trachea and causing lung problems.

In order to talk, the stoma must be covered with one's thumb during exhalation. When the thumb tightly covers the stoma, air will pass from the trachea and into the esophagus. With practice, one can make this air vibrate the walls of the esophagus. This produces a sound that is then modified by the lips and tongue through normal articulation to produce quite normal sounding speech.

Advantages and Disadvantages of Tracheo-Esophageal Speech

Advantages

1. The sound quality with TE speech is very good, probably most closely resembling normal laryngeal speech. In contrast, speech using an electrolarynx has a very mechanical sound.

2. Since the air for the speech is coming from the lungs, one can speak for a fairly long time between breaks. With plain esophageal speech, the air comes from the stomach and speech

segments are short. There also is better control of the air flow with TE speech.

Disadvantages

1. Not everyone can do TE speech. In some cases the walls of the esophagus are too tight to allow passage of air. In those cases, when one exhales and covers the stoma, air just can't escape. It is like trying to blow against a sealed tube. There is a test that a speech pathologist can do prior to placement of a TE fistula to see if the esophagus will tolerate TE speech.

2. The voice prosthesis must be removed and cleaned periodically. This requires a moderate amount of dexterity, especially in putting it back in the right spot. However, there are now prostheses called "in-dwelling" that are designed to stay in for weeks or months at a time.

3. The stoma must be tightly covered during exhalation in order for air to get into the esophagus. This requires good arm and hand movement, and this may be difficult after a spinal cord injury. There are valves that can be placed over the stoma that divert air into the esophagus, but they do not always work.

4. There can be food that leaks into the esophagus.

5. The prosthesis can fall out and the hole will seal over in about 24 hours. If it does seal over, a second operation must usually be done to make a new hole. If the prosthesis falls into the trachea, it must be removed to prevent aspiration.

Chapter 56

Otolaryngologists Recommend Smoking Cessation

Who Can Help Me?

Your physician should be your first stop. Additional help is often available through community health programs that offer group counseling and smoking cessation programs. Many smokers find group counseling encouraging because they are in an environment where everyone shares the same problems, making it easier to discuss them openly. The American Cancer Society, the American Lung Association, American Heart Association, and others offer excellent programs.

Where Do I Start?

Mark Twain once quipped, "It is easy to quit smoking; I've done it hundreds of times." For a few disciplined people it is easy to quit abruptly or cold turkey; but for many others, it is not easy at all.

Since the prospect of never smoking again may seem unbearable to you, promise to quit for just one week. After you have conquered the first smokeless week, then promise another week, and so on, until you stop for good. You have two major hurdles to overcome: the **addiction** to nicotine, and the **habit** of smoking.

Kicking the Addiction

Tobacco contains nicotine, an addictive drug, and smokers become addicted. If you quit abruptly, you will go through the physical and psychological effects of drug-withdrawal. These may include intense food cravings, jittery nerves, anxiety, short temper, depression, and sleeplessness. The addiction-withdrawal symptoms will be worst the first week and less severe during the second. After a month, most of the withdrawal symptoms will be gone. If you quit gradually, the withdrawal may be less intense but more prolonged. This is why many experts recommend quitting abruptly.

Breaking the Habit

You must break that habit of automatically lighting-up and taking a puff before you think of it. So from now on, every time you start to light-up, become conscious of the fact that you are doing so. Next, try to think of why you want to smoke. Are you upset about something? Are you in an environment where you usually smoke? Are you nervous? If you can determine exactly when you smoke and why you smoke at that time, you will have better control of these situations.

Can Nicotine Gum and Patches Help?

Nicotine gum and patches may help you break the habit of smoking and systematically reduce your nicotine addiction. By providing an alternative source of nicotine without the other harmful additives found in tobacco products, they allow you to concentrate on overcoming the psychological and social factors of the smoking habit.

The patches contain nicotine which is slowly released into your bloodstream through the skin; they come in different styles and strengths. Depending on how much you smoke, you may start with a higher dose and reduce to a lower strength.

Warning: when you use the patch you *cannot keep smoking*. If you do, the double amount of nicotine can lead to a very serious condition called *nicotine toxicity* and cause a heart attack. If you continue to smoke while using the patch, you may end up in the hospital.

Nicotine gum also provides an alternative source of nicotine. Once the habit is broken, you stop chewing the gum and go through drug-withdrawal. For some, separating the withdrawal from breaking the habit makes quitting easier.

Although either method can help satisfy your nicotine craving, they are only aids. They are no substitute for willpower and won't work unless you are committed to quitting. The gum or patch should be used in conjunction with a smoking cessation program.

Tips to Quit

- Tell your friends, family, boss, and fellow workers that you have just quit smoking. You may be temporarily irritable, depressed, and anxious for a week or so, but these withdrawal symptoms *will* pass. Ask for everyone's support and understanding.

- Do anything to keep busy and keep your mind off smoking. Exercise; work on that talent or hobby you always wanted to develop, especially if it involves use of your hands (sewing, model building, practicing the piano, etc). Visit your nonsmoking friends, but avoid circumstances you associate with smoking such as cocktail parties, watching television, balancing the checkbook, talking on the telephone, your usual coffee break, etc.

- An excellent time to quit smoking is when you are hospitalized. This controlled environment is very helpful. Physicians often insist that you quit smoking before surgery and anesthesia so you can better resist post-operative pneumonia that smokers are more likely to develop.

- Once you have conquered the addiction, never have a cigarette again—not even just one little puff. Many a successful quitter has stumbled back into a full addiction by having one cigarette to be sociable.

- Instead of having a cigarette, try the following:

  - Keep a pack of chewing gum in the place where your cigarettes would usually be.

  - Drink a glass of water each time the urge to smoke occurs.

  - Start an exercise program to reduce stress and anxiety and burn off those calories you might put on.

- Hide your cigarettes in places where you ordinarily wouldn't look for them.

- Buy cigarettes by the single pack only and not by the carton.

- Avoid sweets and other fattening foods. Eat low calorie, healthy ones instead; e.g. chew carrots or celery sticks. Weight gain can be a problem for some smokers who are quitting.

Did You Know

- Tobacco related illness, including pipe and spit tobacco, is the most preventable cause of death. In the U.S., 340,000 people die each year from these illnesses.

- Half of the adolescents, whether boys or girls, who start smoking and smoke throughout their lives will be killed by tobacco.

- Tobacco is a health risk to unborn babies of mothers who smoke. It increases the risk of miscarriage, low birth weight, complications during pregnancy, and the likelihood of health problems during infancy and childhood.

- Smoking is the cause of about 30% of all cancers and 80–90% of lung cancer. Lung cancer is the leading cause of death for men and has just surpassed breast cancer as the leading cause of death for women.

- Smokers have two times greater risk of dying of heart attacks and three times greater risk of dying of strokes than nonsmokers.

- Pipe and cigar smokers are 3–5 times more likely than nonsmokers to develop cancer of the mouth and esophagus (swallowing passage).

- Smoking is the major cause of cancer of the larynx (voice box), a cancer that can rob you of your natural voice or lead to death.

- Smokers are more likely to catch pneumonia, colds, bronchitis, and sinus infections more often and have greater difficulty recovering than nonsmokers. Even nonsmokers who work or live with smokers (who cannot avoid breathing their secondhand smoke) suffer this decreased resistance to infections. **This is especially true of children who live in a smoker's household.**

Chapter 57

Otolaryngologists Warn against Spit Tobacco

What's in Spit Tobacco?

There are two forms of spit tobacco: chewing tobacco and snuff. Chewing tobacco is usually sold as leaf tobacco (packaged in a pouch) or plug tobacco (in brick form) and both are put between the cheek and gum. Users keep chewing tobacco in their mouths for several hours to get a continuous high from the nicotine in the tobacco.

Snuff is a powdered tobacco (usually sold in cans) that is put between the lower lip and the gum. Just a pinch is all that's needed to release the nicotine, which is then swiftly absorbed into the bloodstream, resulting in a quick high. Sounds ok right? Not exactly, keep reading...

What Is Spit Tobacco?

Chemicals. Keep in mind that the spit tobacco you or your friends are putting into your mouths contains many chemicals that can have a harmful effect on your health. Here are a few of the ingredients found in spit tobacco:

- Polonium 210 (nuclear waste)
- Cyanide

- Arsenic
- N-Nitrosamines (cancer-causing)
- Benzene
- Lead (nerve poison)
- Formaldehyde (embalming fluid)
- Nicotine (addictive drug)
- Cadmium (used in car batteries)

The chemicals contained in chew or snuff are what make you high. They also make it very hard to quit. Why? Every time you use smoke-less tobacco your body adjusts to the amount of tobacco needed to get that high. Then you need a little more tobacco to get the same feeling. You see, your body gets used to the chemicals you give it. Pretty soon you'll need more smokeless tobacco, more often or you'll need stronger spit tobacco to reach the same level. This process is called addiction.

Some people say spit tobacco is ok because there's no smoke, like a cigarette has. Don't believe them. It's not a safe alternative to smoking. You just move health problems from your lungs to your mouth.

Physical and Mental Effects

If you use spit tobacco, here's what you might have to look forward to:

- **Cancer.** Cancer of the mouth (including the lip, tongue, and cheek) and throat. Cancers most frequently occur at the site where tobacco is held in the mouth.

- **Leukoplakia.** Whoa, what's this? When you hold tobacco in one place in your mouth, your mouth becomes irritated by the tobacco juice. This causes a white, leathery like patch to form, and this is called leukoplakia. These patches can be different in size, shape, and appearance. They are also considered pre-cancerous. **If you find one in your mouth, see your doctor immediately!**

- **Heart Disease.** The constant flow of nicotine into your body causes many side effects including: increased heart rate, increased blood pressure, and sometimes irregular heart beats (this leads to a greater risk of heart attacks and strokes). Nicotine in the body also causes constricted blood vessels which can slow down reaction time and cause dizziness—not a good move if you play sports.

- **Gum and Tooth Disease.** Spit tobacco permanently discolors teeth. Chewing tobacco causes halitosis (bad breath). Its direct and repeated contact with the gums causes them to recede, which can cause your teeth to fall out. Spit tobacco contains a lot of sugar which, when mixed with the plaque on your teeth, forms acid that eats away at tooth enamel, causes cavities, and chronic painful sores.

- **Social Effects.** The really bad breath, discolored teeth, gunk stuck in your teeth, and constant spitting can have a very negative effect on your social and love life. An even more serious effect of spit tobacco is oral cancer, and the surgery for this could lead to removal of parts of your face, tongue, cheek or lip.

Early Warning Signs

Check your mouth often, looking closely at the places where you hold the tobacco. See your doctor right away if you have any of the following:

- a sore that bleeds easily and doesn't heal
- a lump or thickening anywhere in your mouth or neck
- soreness or swelling that doesn't go away
- a red or white patch that doesn't go away
- trouble chewing, swallowing, or moving your tongue or jaw

Even if you don't find a problem today, see your doctor or dentist every three months to have your mouth checked. Your chances for a cure are higher if oral cancer is found early.

Tips To Quit

You've just read the bad news, but there is good news. Even though it is very difficult to quit using spit tobacco, it can be done. Read the following tips to quit for some helpful ideas to kick the habit. Remember, most people don't start chewing on their own, so don't try quitting on your own. Ask for help and positive reinforcement from your support groups (friends, parents, coaches, teachers, whomever...).

461

Think of reasons why you want to quit. You may want to quit because:

- You don't want to risk getting cancer.
- The people around you find it offensive.
- You don't like having bad breath after chewing and dipping.
- You don't want stained teeth or no teeth.
- You don't like being addicted to nicotine.
- You want to start leading a healthier life.

Pick a quit date and throw out all your chewing tobacco and snuff. Tell yourself out loud every day that you're going to quit.

Ask your friends, family, teachers, and coaches to help you kick the habit by giving you support and encouragement. Tell friends not to offer you smokeless tobacco. You may want to ask a friend to quit with you.

Ask your doctor about a nicotine chewing gum tobacco cessation program.

Find alternatives to spit tobacco. A few good examples are sugarless gum, pumpkin or sunflower seeds, apple slices, raisins, or dried fruit.

Find activities to keep your mind off of spit tobacco. You could ride a bike, talk or write a letter to a friend, work on a hobby, or listen to music. Exercise can help relieve tension caused by quitting.

Remember that everyone is different, so develop a personalized plan that works best for you. Set realistic goals and achieve them.

Reward yourself. You could save the money that would have been spent on spit tobacco products and buy something nice for yourself.

Part Six

Cancers Related to the Ears, Nose, and Throat

Chapter 58

Head and Neck Cancer

Here's what you should watch for:

A lump in the neck. Cancers that begin in the head or neck usually spread to lymph nodes in the neck before they spread elsewhere. A lump in the neck that lasts more than two weeks should be seen by a physician as soon as possible. Of course, not all lumps are cancer. But a lump (or lumps) in the neck can be the first sign of cancer of the mouth, throat, voicebox (larynx), thyroid gland, or of certain lymphomas or blood cancers. Such lumps are generally painless and continue to enlarge steadily.

Change in the voice. Most cancers in the larynx cause some change in voice. Any hoarseness or other voice change lasting more than two weeks should alert you to see your physician. An otolaryngologist is a head and neck specialist who can examine your vocal cords easily and painlessly. While most voice changes are not caused by cancer, you shouldn't take chances. If you are hoarse more than two weeks, make sure you don't have cancer of the larynx. See your doctor.

A growth in the mouth. Most cancers of the mouth or tongue cause a sore or swelling that doesn't go away. These sores and swellings may be painless unless they become infected. Bleeding may occur, but

©1994. American Academy of Otolaryngology–Head and Neck Surgery, Inc., One Prince Street, Alexandria, VA 22314-3357. For more information, visit our home page at http://www.entnet.org.

465

often not until late in the disease. If an ulcer or swelling is accompanied by lumps in the neck, be very concerned. Your dentist or doctor can determine if a biopsy (tissue sample test) is needed and can refer you to a head and neck surgeon to perform this procedure.

Bringing up blood. This is often caused by something other than cancer. However, tumors in the nose, mouth, throat or lungs can cause bleeding. If blood appears in your saliva or phlegm for more than a few days, you should see your physician.

Swallowing problems. Cancer of the throat or esophagus (swallowing tube) may make swallowing solid foods difficult. Sometimes liquids can also be troublesome. The food may "stick" at a certain point and then either go through to the stomach or come back up. If you have trouble almost every time you try to swallow something, you should be examined by a physician. Usually a barium swallow x-ray or an esophagoscopy (direct examination of the swallowing tube with a telescope) will be performed to find the cause.

Changes in the skin. The most common head and neck cancer is basal cell cancer of the skin. Fortunately this is rarely a major problem if treated early. Basal cell cancers appear most often on sun-exposed areas like the forehead, face, and ears, although they can occur almost anywhere on the skin. Basal cell cancer often begins as a small, pale patch that enlarges slowly, producing a central "dimple" and eventually an ulcer. Parts of the ulcer may heal, but the major portion remains ulcerated. Some basal cell cancers show color changes.

Other kinds of cancer, including squamous cell cancer and malignant melanoma, also occur on the skin of the head and neck. Most squamous cell cancers occur on the lower lip and ear. They may look like basal cell cancers and, if caught early and properly treated, usually are not much more dangerous. If there is a sore on the lip, lower face, or ear that does not heal, consult a physician.

Malignant melanoma classically produces dense blue-black or black discolorations of the skin. However, any mole that changes size, color, or begins to bleed may be trouble. A black or blue-black spot on the face or neck, particularly if it changes size or shape, should be seen as soon as possible by a dermatologist or other physician.

Persistent Earache. Constant pain in or around the ear when you swallow can be a sign of infection or tumor growth in the throat. This is particularly serious if it is associated with difficulty in swallowing,

466

hoarseness or a lump in the neck. These symptoms are best evaluated by an otolaryngologist.

Identifying High Risk of Head and Neck Cancer

As many as 90 percent of head and neck cancers arise after prolonged exposure to specific factors. Use of tobacco (cigarettes, cigars, chewing tobacco or snuff) and alcoholic beverages are closely linked with cancers of the mouth, throat, voice box and tongue. (*In adults who neither smoke nor drink, cancer of the mouth and throat are nearly nonexistent.*) Prolonged exposure to sunlight is linked with cancer of the lip and is also an established major cause of skin cancer.

What You Should Do

All of the symptoms and signs described here can occur with no cancer present. In fact, many times complaints of this type will be due to some other condition. But you can't tell without an examination. So, if they do occur, see your doctor—and be sure.

Remember: When found early, most cancers in the head and neck can be cured with relatively little difficulty. Cure rates for these cancers could be greatly improved if people would seek medical advice as soon as possible. So play it safe. If you think you have one of the warning signs of head and neck cancer, see your doctor right away.

Be sure to be safe—see your doctor early! And practice health habits which will make these diseases unlikely to occur.

Chapter 59

Metastatic Squamous Neck Cancer

What Is Metastatic Squamous Neck Cancer with Occult Primary?

Cancer is a disease in which certain cells begin to divide too quickly and without any order. Cancer can spread to tissues and organs near the place where it started (called the primary site). Cancer cells can also spread through the bloodstream and the lymph system to other parts of the body to form new tumors. Cancer that started in one place, but has spread to another part of the body is called metastatic cancer.

Squamous cells line the outside of many body organs, including your mouth, nose, skin, throat, and lungs. Cancer can begin in the squamous cells and spread (metastasize) from its original site to the lymph nodes in the neck or around the collarbone. Lymph nodes are small bean-shaped structures that are found throughout the body. They produce and store infection-fighting cells. When the lymph nodes in the neck are found to contain squamous cell cancer, your doctor will try to find out where the cancer started (the primary tumor). If your doctor cannot find a primary tumor, the cancer is called a metastatic cancer with unseen (occult) primary.

Like most cancers, metastatic squamous neck cancer with occult primary is best treated when it is found (diagnosed) early. You should

National Cancer Institute PDQ Database, http://cancernet.nci.nih.gov/ clinpdq/pif/Metastatic_squamous_neck_cancer_with_occult_primary_Patient. html; last updated September 1997.

see your doctor if you have a lump or pain in your neck or throat that doesn't go away. If tissue that is not normal is found, your doctor will need to cut out a small piece and look at it under the microscope to see if there are any cancer cells. This is called a biopsy. If the biopsy shows that you have squamous cell cancer, your doctor will do many kinds of tests to see whether a primary site can be found. If the primary site cannot be found, your doctor will treat the cancer in the neck.

Your chance of recovery (prognosis) depends on how many lymph nodes contain cancer, where the cancer is found in the neck, whether or not a primary tumor is found, and your general state of health.

Stage Explanation

Stages of Metastatic Squamous Neck Cancer with Occult Primary

Once metastatic squamous neck cancer with occult primary is found, more tests will be done to find out how far the cancer cells have spread. This is called staging. Your doctor needs to know the stage of your disease to plan treatment. The following stages are used for metastatic squamous neck cancer with occult primary:

Untreated

Untreated metastatic squamous neck cancer with occult primary means no treatment has been given for the cancer except to treat symptoms.

Recurrent

Recurrent disease means that the cancer has come back (recurred) after it has been treated. It may come back in the neck or in another part of the body.

Treatment Option Overview

How Metastatic Squamous Neck Cancer with Occult Primary Is Treated

There are treatments for all patients with metastatic squamous neck cancer with occult primary. Two kinds of treatment are used:

- surgery (taking out the cancer)
- radiation therapy (using high-dose x-rays or other high-energy rays to kill cancer cells).

Chemotherapy is being studied in clinical trials.

Surgery is a common treatment for metastatic neck cancer. Your doctor may cut out the lymph nodes that contain cancer and some of the healthy lymph nodes around them (lymph node dissection).

Radiation therapy uses high-energy x-rays to kill cancer cells and shrink tumors. Radiation may come from a machine outside the body (external radiation therapy) or from putting materials that produce radiation (radioisotopes) through thin plastic tubes that are put into the area where the cancer cells are found (internal radiation therapy). External radiation to the thyroid or the pituitary gland may change the way your thyroid gland works. Your doctor may wish to test your thyroid gland before and after therapy to make sure it is working properly.

Chemotherapy uses drugs to kill cancer cells. Chemotherapy may be taken by pill, or it may be put into the body by a needle in a vein or muscle. Chemotherapy is called a systemic treatment because the drug enters the bloodstream, travels through the body, and can kill cancer cells outside the neck.

Treatment by Stage

Treatment for metastatic squamous neck cancer with occult primary depends on how many lymph nodes contain cancer, whether or not an original (primary) tumor is found, your age, and your overall condition.

You may receive treatment that is considered standard based on its effectiveness in a number of patients in past studies, or you may choose to go into a clinical trial. Not all patients are cured with standard therapy and some standard treatments may have more side effects than are desired. For these reasons, clinical trials are designed to find better ways to treat cancer patients and are based on the most up-to-date information. Clinical trials are going on in some parts of the country for metastatic squamous neck cancer. If you want more information, call the Cancer Information Service at 1-800-4-CANCER (1-800-422-6237); TTY at 1-800-332-8615.

Untreated Metastatic Squamous Neck Cancer with Occult Primary

Your treatment may be one of the following:

1. Surgery to remove the lymph nodes in the neck (lymph node dissection).

2. Radiation therapy.

3. Radiation therapy plus surgery.

4. A clinical trial that includes chemotherapy, radiation therapy, and/or surgery.

Recurrent Metastatic Squamous Neck Cancer with Occult Primary

Your treatment depends on the type of treatment you had before, where the cancer came back, and your health. You may want to take part in a clinical trial of new treatments.

To Learn More

To Learn More..... Call 1-800-4-CANCER

To learn more about metastatic squamous neck cancer with occult primary, call the National Cancer Institute's Cancer Information Service at 1-800-4-CANCER (1-800-422-6237); TTY at 1-800-332-8615. By dialing this toll-free number, you can speak with someone who can answer your questions.

You can also write to the National Cancer Institute at this address:

National Cancer Institute
Office of Cancer Communications
31 Center Drive, MSC 2580
Bethesda, MD 20892-2580

Chapter 60

Cancer of the Oral Cavity and Upper Throat

What You Need to Know about Oral Cancer

The National Cancer Institute (NCI) has written this to help people with *oral cancer* and their families and friends better understand this disease. We hope others will also read it to learn more about oral cancer.

This chapter describes symptoms, diagnosis, and treatment. It also has information about rehabilitation and about sources of support to help patients cope with oral cancer.

Our knowledge about oral cancer keeps increasing. For up-to-date information, call the National Cancer Institute's Cancer Information Service (CIS), described at the end of this chapter. The toll-free number is 1-800-4-CANCER (1-800-422-6237).

The CIS uses a National Cancer Institute cancer information database called PDQ and other NCI resources to answer callers' questions. Cancer information specialists can also send information from PDQ and other NCI materials about cancer, its treatment, and living with the disease.

The Oral Cavity

This chapter deals with cancer of the oral cavity (mouth) and the *oropharynx* (the part of the throat at the back of the mouth). The oral cavity includes many parts: the lips; the lining inside the lips and

National Cancer Institute, NIH Pub. No. 97-1574, Revised November 1996.

cheeks, called the *buccal mucosa*; the teeth; the bottom (floor) of the mouth under the tongue; the front two-thirds of the tongue; the bony top of the mouth (hard *palate*); the gums; and the small area behind the wisdom teeth. The oropharynx includes the back one-third of the tongue, the soft palate, the *tonsils*, and the part of the throat behind the mouth. *Salivary glands* throughout the oral cavity make saliva, which keeps the mouth moist and helps digest food.

What Is Cancer?

Cancer is a group of diseases. It occurs when cells become abnormal and divide without control or order. More than 100 different types of cancer are known.

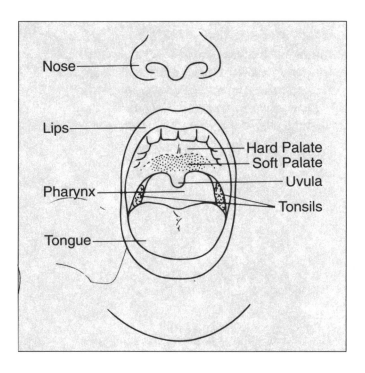

Figure 60.1. The oral cavity and upper throat.

Like all organs of the body, the mouth and throat are made up of many kinds of cells. Cells normally divide in an orderly way to produce more cells only when the body needs them. This process helps keep the body healthy.

Cells that divide when new cells are not needed form too much tissue. The mass of extra tissue, called a *tumor*, can be *benign* or *malignant*.

- Benign tumors are not cancer. They can usually be removed, and in most cases, they don't grow back. Most important, the cells in benign tumors do not invade other tissues and do not spread to other parts of the body. Benign tumors usually are not a threat to life.

- Malignant tumors are cancer. They can invade and damage nearby tissues and organs. Also, cancer cells can break away from a malignant tumor and enter the bloodstream or the *lymphatic system*. This is how cancer spreads and forms secondary tumors in other parts of the body. The spread of cancer is called *metastasis*.

When oral cancer spreads, it usually travels through the lymphatic system. Cancer cells that enter the lymphatic system are carried along by *lymph*, an almost colorless, watery fluid containing cells that help the body fight infection and disease. Along the lymphatic channels are groups of small, bean-shaped organs called *lymph nodes* (sometimes called lymph glands). Oral cancer that spreads usually travels to the lymph nodes in the neck. It can also spread to other parts of the body. Cancer that spreads is the same disease and has the same name as the original (primary) cancer.

Early Detection

Regular checkups that include an examination of the entire mouth can detect *precancerous* conditions or the early stages of oral cancer. Your doctor and dentist should check the tissues in your mouth as part of your routine exams.

Symptoms

Oral cancer usually occurs in people over the age of 45 but can develop at any age. These are some symptoms to watch for:

- A sore on the lip or in the mouth that does not heal;

- A lump on the lip or in the mouth or throat;

- A white or red patch on the gums, tongue, or lining of the mouth;

- Unusual bleeding, pain, or numbness in the mouth;

- A sore throat that does not go away, or a feeling that something is caught in the throat;

- Difficulty or pain with chewing or swallowing;

- Swelling of the jaw that causes dentures to fit poorly or become uncomfortable;

- A change in the voice; and/or

- Pain in the ear.

These symptoms may be caused by cancer or by other, less serious problems. It is important to see a dentist or doctor about any symptoms like these, so that the problem can be diagnosed and treated as early as possible.

Diagnosis and Staging

If an abnormal area has been found in the oral cavity, a *biopsy* is the only way to know whether it is cancer. Usually, the patient is referred to an *oral surgeon* or an ear, nose, and throat surgeon, who removes part or all of the lump or abnormal-looking area. A *pathologist* examines the tissue under a microscope to check for cancer cells.

Almost all oral cancers are *squamous cell carcinomas*. Squamous cells line the oral cavity.

A patient who needs a biopsy may want to ask the doctor these questions:

- How much tissue will be removed for the biopsy?
- How long will the biopsy take? Will I be awake? Will it hurt?
- How should I care for the biopsy site afterward?
- How soon will I know the results?
- If I do have cancer, who will talk with me about treatment? When?

If the pathologist finds oral cancer, the patient's doctor needs to know the stage, or extent, of the disease in order to plan the best treatment.

Staging tests and exams help the doctor find out whether the cancer has spread and what parts of the body are affected.

Staging generally includes dental x-rays and x-rays of the head and chest. The doctor may also want the patient to have a *CT* (or *CAT*) *scan*. A CT scan is a series of x-rays put together by a computer to form detailed pictures of areas inside the body.

Ultrasonography is another way to produce pictures of areas in the body. High-frequency sound waves (ultrasound), which cannot be heard by humans, are bounced off organs and tissue. The pattern of echoes produced by these waves creates a picture called a sonogram. Sometimes the doctor asks for *MRI* (magnetic resonance imaging), a procedure in which pictures are created using a magnet linked to a computer. The doctor also feels the lymph nodes in the neck to check for swelling or other changes. In most cases, the patient will have a complete physical examination before treatment begins.

Treatment

After diagnosis and staging, the doctor develops a treatment plan to fit each patient's needs. Treatment for oral cancer depends on a number of factors. Among these are the location, size, type, and extent of the tumor and the stage of the disease. The doctor also considers the patient's age and general health. Treatment involves surgery, *radiation therapy*, or, in many cases, a combination of the two. Some patients receive *chemotherapy*, treatment with anticancer drugs.

For most patients, it is important to have a complete dental exam before cancer treatment begins. Because cancer treatment may make the mouth sensitive and more easily infected, doctors often advise patients to have any needed dental work done before treatment begins.

Most people with cancer want to learn all they can about their disease and their treatment choices so they can take an active part in decisions about their medical and dental care. The doctor is the best person to answer their questions. Also, the patient may want to talk with the doctor about taking part in a research study of new treatment methods. Such studies, called *clinical trials*, are designed to improve cancer treatment. More information about clinical trials can be found in the section titled "Clinical Trials."

Many patients find it useful to make a list of questions before seeing the doctor. Taking notes can make it easier to remember what the doctor says. Some patients also find that it helps to have a family member or friend with them—to take part in the discussion, to take notes, or just to listen.

Before treatment begins, the patient may want to ask the doctor these questions:

- What are my treatment choices? Which do you recommend for me? Why?

- What are the risks and possible side effects of each treatment?

- What are the expected benefits of each kind of treatment?

- What can be done about side effects?

- Would a clinical trial be appropriate for me?

There is a lot to learn about cancer and its treatment. Patients do not need to ask all their questions or understand all the answers at once. They will have many chances to ask the doctor to explain things that are not clear and to ask for more information.

Planning Treatment

Treatment decisions can be complex. Before starting treatment, the patient may want to have another doctor review the diagnosis and treatment plan. A short delay will not reduce the chance that treatment will be successful. There are a number of ways to find a doctor for a second opinion:

- The patient's doctor or dentist may suggest a specialist who treats oral cancer.

- The Cancer Information Service, at 1-800-4-CANCER, can tell callers about cancer centers and other NCI-supported programs in their area.

- Patients can get the names of specialists from their local medical or dental society, a nearby hospital, or a medical or dental school.

- The *Directory of Medical Specialists* lists doctors' names along with their specialty and their background. This resource is available in most public libraries.

Methods of Treatment

Patients with oral cancer may be treated by a team of specialists. The medical team may include an oral surgeon; an ear, nose, and throat surgeon; a medical *oncologist*; a radiation oncologist; a *prosthodontist*; a general dentist; a plastic surgeon; a dietitian; a social worker; a nurse; and a speech therapist.

Surgery. Surgery to remove the tumor in the mouth is the usual treatment for patients with oral cancer. If there is evidence that the cancer has spread, the surgeon may also remove lymph nodes in the neck. If the disease has spread to muscles and other tissues in the neck, the operation may be more extensive.

Before surgery, the patient may want to ask the doctor these questions:

- What kind of operation will it be?
- How will I feel after the operation? If I have pain, how will you help me?
- Will I have trouble eating?
- Where will the scars be? What will they look like?
- Do you expect that there will be long-term effects from the surgery?
- Will there be permanent changes in my appearance?
- Will I lose any teeth? Can they be replaced? How soon?
- If I need to have plastic surgery, when can that be done?
- Will I need to see a specialist for help with my speech?
- When can I get back to my normal activities?

Radiation therapy. Radiation therapy (also called radiotherapy) is the use of high-energy rays to damage cancer cells and stop them from growing. Like surgery, radiation therapy is *local therapy*; it affects only the cells in the treated area. The energy may come from a large machine (*external radiation*). It can also come from radioactive materials placed directly into or near the tumor (*internal radiation*). Radiation therapy is sometimes used instead of surgery for small tumors in the mouth. Patients with large tumors may need both surgery and radiation therapy.

Radiation therapy may be given before or after surgery. Before surgery, radiation can shrink the tumor so that it can be removed. Radiation after surgery is used to destroy cancer cells that may remain.

For external radiation therapy, the patient goes to the hospital or clinic each day for treatments. Usually, treatment is given 5 days a week for 5 to 6 weeks. This schedule helps protect healthy tissues by dividing the total amount of radiation into small doses.

Implant radiation therapy puts tiny "seeds" containing radioactive material directly into the tumor or in tissue near it. Generally, an implant is left in place for several days, and the patient will stay in the hospital in a private room. The length of time nurses and other caregivers, as well as visitors, can spend with the patient will be limited. The implant is removed before the patient goes home.

Before radiation therapy, a patient may want to ask the doctor these questions:

- When will the treatments begin? When will they end?
- How will I feel during therapy?
- What can I do to take care of myself during therapy?
- Can I continue my normal activities?
- How will my mouth and face look afterward?
- Will I need a special diet? For how long?
- If my mouth becomes dry, what can I do about it?

Chemotherapy. Chemotherapy is the use of drugs to kill cancer cells. Researchers are looking for effective drugs or drug combinations to treat oral cancer. They are also exploring ways to combine chemotherapy with other forms of cancer treatment to help destroy the tumor and prevent the disease from spreading.

Clinical Trials

Researchers are developing treatment methods that are more effective against oral cancer, and they are also finding ways to reduce side effects of treatment. When laboratory research shows that a new method has promise, doctors use it to treat cancer patients in clinical trials. These trials are designed to answer scientific questions about the new approach and to find out whether it is both safe and effective. Patients who take part in clinical trials make an important contribution to medical science and may have the first chance to benefit from improved treatment methods.

Clinical trials to study new treatments for oral cancer are under way in hospitals throughout the country. Some trials involve ways to shrink or destroy the primary tumor. In others, scientists are testing ways to prevent the cancer from coming back in the mouth or spreading to other parts of the body. Still others involve treatments to slow or stop cancer that has already spread.

Researchers are studying the timing of treatments and new ways to combine various types of treatment. For example, they are trying to increase the effectiveness of radiation therapy by giving treatments twice a day instead of once a day. They are also working with *hyperthermia* (heat) and with drugs called radiosensitizers to try to make cancer cells more sensitive to radiation. Researchers are also using drugs to help protect normal cells from radiation damage. In addition, they are exploring various new anticancer drugs and drug combinations.

People who have had oral cancer have an increased risk of getting a new cancer of the mouth or another part of the head or neck. Doctors are trying to find ways to prevent these new cancers. Some research has shown that a substance related to vitamin A may prevent a new cancer from developing in someone who has already been successfully treated for oral cancer.

Oral cancer patients who are interested in taking part in a trial should talk with their doctor. They may want to read *What Are Clinical Trials All About?*, a booklet that explains what treatment studies are and outlines some of their possible benefits and risks.

One way to learn about clinical trials is through PDQ, a computerized resource developed by the National Cancer Institute. PDQ contains information about cancer treatment and an up-to-date list of trials all over the country. The Cancer Information Service, at 1-800-4-CAN-CER, can provide PDQ information to patients and the public.

Side Effects of Treatment

It is hard to limit the effects of cancer treatment so that only cancer cells are removed or destroyed. Because healthy cells and tissues may also be damaged, treatment often causes side effects.

The side effects of cancer treatment vary. They depend mainly on the type and extent of the treatment and the specific area being treated. Also, each person reacts differently. Some side effects are temporary; others are permanent. Doctors try to plan the patient's therapy to keep side effects to a minimum. They also watch patients very carefully so they can help with any problems that occur.

Surgery to remove a small tumor in the mouth usually does not cause any lasting problems. For a larger tumor, however, the surgeon may need to remove part of the palate, tongue, or jaw. Such surgery is likely to change the patient's ability to chew, swallow, or talk. The patient may also look different.

After surgery, the patient's face may be swollen. This swelling usually goes away within a few weeks. However, removing lymph nodes can slow the flow of lymph, which may collect in the tissues; this swelling may last for a long time.

Before starting radiation therapy, a patient should see a dentist who is familiar with the changes this therapy can cause in the mouth. Radiation therapy can make the mouth sore. It can also cause changes in the saliva and may reduce the amount of saliva, making it hard to chew and swallow. Because saliva normally protects the teeth, mouth dryness can promote tooth decay. Good mouth care can help keep the teeth and gums healthy and can make the patient feel more comfortable. The health care team may suggest the use of a special kind of toothbrush or mouthwash. The dentist usually suggests a special fluoride program to keep the teeth healthy. To help relieve mouth dryness, the health care team may suggest the use of artificial saliva and other methods to keep the mouth moist. Mouth dryness from radiation therapy goes away in some patients, but it can be permanent.

Weight loss can be a serious problem for patients being treated for oral cancer because a sore mouth may make eating difficult. Your doctor may suggest ways to maintain a healthy diet. In many cases, it helps to have food and beverages in very small amounts. Many patients find that eating several small meals and snacks during the day works better than trying to have three large meals. Often, it is easier to eat soft, bland foods that have been moistened with sauces or gravies; thick soups, puddings, and high-protein milkshakes are nourishing and easy to swallow. It may be helpful to prepare other foods in a blender. The doctor may also suggest special liquid dietary supplements for patients who have trouble chewing. Drinking lots of fluids helps keep the mouth moist and makes it easier to eat.

Some patients are able to wear their dentures during radiation therapy. Many, however, will not be able to wear dentures for up to a year after treatment. Because the tissues in the mouth that support the denture may change during or after treatment, dentures may no longer fit properly. After treatment is over, a patient may need to have dentures refitted or replaced.

Radiation therapy can also cause sores in the mouth and cracked and peeling lips. These usually heal in the weeks after treatment is completed. Often, good mouth care can help prevent these sores. Dentures should not be worn until the sores have healed.

During radiation therapy, patients may become very tired, especially in the later weeks of treatment. Resting is important, but doctors usually advise their patients to try to stay reasonably active. Patients should match their activities to their energy level. It's common for radiation to cause the skin in the treated area to become red and dry, tender, and itchy. Toward the end of treatment, the skin may become moist and "weepy." There may be permanent darkening or "bronzing" of the skin in the treated area. This area should be exposed to the air as much as possible but should also be protected from the sun. Good skin care is important at this time, but patients should not use any lotions or creams without the doctor's advice. Men may lose all or part of their beard, but facial hair generally grows back after treatment is done. Usually, men shave with an electric razor during treatment to prevent cuts that may lead to infection. Most effects of radiation therapy on the skin are temporary. The area will heal when the treatment is over.

The side effects of chemotherapy depend on the drugs that are given. In general, anticancer drugs affect rapidly growing cells, such as blood cells that fight infection, cells that line the mouth and the digestive tract, and cells in *hair follicles*. As a result, patients may have side effects such as lower resistance to infection, loss of appetite, nausea, vomiting, or mouth sores. They also may have less energy and may lose their hair.

The side effects of cancer treatment are different for each person, and they may even be different from one treatment to the next. Doctors, nurses, and dietitians can explain the side effects of cancer treatment and can suggest ways to deal with them. The booklets *Radiation Therapy and You* and *Eating Hints* contain helpful information about cancer treatment and coping with side effects. Patients receiving anticancer drugs will find useful information in *Chemotherapy and You*.

Rehabilitation

Rehabilitation is a very important part of treatment for patients with oral cancer. The goals of rehabilitation depend on the extent of the disease and the treatment a patient has received. The health care team makes every effort to help the patient return to normal activities as soon as possible. Rehabilitation may include dietary counseling, surgery, a dental *prosthesis*, speech therapy, and other services.

Sometimes, a patient needs reconstructive and plastic surgery to rebuild the bones or tissues of the mouth. If this is not possible, a prosthodontist may be able to make an artificial dental and/or facial part (prosthesis). Patients may need special training to use the device.

Speech therapy generally begins as soon as possible for a patient who has trouble speaking after treatment. Often, a speech therapist visits the patient in the hospital to plan therapy and teach speech exercises. Speech therapy usually continues after the patient returns home.

Followup Care

Regular followup exams are very important for anyone who has been treated for oral cancer. The physician and the dentist watch the patient closely to check the healing process and to look for signs that the cancer may have returned. Patients with mouth dryness from radiation therapy should have dental exams three times a year.

The patient may need to see a dietitian if weight loss or eating problems continue. Most doctors urge their oral cancer patients to stop using tobacco and alcohol to reduce the risk of developing a new cancer.

Support for Cancer Patients

Living with a serious disease isn't easy. Cancer patients and those who care about them face many problems and challenges. Finding the strength to cope with these difficulties is easier when people have helpful information and support services. Several useful booklets, including *Taking Time: Support for People With Cancer and the People Who Care About Them*, are available from the Cancer Information Service.

Cancer patients may worry about holding a job, caring for their family, or starting new relationships. Worries about tests, treatments, hospital stays, and medical bills are common. Doctors, nurses, and other members of the health care team can help calm fears and ease confusion about treatment, working, or daily activities. Also, meeting with a nurse, social worker, counselor, or member of the clergy can be helpful for patients who want to talk about their feelings or discuss their concerns.

Friends and relatives, especially those who have had personal experience with cancer, can be very supportive. Also, many patients find it helpful to discuss their concerns with others who are facing similar problems. Cancer patients often get together in support groups, where they can share what they have learned about cancer and its treatment and about coping with the disease. It is important to keep in mind, however, that each patient is different. Treatments and ways of dealing with cancer that work for one person may not be right for another—even if they both have the same kind of cancer. It is always a good idea to discuss the advice of friends and family members with the doctor.

Often, a social worker at the hospital or clinic can suggest groups that can help with rehabilitation, emotional support, financial aid, transportation, or home care. The American Cancer Society is one such group. This nonprofit organization has many services for patients and their families. Local offices of the American Cancer Society are listed in the white pages of the telephone directory. More information about this resource is included in the "Resources" section at the end of this chapter.

Information about other programs and services is available through the Cancer Information Service. The toll-free number is 1-800-4-CANCER.

The public library is a good place to find books and articles on living with cancer. Cancer patients and their families and friends also can find helpful suggestions in the booklets listed at the end of this chapter.

What the Future Holds

Patients and their families are naturally concerned about what the future holds. Sometimes they use statistics to try to figure out whether the patient will be cured or how long he or she will live. It is important to remember, however, that statistics are averages based on large numbers of patients. They cannot be used to predict what will happen to a certain patient because no two cancer patients are alike. The doctor who takes care of the patient knows his or her medical history and is in the best position to discuss the person's outlook (*prognosis*).

People should feel free to ask the doctor about their chance of recovery, but not even the doctor knows for sure what will happen. When doctors talk about surviving cancer, they may use the term *remission* rather than cure. Even though many patients with oral cancer recover completely, doctors use this term because oral cancer can recur.

Causes and Prevention

Scientists at hospitals and medical centers all across the country are studying this disease to learn more about what causes it and how to prevent it. Doctors do know that no one can "catch" cancer from another person: it is not contagious. Two known causes of oral cancer are tobacco and alcohol use.

Tobacco use—smoking cigarettes, cigars, or pipes; chewing tobacco; or dipping snuff—accounts for 80 to 90 percent of oral cancers. A number of studies have shown that cigar and pipe smokers have the same risk as cigarette smokers. Studies indicate that smokeless tobacco users are at particular risk of developing oral cancer. For long-time users, the risk is much greater, making the use of snuff or chewing tobacco among young people a special concern.

People who stop using tobacco—even after many years of use—can greatly reduce their risk of oral cancer. Special counseling or self-help groups may be useful for those who are trying to give up tobacco. Some hospitals have groups for people who want to quit. Also, the Cancer Information Service and the American Cancer Society may have information about groups in local areas to help people quit using tobacco.

Chronic and/or heavy use of alcohol also increases the risk of oral cancer, even for people who do not use tobacco. However, people who use both alcohol and tobacco have an especially high risk of oral cancer. Scientists believe that these substances increase each other's harmful effects.

Cancer of the lip can be caused by exposure to the sun. The risk can be avoided with the use of a lotion or lip balm containing a sunscreen. Wearing a hat with a brim can also block the sun's harmful rays. Pipe smokers are especially prone to cancer of the lip.

Some studies have shown that many people who develop oral cancer have a history of *leukoplakia*, a whitish patch inside the mouth. The causes of leukoplakia are not well understood, but it is commonly associated with heavy use of tobacco and alcohol. The condition often occurs in irritated areas, such as the gums and mouth lining of smokeless tobacco users and the lower lip of pipe smokers.

Another condition, *erythroplakia*, appears as a red patch in the mouth. Erythroplakia occurs most often in people 60 to 70 years of age. Early diagnosis and treatment of leukoplakia and erythroplakia are important because cancer may develop in these patches.

People who think they might be at risk for developing oral cancer should discuss this concern with their doctor or dentist, who may be able to suggest ways to reduce the risk and plan an appropriate schedule for checkups.

Resources

Information about oral cancer is available from several sources, including the ones listed below. You may wish to check for additional information at your local library or bookstore or from support groups in your community.

Cancer Information Service (CIS)
1-800-4-CANCER

The Cancer Information Service, a program of the National Cancer Institute, provides a nationwide telephone service for cancer patients and their families and friends, the public, and health professionals. Cancer information specialists can answer questions in English or Spanish. They can send booklets about cancer and can also provide information from the National Cancer Institute's PDQ database. In addition, CIS staff have information about national and local resources, and can suggest ways to find support groups and other services. One toll-free number, 1-800-4-CANCER (1-800-422-6237), connects callers all over the country with the office that serves their area. The number for callers with TTY equipment is 1-800-332-8615.

American Cancer Society (ACS)
1-800-ACS-2345

The American Cancer Society is a voluntary organization with local units all over the country. It supports research, conducts educational programs, and offers many services to patients and their families. It provides free booklets on cancer. To obtain booklets or to learn about services and activities in local areas, call the Society's toll-free number, 1-800 -ACS-2345 (1-800 -227-2345), or the number listed under American Cancer Society in the white pages of the telephone book.

National Institute of Dental Research
Building 31, Room 2C35
9000 Rockville Pike
Bethesda, MD 20892

The National Institute of Dental Research, an agency of the Federal Government, is concerned with the causes, prevention, diagnosis, and treatment of oral and dental diseases. It can supply free printed material about oral health during and after cancer treatment.

Other Booklets

The NCI booklets listed below are available free of charge by calling the Cancer Information Service at 1-800-4-CANCER.

Booklets about Cancer Treatment

- *Radiation Therapy and You: A Guide to Self-Help During Treatment*

- _Chemotherapy and You: A Guide to Self-Help During Treatment_
- _Eating Hints for Cancer Patients_
- _Helping Yourself During Chemotherapy: 4 Steps for Cancer Patients_
- _What Are Clinical Trials All About?_
- _Questions and Answers About Pain Control_
- _Get Relief from Cancer Pain_

Booklets about Living with Cancer

- _Taking Time: Support for People With Cancer and the People Who Care About Them_
- _Facing Forward: A Guide for Cancer Survivors_
- _When Cancer Recurs: Meeting the Challenge Again_
- _Advanced Cancer: Living Each Day_

Chapter 61

Paranasal Sinus and Nasal Cavity Cancer

What Is Cancer of the Paranasal Sinus and Nasal Cavity?

Cancer of the paranasal sinus and nasal cavity is a disease in which cancer (malignant) cells are found in the tissues of the paranasal sinuses or nasal cavity. Your paranasal sinuses are small hollow spaces around your nose. The sinuses are lined with cells that make mucus, which keeps the nose from drying out; the sinuses are also a space through which your voice can echo to make sounds when you talk or sing. Your nasal cavity is the passageway just behind your nose through which air passes on the way to your throat when you breathe. The area inside your nose is called the nasal vestibule.

There are several paranasal sinuses, including the frontal sinuses above your nose, the maxillary sinuses in the upper part of either side of your upper jawbone, the ethmoid sinuses just behind either side of your upper nose, and the sphenoid sinus behind the ethmoid sinus in the center of your skull.

Cancer of the paranasal sinus and nasal cavity most commonly starts in the cells that line the oropharynx, called squamous cells. Much less often, cancer of the paranasal sinus and nasal cavity starts in the color-making cells called melanocytes, and is called a melanoma.

National Cancer Institute PDQ Database, http://cancernet.nci.nih.gov/clinpdq/pif/Paranasal_sinus_and_nasal_cavity_cancer_Patient.html; last updated September 1997.

If the cancer starts in the muscle or connecting tissue, it is called a sarcoma. Another type of cancer that can occur here, called an inverting papilloma, grows more slowly than other cancers that start here. Cancers called midline granulomas may also occur in the paranasal sinuses or nasal cavity, and they cause the tissue around them to break down.

Like most cancers, cancer of the paranasal sinus and nasal cavity is best treated when it is found (diagnosed) early. You should see your doctor if you have blocked sinuses that don't clear, sinus infection, bleeding through your nose, a lump or sore that doesn't heal inside your nose, frequent headaches or pain in the sinus region, swelling or other trouble with your eyes, pain in your upper teeth, or problems with dentures.

If you have symptoms, your doctor will examine your nose using a mirror and lights. Your doctor may order a CT scan (a special x-ray that uses a computer) or an MRI scan (an x-ray-like procedure that uses magnetic energy) to make a picture of the inside of parts of your body. A special instrument (called a rhinoscope or a nasoscope) may be put into your nose to see inside. If tissue that is not normal is found, your doctor will need to cut out a small piece and look at it under the microscope to see if there are any cancer cells. This is called a biopsy. Sometimes your doctor will need to cut into your sinus in order to do a biopsy.

Your chance of recovery (prognosis) depends on where the cancer is in your sinuses, whether the cancer is just in the area where it started or has spread to other tissues (the stage), and your general state of health.

Stage Explanation

Stages of Cancer of the Paranasal Sinus and Nasal Cavity

Once cancer of the paranasal sinus and nasal cavity is found, more tests will be done to find out if cancer cells have spread to other parts of the body. This is called staging. Your doctor needs to know the stage of your disease to plan treatment. There is no staging system for cancer of the nasal cavity or for some of the less common paranasal sinus cancers. The following stages are used for cancer of the maxillary sinus, the most common type of paranasal sinus cancer:

Stage I

The cancer is in only the maxillary sinus and has not destroyed any of the bone in the sinus. The cancer has not spread to lymph nodes in the area (lymph nodes are small bean-shaped structures that are found throughout the body; they produce and store infection-fighting cells).

Stage II

The cancer has begun to destroy the bones around the sinus, but has not spread to lymph nodes in the area.

Stage III

Either of the following may be true:

- The cancer has spread no further than the bones around the sinus and to only one lymph node on the same side of the neck as the cancer. The lymph node that contains cancer measures no more than 3 centimeters (just over one inch).

- The cancer has spread to the cheek, the back of the maxillary sinus, the eye socket, or the ethmoid sinus in front of the maxillary sinus. The cancer may or may not have spread to one lymph node on the same side of the neck as the cancer.

Stage IV

Any of the following may be true:

- The cancer has spread to the eye or to other sinuses or places around the sinuses. The lymph nodes in the area may or may not contain cancer.

- The cancer is in only the sinuses or has spread to the areas around it. The cancer has spread to more than one lymph node on the same side of the neck as the cancer, to lymph nodes on one or both sides of the neck, or to any lymph node that measures more than 6 centimeters (over 2 inches).

- The cancer has spread to other parts of the body.

Recurrent

Recurrent disease means that the cancer has come back (recurred) after it has been treated. It may come back in the paranasal sinuses or nasal cavity or in another part of the body.

Treatment Option Overview

How Cancer of the Paranasal Sinus and Nasal Cavity Is Treated

There are treatments for all patients with cancer of the paranasal sinus and nasal cavity. Three kinds of treatment are used:

- Surgery (taking out the cancer)

- Radiation therapy (using high-dose x-rays or other high-energy rays to kill cancer cells)

- Chemotherapy (using drugs to kill cancer cells).

Surgery is commonly used to remove cancers of the paranasal sinus or nasal cavity. Depending on where the cancer is and how far it has spread, your doctor may need to cut out bone or tissue around the cancer. If cancer has spread to lymph nodes in the neck, the lymph nodes may be removed (lymph node dissection).

Radiation therapy is also a common treatment for cancer of the paranasal sinus and nasal cavity. Radiation therapy uses high-energy x-rays to kill cancer cells and shrink tumors. Radiation may come from a machine outside the body (external radiation therapy) or from putting materials that produce radiation (radioisotopes) through thin plastic tubes in the area where the cancer cells are found (internal radiation therapy). External radiation to the thyroid or the pituitary gland may change the way your thyroid gland works. Your doctor may wish to test your thyroid gland before and after therapy to make sure it is working properly.

Chemotherapy uses drugs to kill cancer cells. Chemotherapy may be taken by pill, or it may be put into the body by a needle in a vein or muscle. Chemotherapy is called a systemic treatment because the drug enters the bloodstream, travels through the body, and can kill cancer cells throughout the body.

Because your paranasal sinuses and nasal cavity help you to talk and breathe and are close to your face, you may need special help adjusting to the side effects of the cancer and its treatment. Your doctor will consult with several kinds of doctors who can help determine the best treatment for you. Trained medical staff can also help you to recover from treatment. You may need plastic surgery if a large amount of tissue or bone around your paranasal sinuses or nasal cavity is taken out.

Treatment by Stage

Treatment for cancer of the paranasal sinus and nasal cavity depends on where the cancer is, the stage of your disease, your age, and your overall health.

You may receive treatment that is considered standard based on its effectiveness in a number of patients in past studies, or you may choose to go into a clinical trial. Not all patients are cured with standard therapy and some standard treatments may have more side effects than are desired. For these reasons, clinical trials are designed to find better ways to treat cancer patients and are based on the most up-to-date information. Clinical trials are going on in some parts of the country for patients with cancer of the paranasal sinus and nasal cavity. If you want more information, call the Cancer Information Service at 1-800-4-CANCER (1-800-422-6237); TTY at 1-800-332-8615.

Stage I Paranasal Sinus and Nasal Cavity Cancer

Your treatment depends on the type of cancer and where the cancer is found.

- If you have cancer in the **maxillary sinus**, your treatment will probably be surgery to remove the cancer. Radiation therapy may be given after surgery.

- If you have cancer in the **ethmoid sinus**, your treatment may be one of the following:

  1. Radiation therapy if the cancer cannot be removed with surgery.

  2. Surgery followed by radiation therapy.

- If you have cancer in the **sphenoid sinus**, your treatment will probably be radiation therapy.

- If you have cancer in the **nasal cavity**, your treatment may be surgery, radiation therapy, or both.

- If you have a cancer called an **inverting papilloma**, your treatment will probably be surgery.

- If you have a cancer called a **melanoma** or **sarcoma**, your treatment will probably be surgery. For certain types of sarcoma, surgery, radiation therapy, and chemotherapy may be given.

- If you have a cancer called a **midline granuloma**, your treatment will probably be radiation therapy.

- If you have a cancer of the **nose** (**nasal vestibule**), your treatment may be surgery or radiation therapy.

Stage II Paranasal Sinus and Nasal Cavity Cancer

Your treatment depends on the type of cancer and where the cancer is found.

- If you have cancer in the **maxillary sinus**, your treatment will probably be surgery to remove the cancer. Radiation therapy is given before or after surgery.

- If you have cancer in the **ethmoid sinus**, your treatment may be one of the following:

  1. External beam radiation therapy.
  2. Surgery followed by radiation therapy.

- If you have cancer in the **sphenoid sinus**, your treatment will probably be radiation therapy.

- If you have cancer in the **nasal cavity**, your treatment may be surgery, radiation therapy, or both.

- If you have a cancer called an **inverting papilloma**, your treatment will probably be surgery. If the cancer comes back after surgery, you may receive radiation therapy.

- If you have a cancer called a **melanoma** or **sarcoma**, your treatment will probably be surgery. For certain types of sarcoma, surgery, radiation therapy, and chemotherapy may be given.

- If you have a cancer called a **midline granuloma**, your treatment will probably be radiation therapy.

- If you have a cancer of the inside of the **nose** (**nasal vestibule**), your treatment may be surgery or radiation therapy.

Stage III Paranasal Sinus and Nasal Cavity Cancer

Your treatment depends on the type of cancer and where the cancer is found.

- If you have cancer in the **maxillary sinus**, your treatment may be one of the following:
    1. Surgery to remove the cancer. Radiation therapy is given before or after surgery.
    2. A clinical trial of a special type of radiation therapy given before or after surgery.
    3. A clinical trial of chemotherapy combined with radiation therapy.

- If you have cancer in the **ethmoid sinus**, your treatment may be one of the following:
    1. Surgery followed by radiation therapy.
    2. A clinical trial of chemotherapy before surgery or radiation therapy.
    3. A clinical trial of chemotherapy following surgery with or without radiation therapy.
    4. A clinical trial of chemotherapy combined with radiation therapy.

- If you have cancer in the **sphenoid sinus**, your treatment will probably be radiation therapy.

- If you have cancer in the **nasal cavity**, your treatment may be one of the following:
    1. Surgery.
    2. Radiation therapy.
    3. Surgery plus radiation therapy.
    4. A clinical trial of chemotherapy before surgery or radiation therapy.
    5. A clinical trial of chemotherapy following surgery with or without radiation therapy.
    6. A clinical trial of chemotherapy combined with radiation therapy.

- If you have a cancer called an **inverting papilloma**, your treatment will probably be surgery. If the cancer comes back after surgery, you may receive radiation therapy.

- If you have a cancer called a **melanoma** or **sarcoma**, your treatment will probably be surgery. Radiation therapy may be given if the cancer cannot be removed with surgery. For certain types of sarcoma, surgery, radiation therapy, and chemotherapy may be given.

- If you have a cancer called a **midline granuloma**, your treatment will probably be radiation therapy.

- If you have a cancer of the inside of the **nose (nasal vestibule)**, your treatment may be one of the following:

  1. External beam and/or internal radiation therapy.

  2. Surgery if the cancer comes back following treatment.

  3. A clinical trial of chemotherapy before surgery or radiation therapy.

  4. A clinical trial of chemotherapy following surgery with or without radiation therapy.

  5. A clinical trial of chemotherapy combined with radiation therapy.

Stage IV Paranasal Sinus and Nasal Cavity Cancer

Your treatment depends on the type of cancer and where the cancer is found.

- If you have cancer in the **maxillary sinus**, your treatment will probably be one of the following:

  1. Radiation therapy.

  2. A clinical trial of chemotherapy before surgery or radiation therapy.

  3. A clinical trial of chemotherapy following radiation therapy.

  4. A clinical trial of chemotherapy combined with radiation therapy.

- If you have cancer in the **ethmoid sinus**, your treatment may be one of the following:

1. Surgery followed by radiation therapy.
2. Radiation therapy followed by surgery.
3. A clinical trial of chemotherapy before surgery or radiation therapy.
4. A clinical trial of chemotherapy following surgery with or without radiation therapy.
5. A clinical trial of chemotherapy combined with radiation therapy.

- If you have cancer in the **sphenoid sinus**, your treatment will probably be radiation therapy.

- If you have cancer in the **nasal cavity**, your treatment may be one of the following:

1. Surgery.
2. Radiation therapy.
3. Surgery plus radiation therapy.
4. A clinical trial of chemotherapy before surgery or radiation therapy.
5. A clinical trial of chemotherapy following surgery with or without radiation therapy.
6. A clinical trial of chemotherapy combined with radiation therapy.

- If you have a cancer called an **inverting papilloma**, your treatment will probably be surgery. If the cancer comes back after surgery, you may receive radiation therapy.

- If you have a cancer called a **melanoma** or **sarcoma**, your treatment will probably be surgery, if possible. Radiation therapy or chemotherapy may be given if the cancer cannot be removed with surgery.

- If you have a cancer called a **midline granuloma**, your treatment will probably be radiation therapy.

- If you have a cancer of the inside of the **nose (nasal vestibule)**, your treatment may be one of the following:

1. External beam and/or internal radiation therapy.

2. Surgery if the cancer comes back following treatment.

3. A clinical trial of chemotherapy before surgery or radiation therapy.

4. A clinical trial of chemotherapy following surgery with or without radiation therapy.

5. A clinical trial of chemotherapy combined with radiation therapy.

Recurrent Paranasal Sinus and Nasal Cavity Cancer

Your treatment depends on the type of cancer, where the cancer is found, and the type of treatment you received before.

- If you have cancer in the **maxillary sinus**, your treatment will probably be one of the following:

  1. If surgery was done before, more extensive surgery followed by radiation therapy or radiation therapy alone.

  2. If radiation therapy was given before, surgery.

  3. Chemotherapy. Clinical trials are testing new chemotherapy drugs.

- If you have cancer in the **ethmoid sinus**, your treatment may be one of the following:

  1. If limited surgery was done before, more extensive surgery followed by radiation therapy or radiation therapy alone.

  2. If radiation therapy was given before, surgery.

  3. Chemotherapy. Clinical trials are testing new chemotherapy drugs.

- If you have cancer in the **sphenoid sinus**, your treatment will probably be radiation therapy. Chemotherapy is given if radiation therapy does not work.

- If you have cancer in the **nasal cavity**, your treatment may be one of the following:

  1. If limited surgery was done before, radiation therapy alone or more extensive surgery followed by radiation therapy.

  2. If radiation therapy was given before, surgery.

3. Chemotherapy. Clinical trials are testing new chemotherapy drugs.

- If you have a cancer called an **inverting papilloma**, your treatment will probably be surgery. If the cancer comes back after surgery, you may receive more surgery or radiation therapy.

- If you have a cancer called a **melanoma** or **sarcoma**, your treatment may be surgery or chemotherapy.

- If you have a cancer called a **midline granuloma**, your treatment will probably be radiation therapy.

- If you have a cancer of the inside of the **nose** (**nasal vestibule**), your treatment may be one of the following:

  1. If radiation therapy was given before, surgery.

  2. If surgery was done before, radiation therapy alone or more extensive surgery followed by radiation therapy.

  3. Chemotherapy. Clinical trials are testing new chemotherapy drugs.

To Learn More

To Learn More..... Call 1-800-4-CANCER

To learn more about cancer of the paranasal sinus and nasal cavity, call the National Cancer Institute's Cancer Information Service at 1-800-4-CANCER (1-800-422-6237); TTY at 1-800-332-8615. By dialing this toll-free number, you can speak with someone who can answer your questions.

You can also write to the National Cancer Institute at this address:

National Cancer Institute
Office of Cancer Communications
31 Center Drive, MSC 2580
Bethesda, MD 20892-2580

Chapter 62

Nasopharyngeal Cancer

What Is Cancer of the Nasopharynx?

Cancer of the nasopharynx is a disease in which cancer (malignant) cells are found in the tissues of the nasopharynx. The nasopharynx is behind the nose and is the upper part of the throat (also called the pharynx). The pharynx is a hollow tube about 5 inches long that starts behind the nose and goes down to the neck to become part of the tube that goes to the stomach (the esophagus). Air and food pass through the pharynx on the way to the windpipe (trachea) or the esophagus. The holes in the nose through which you breathe (the nares) lead into the nasopharynx. Two openings on the side of the nasopharynx lead into the ear.

Cancer of the nasopharynx most commonly starts in the cells that line the oropharynx, called squamous cells. If you have a cancer that started in the lymph cells of the nasopharynx (a lymphoma), see the PDQ patient information statement on non-Hodgkin's lymphoma.

Like most cancers, cancer of the nasopharynx is best treated when it is found (diagnosed) early. You should see your doctor if you have trouble breathing or speaking, frequent headaches, a lump in your nose or neck, pain or ringing in your ear, or trouble hearing.

If you have symptoms, your doctor will examine your throat using a mirror and lights. A special instrument (called a nasoscope) may be

National Cancer Institute PDQ Database, http://cancernet.nci.nih.gov/clinpdq/pif/Nasopharyngeal_cancer_Pa tient.html; last updated September 1997.

put into your nose to see into the nasopharynx. Your doctor will also feel your neck for lumps. If tissue that is not normal is found, your doctor will need to cut out a small piece and look at it under the microscope to see if there are any cancer cells. This is called a biopsy.

Your chance of recovery (prognosis) depends on where the cancer is in your throat, whether the cancer is just in your throat or has spread to other tissues (the stage), and your general state of health.

Stage Explanation

Stages of Cancer of the Nasopharynx

Once cancer of the nasopharynx is found, more tests will be done to find out if cancer cells have spread to other parts of the body. This is called staging. Your doctor needs to know the stage of your disease to plan treatment. The following stages are used for cancer of the nasopharynx:

Stage I

The cancer is in only one part of the nasopharynx and has not spread to lymph nodes in the area (lymph nodes are small bean-shaped structures that are found throughout the body; they produce and store infection-fighting cells).

Stage II

The cancer is in more than one part of the nasopharynx and has not spread to lymph nodes in the area.

Stage III

Either of the following may be true:

- The cancer has spread into the nose or to the part of the throat behind the mouth (the oropharynx).

- The cancer is in the nasopharynx or has spread to the nose or the oropharynx. The cancer has spread to only one lymph node on the same side of the neck as the cancer. The lymph node that contains cancer measures no more than 3 centimeters (just over one inch).

Stage IV

Any of the following may be true:

- The cancer has spread to the bones or nerves in the head. The lymph nodes in the area may or may not contain cancer.

- The cancer is in the nasopharynx or has spread to the nose, the nasopharynx, or the bone or nerves in the head. The cancer has spread to more than one lymph node on the same side of the neck as the cancer, to lymph nodes on one or both sides of the neck, or to any lymph node that measures more than 6 centimeters (over 2 inches).

- The cancer has spread to other parts of the body.

Recurrent

Recurrent disease means that the cancer has come back (recurred) after it has been treated. It may come back in the nasopharynx or in another part of the body.

Treatment Option Overview

How Cancer of the Nasopharynx Is Treated

There are treatments for all patients with cancer of the nasopharynx. Three kinds of treatment are used:

- Radiation therapy (using high-dose x-rays or other high-energy rays to kill cancer cells).

- Surgery (taking out the cancer).
- Chemotherapy (using drugs to kill cancer cells).

Biological therapy (using the body's immune system to fight cancer) is being tested in clinical trials.

Radiation therapy is the most common treatment for cancer of the nasopharynx. Radiation therapy uses high-energy x-rays to kill cancer cells and shrink tumors. Radiation may come from a machine outside the body (external radiation therapy) or from putting materials that produce radiation (radioisotopes) through thin plastic tubes in the area where the cancer cells are found (internal radiation therapy). External radiation to the thyroid or the pituitary gland may change the way your thyroid gland works. Your doctor may wish to test your thyroid gland before and after therapy to make sure it is working properly.

Surgery is sometimes used for cancer of the nasopharynx that does not respond to radiation. If cancer has spread to lymph nodes, the lymph nodes may be removed (lymph node dissection).

Chemotherapy uses drugs to kill cancer cells. Chemotherapy may be taken by pill, or it may be put into the body by a needle in the vein or muscle. Chemotherapy is called a systemic treatment because the drug enters the bloodstream, travels through the body, and can kill cancer cells throughout the body.

Biological therapy tries to get your own body to fight cancer. It uses materials made by your own body or made in a laboratory to boost, direct, or restore your body's natural defenses against disease. Biological therapy is sometimes called biological response modifier (BRM) therapy or immunotherapy.

Because the nasopharynx helps you to breathe and is close to your face, you may need special help adjusting to the side effects of the cancer and its treatment. Your doctor will consult with several kinds of doctors who can help determine the best treatment for you. Trained medical staff can also help you to recover from treatment. You may need plastic surgery if a large part of your nasopharynx is taken out.

Treatment by Stage

Treatment for cancer of the nasopharynx depends on where the cancer is in the nasopharynx, the stage of your disease, your age, and your overall health.

You may receive treatment that is considered standard based on its effectiveness in a number of patients in past studies, or you may choose to go into a clinical trial. Not all patients are cured with standard therapy and some standard treatments may have more side effects than are desired. For these reasons, clinical trials are designed to find better ways to treat cancer patients and are based on the most up-to-date information. Clinical trials are going on in many parts of the country for patients with cancer of the nasopharynx. If you want more information, call the Cancer Information Service at 1-800-4-CANCER (1-800-422-6237); TTY at 1-800-332-8615.

Stage I Nasopharyngeal Cancer

Your treatment will probably be radiation therapy to the cancer and the lymph nodes in the neck.

Stage II Nasopharyngeal Cancer

Your treatment will probably be radiation therapy to the cancer and the lymph nodes in the neck.

Stage III Nasopharyngeal Cancer

Your treatment may be one of the following:

1. Radiation therapy to the cancer and the lymph nodes in the neck.
2. Radiation therapy followed by surgery to remove lymph nodes in the neck that remain large after radiation.
3. A clinical trial of chemotherapy followed by surgery or radiation therapy.
4. A clinical trial of radiotherapy followed by chemotherapy.
5. A clinical trial of surgery, radiation therapy, and chemotherapy.
6. A clinical trial of chemotherapy combined with radiation therapy.

Stage IV Nasopharyngeal Cancer

Your treatment may be one of the following:

1. Radiation therapy to the cancer and the lymph nodes in the neck.
2. Radiation therapy followed by surgery to remove lymph nodes in the neck that remain large after radiation.
3. A clinical trial of chemotherapy followed by surgery or radiation therapy.
4. A clinical trial of surgery, radiation therapy, and chemotherapy.
5. A clinical trial of chemotherapy combined with radiation therapy.

Recurrent Nasopharyngeal Cancer

Your treatment may be one of the following:

1.   Radiation therapy.

2.   Surgery to remove the cancer.

3.   Chemotherapy.

4.   A clinical trial of chemotherapy and/or biological therapy.

To Learn More

To Learn More..... Call 1-800-4-CANCER

To learn more about cancer of the nasopharynx, call the National Cancer Institute's Cancer Information Service at 1-800-4-CANCER (1-800-422-6237); TTY at 1-800-332-8615. By dialing this toll-free number, you can speak with someone who can answer your questions.

You can also write to the National Cancer Institute at this address:

National Cancer Institute
Office of Cancer Communications
31 Center Drive, MSC 2580
Bethesda, MD 20892-2580

Chapter 63

Esophageal Cancer

What Is Cancer of the Esophagus?

Cancer of the esophagus is a disease in which cancer (malignant) cells are found in the tissues of the esophagus. The esophagus is the hollow tube that carries food and liquid from the throat to the stomach.

The most common sign of cancer of the esophagus is difficulty swallowing. Pain may be felt when swallowing or pain may be felt from behind the breastbone.

If there are symptoms, a doctor will usually do a special x-ray called a barium swallow. For this test the patient drinks a liquid containing barium, which makes the esophagus easier to see in the x-ray. This test is usually done in a doctor's office.

A doctor may also look at the inside of the esophagus with a thin, lighted tube called a esophagoscope. This test is called an esophagoscopy. For the test, the esophagoscope is passed through the mouth and down the throat into the esophagus. Before the test, a local anesthetic (a substance that causes temporary loss of feeling) is applied to the throat so no pain is felt. This test is usually done in a doctor's office. If the doctor sees tissue that does not look normal, he or she will remove a small piece of tissue so it can be looked at under a microscope to see if there are any cancer cells. This is called a biopsy. Biopsies are usually done during the esophagoscopy while the anesthetic is still working so no pain is felt. Sometimes a biopsy may show changes in the esophagus that are not cancer but may lead to cancer.

National Cancer Institute PDQ Database, http://cancernet.nci.nih.gov/clinpdq/pif/Esophageal_cancer_Patien t.html; last updated January 1998.

The chance of recovery (prognosis) and choice of treatment depend on the stage of the cancer (whether it is just in the esophagus or if it has spread to other places) and the patient's general state of health.

Stage Explanation

Stages of Cancer of the Esophagus

Once esophageal cancer is found, more tests will be done to find out if cancer cells have spread to other parts of the body (staging). A doctor needs to know the stage of the disease to plan treatment. The following stages are used for esophageal cancer:

Stage 0 or Carcinoma In Situ

Stage 0 cancer of the esophagus is very early cancer. Cancer is found only in the first layer of cells in the lining of the esophagus.

Stage I

Cancer is found in only a small part of the esophagus and has not spread to nearby tissues, lymph nodes, or other organs. (Lymph nodes are small, bean-shaped structures that are found throughout the body. They produce and store infection-fighting cells.)

Stage II

Cancer is found in a large portion of the esophagus and has spread to all sides of the esophagus, and may have spread to local lymph nodes, but has not spread to other tissues.

Stage III

Cancer has spread to tissues or lymph nodes near the esophagus, but has not spread to other parts of the body.

Stage IV

Cancer has spread to other parts of the body.

Recurrent

Recurrent disease means that the cancer has come back (recurred) after it has been treated. It may come back in the esophagus or in another part of the body.

Treatment Option Overview

How Cancer of the Esophagus Is Treated

There are treatments for all patients with cancer of the esophagus. Three kinds of treatment are used:

- surgery (taking out the cancer in an operation)
- radiation therapy (using high-dose x-rays to kill cancer cells)
- chemotherapy (using drugs to kill cancer cells)

Surgery is the most common treatment for cancer of the esophagus. A doctor may remove the esophagus in an operation called an esophagectomy. The doctor will connect the remaining healthy part of the esophagus to the stomach so the patient can still swallow. A plastic tube or part of the intestine may sometimes be used to make the connection. The doctor may also remove lymph nodes around the esophagus and look at them under a microscope to see if they contain cancer.

Radiation therapy uses x-rays or other high-energy rays to kill cancer cells and shrink tumors. Radiation may come from a machine outside the body (external radiation therapy) or from putting materials that contain radiation through thin plastic tubes (internal radiation therapy) in the area where the cancer cells are found. When radiation therapy is used to treat cancer of the esophagus, a plastic tube is sometimes inserted into the esophagus to keep it open. This is called intraluminal intubation and dilation.

Chemotherapy uses drugs to kill cancer cells. Chemotherapy may be taken by pill, or it may be put into the body by a needle in the vein or muscle. Chemotherapy is called a systemic treatment because the drug enters the bloodstream, travels through the body, and can kill cancer cells throughout the body. Chemotherapy with or without radiation is being tested in clinical trials. The use of chemotherapy and radiation therapy before surgery (neoadjuvant therapy) is also being tested in clinical trials.

Treatment by Stage

Treatments for cancer of the esophagus depend on the stage of the disease and the patient's general health.

Standard treatment may be considered because of its effectiveness in patients in past studies, or participation in a clinical trial may be considered. Not all patients are cured with standard therapy and some standard treatments may have more side effects than are desired. For these reasons, clinical trials are designed to find better ways to treat cancer patients and are based on the most up-to-date information. Clinical trials are ongoing in most parts of the country for most stages of cancer of the esophagus. To learn more about clinical trials, call the Cancer Information Service at 1-800-4-CANCER (1-800-422-6237); TTY at 1-800-332-8615.

Stage 0 Esophageal Cancer

Treatment is usually surgery to remove the tumor.

Stage I Esophageal Cancer

Treatment may be one of the following:

1. Surgery to remove the tumor and all or part of the esophagus (esophagectomy).

2. Chemotherapy plus radiation therapy. Surgery may be performed after other therapy is completed. Clinical trials are testing changes in the timing of when chemotherapy and radiation therapy are given.

3. A clinical trial of surgery with or without radiation therapy.

4. Clinical trials of chemotherapy and radiation therapy with surgery.

Stage II Esophageal Cancer

Treatment may be one of the following:

1. Surgery to remove the tumor and all or part of the esophagus (esophagectomy).

2. Chemotherapy plus radiation therapy. Surgery may be performed after other therapy is completed. Clinical trials are testing changes in the timing of when chemotherapy and radiation therapy are given.

3. A clinical trial of surgery with or without radiation therapy.

4. Clinical trials of chemotherapy and radiation therapy with surgery.

Stage III Esophageal Cancer

Treatment may be one of the following:

1. Surgery to remove the tumor to relieve pain or discomfort.

2. Chemotherapy plus radiation therapy. Surgery may be performed after other therapy is completed.

3. Clinical trials of chemotherapy plus radiation therapy.

Stage IV Esophageal Cancer

Treatment may be one of the following:

1. Radiation therapy with or without insertion of a tube to keep the esophagus open (intraluminal intubation and dilation).

2. Clinical trials of chemotherapy plus radiation therapy.

Recurrent Esophageal Cancer

Surgery or radiation therapy may be used to relieve pain or discomfort. A patient may choose to take part in a clinical trial.

To Learn More

To Learn More..... Call 1-800-4-CANCER

To learn more about cancer of the esophagus, call the National Cancer Institute's Cancer Information Service at 1-800-4-CANCER (1-800-422-6237); TTY at 1-800-332-8615. By dialing this toll-free number, trained information specialists can answer your questions.

The Cancer Information Service also has booklets about cancer that are available to the public and can be sent on request. The following booklet about cancer of the esophagus may be helpful: *What You Need To Know About Cancer of the Esophagus*

For more information from the National Cancer Institute, please write to this address:

National Cancer Institute
Office of Cancer Communications
31 Center Drive, MSC 2580
Bethesda, MD 20892-2580

Chapter 64

Oropharyngeal Cancer

What Is Cancer of the Oropharynx?

Cancer of the oropharynx is a disease in which cancer (malignant) cells are found in the tissues of the oropharynx. The oropharynx is the middle part of the throat (also called the pharynx). The pharynx is a hollow tube about 5 inches long that starts behind the nose and goes down to the neck to become part of the tube that goes to the stomach (the esophagus). Air and food pass through the pharynx on the way to the windpipe (trachea) or the esophagus. The oropharynx includes the soft palate (the back of the mouth), the base of the tongue, and the tonsils.

Cancer of the oropharynx most commonly starts in the cells that line the oropharynx, called squamous cells. If you have a cancer that started in the lymph cells of the oropharynx (a lymphoma), see the PDQ patient information statement on non-Hodgkin's lymphoma.

Like most cancers, cancer of the oropharynx is best treated when it is found (diagnosed) early. You should see your doctor if you have a sore throat that does not go away, trouble swallowing, a lump in the back of your mouth or throat, a change in your voice, or pain in your ear.

If you have symptoms, your doctor will examine your throat using a mirror and lights. Your doctor will also feel your throat for lumps. If tissue that is not normal is found, your doctor will need to cut out a small piece and look at it under the microscope to see if there are any cancer cells. This is called a biopsy.

National Cancer Institute PDQ Database, http://cancernet.nci.nih.gov/clinpdq/pif/Oropharyngeal_cancer_Patient.html; last updated September 1997.

513

Your chance of recovery (prognosis) depends on where the cancer is in your throat, whether the cancer is just in your throat or has spread to other tissues (the stage), and your general state of health. After your treatment you should see your doctor regularly because you have a chance of having a second cancer in the head or neck region.

Stage Explanation

Stages of Cancer of the Oropharynx

Once cancer of the oropharynx is found, more tests will be done to find out if cancer cells have spread to other parts of the body. This is called staging. Your doctor needs to know the stage of your disease to plan treatment. The following stages are used for cancer of the oropharynx.

Stage I

The cancer is no more than 2 centimeters (about 1 inch) and has not spread to lymph nodes in the area (lymph nodes are small bean-shaped structures that are found throughout the body; they produce and store infection-fighting cells).

Stage II

The cancer is more than 2 centimeters, but less than 4 centimeters (less than 2 inches), and has not spread to lymph nodes in the area.

Stage III

Either of the following may be true:

- The cancer is more than 4 centimeters.

- The cancer is any size but has spread to only one lymph node on the same side of the neck as the cancer. The lymph node that contains cancer measures no more than 3 centimeters (just over one inch).

Stage IV

Any of the following may be true:

- The cancer has spread to tissues around the oropharynx. The lymph nodes in the area may or may not contain cancer.

- The cancer is any size and has spread to more than one lymph node on the same side of the neck as the cancer, to lymph nodes on one or both sides of the neck, or to any lymph node that measures more than 6 centimeters (over 2 inches).

- The cancer has spread to other parts of the body.

Recurrent

Recurrent disease means that the cancer has come back (recurred) after it has been treated. It may come back in the oropharynx or in another part of the body.

Treatment Option Overview

How Cancer of the Oropharynx is Treated

There are treatments for all patients with cancer of the oropharynx. Three kinds of treatment are used:

- Surgery (taking out the cancer)

- Radiation therapy (using high-dose x-rays or other high-energy rays to kill cancer cells)

- Chemotherapy (using drugs to kill cancer cells).

Hyperthermia (warming the body to kill cancer cells) is being tested in clinical trials.

Surgery is a common treatment for cancer of the oropharynx. Your doctor may remove the cancer and some of the healthy tissue around the cancer. If cancer has spread to lymph nodes, the lymph nodes will be removed (lymph node dissection). A new type of surgery called micrographic surgery is being tested in clinical trials for early cancers of the oropharynx. Micrographic surgery removes the cancer and as little normal tissue as possible. During this surgery, the doctor removes the cancer and then uses a microscope to look at the cancerous area to make sure there are no cancer cells remaining.

Radiation therapy uses high-energy x-rays to kill cancer cells and shrink tumors. Radiation may come from a machine outside the body (external radiation therapy) or from putting materials that produce radiation (radioisotopes) through thin plastic tubes in the area where the cancer cells are found (internal radiation therapy). External radiation to the thyroid or the pituitary gland may change the way your thyroid gland works. Your doctor may wish to test your thyroid gland before and after therapy to make sure it is working properly. Giving drugs with the radiation therapy to make the cancer cells more sensitive to radiation (radiosensitization) is being tested in clinical trials. If you stop smoking before you start radiation therapy, you have a better chance of surviving longer.

Chemotherapy uses drugs to kill cancer cells. Chemotherapy may be taken by pill, or it may be put into the body by a needle in the vein or muscle. Chemotherapy is called a systemic treatment because the drug enters the bloodstream, travels through the body, and can kill cancer cells throughout the body.

People with oropharyngeal cancer have a higher risk of getting other cancers in the head and neck area. Clinical trials of **chemoprevention therapy** are testing whether certain drugs can prevent second cancers from developing in your mouth, throat, windpipe, nose, or esophagus (the tube that connects your throat to your stomach).

Hyperthermia uses a special machine to heat your body for a certain period of time to kill cancer cells. Because cancer cells are often more sensitive to heat than normal cells, the cancer cells die and the cancer shrinks.

Because the oropharynx helps you to breath, eat, and talk, you may need special help adjusting to the side effects of the cancer and its treatment. Your doctor will consult with several kinds of doctors who can help determine the best treatment for you. Trained medical staff can also help you recover from treatment and adjust to new ways of eating and talking. You may need plastic surgery or help learning to eat and speak if a large part of your oropharynx is taken out.

Treatment by Stage

Treatment for cancer of the oropharynx depends on where the cancer is in the oropharynx, the stage of your disease, your age, and your overall health.

You may receive treatment that is considered standard based on its effectiveness in a number of patients in past studies, or you may choose to go into a clinical trial. Not all patients are cured with standard therapy and some standard treatments may have more side effects than are desired. For these reasons, clinical trials are designed to find better ways to treat cancer patients and are based on the most up-to-date information. Clinical trials are going on in many parts of the country for patients with cancer of the oropharynx. If you want more information, call the Cancer Information Service at 1-800-4-CANCER (1-800-422-6237); TTY at 1-800-332-8615.

Stage I Oropharyngeal Cancer

Your treatment may be one of the following:

1. Surgery to remove the cancer.

2. Radiation therapy. Clinical trials are testing new ways of giving radiation therapy.

3. A clinical trial of microsurgery followed by radiation therapy.

Stage II Oropharyngeal Cancer

Your treatment may be one of the following:

1. Surgery to remove the cancer.

2. Radiation therapy. Clinical trials are testing new ways of giving radiation therapy.

3. A clinical trial of microsurgery followed by radiation therapy.

4. A clinical trial of chemoprevention therapy to prevent a second cancer in your mouth, throat, windpipe, nose, or esophagus.

Stage III Oropharyngeal Cancer

Your treatment may be one of the following:

1. Surgery to remove the cancer followed by radiation therapy.

2. A clinical trial of chemotherapy followed by surgery or radiation therapy.

3. A clinical trial of chemotherapy combined with radiation therapy.

4. A clinical trial of new ways of giving radiation therapy.

5. A clinical trial of microsurgery followed by radiation therapy.

6. A clinical trial of chemoprevention therapy to prevent a second cancer in your mouth, throat, windpipe, nose, or esophagus.

Stage IV Oropharyngeal Cancer

If the cancer *can be removed by surgery*, your treatment may be one of the following:

1. Surgery to remove the cancer followed by radiation therapy.

2. A clinical trial of radiation therapy combined with chemotherapy.

3. A clinical trial of new ways of giving radiation therapy.

4. A clinical trial of microsurgery followed by radiation therapy.

If the cancer *cannot be removed by surgery*, your treatment may be one of the following:

1. Radiation therapy. Clinical trials are testing new ways of giving radiation therapy.

2. A clinical trial of chemotherapy followed by surgery or radiation therapy.

3. A clinical trial of radiation therapy given with chemotherapy or with drugs to make the cancer cells more sensitive to radiation therapy (radiosensitizers).

4. A clinical trial of hyperthermia plus radiation therapy.

Recurrent Oropharyngeal Cancer

Your treatment may be one of the following:

1. Surgery to remove the cancer.

2. Radiation therapy.

3. A clinical trial of chemotherapy.

4. A clinical trial of hyperthermia plus radiation therapy.

To Learn More

To Learn More..... Call 1-800-4-CANCER

To learn more about cancer of the oropharynx, call the National Cancer Institute's Cancer Information Service at 1-800-4-CANCER (1-800-422-6237); TTY at 1-800-332-8615. By dialing this toll-free number, you can speak with someone who can answer your questions.

The Cancer Information Service can also send you booklets. The following booklet about oral cancer may be helpful to you: *What You Need To Know About Oral Cancer*.

You can also write to the National Cancer Institute at this address:

National Cancer Institute
Office of Cancer Communications
31 Center Drive, MSC 2580
Bethesda, MD 20892-2580

Chapter 65

Hypopharyngeal Cancer

What Is Cancer of the Hypopharynx?

Cancer of the hypopharynx is a disease in which cancer (malignant) cells are found in the tissues of the hypopharynx. The hypopharynx is the bottom part of the throat (also called the pharynx). The pharynx is a hollow tube about 5 inches long that starts behind the nose and goes down to the neck to become part of the esophagus, the tube that goes to the stomach. Air and food pass through the pharynx on the way to the windpipe (trachea) or the esophagus.

Cancer of the hypopharynx most commonly starts in the cells that line the hypopharynx, called squamous cells. If cancer has started in the lymph cells of the hypopharynx (a lymphoma), see the PDQ patient information summary on non-Hodgkin's lymphoma.

A doctor should be seen if a person has a sore throat that does not go away, trouble swallowing, a lump in the neck, a change in voice, or ear pain.

If there are symptoms, a doctor will examine the throat using a mirror and lights. A thin lighted tube called an endoscope may be put down the throat so the doctor can see if there is tissue that is not normal. The doctor will also feel the throat for lumps. If tissue that is not normal is found, the doctor will need to cut out a small piece and look at it under the microscope to see if there are any cancer cells. This is called a biopsy.

National Cancer Institute PDQ Database, http://cancernet.nci.nih.gov/clinpdq/pif/Hypopharyngeal_cancer_Patient.html; last updated February 1998.

The chance of recovery (prognosis) depends on where the cancer is in the throat, whether the cancer is just in the throat or has spread to other tissues (the stage), and the patient's general state of health.

Stage Explanation

Stages of Cancer of the Hypopharynx

Once cancer of the hypopharynx is found, more tests will be done to find out if cancer cells have spread to other parts of the body. This is called staging. A doctor needs to know the stage of the disease to plan treatment. The following stages are used for cancer of the hypopharynx:

Stage I

The cancer is in only one part of the hypopharynx and has not spread to lymph nodes in the area (lymph nodes are small bean-shaped structures that are found throughout the body; they produce and store infection-fighting cells).

Stage II

The cancer is in more than one part of the hypopharynx or has spread to tissue next to the hypopharynx, but has not grown into the voice box (larynx). The cancer has not spread to lymph nodes in the area.

Stage III

Either of the following may be true:

- The cancer is in more than one part of the hypopharynx or has spread to tissue next to the hypopharynx. The cancer has grown into the larynx.
- The cancer is in the hypopharynx or has spread to the tissue around the hypopharynx. The cancer has spread to only one lymph node on the same side of the neck as the cancer. The lymph node that contains cancer measures no more than 3 centimeters (just over one inch).

Stage IV

Any of the following may be true:

- The cancer has spread to the connecting tissue or soft tissues of the neck. The lymph nodes in the area may or may not contain cancer.

- The cancer is in the hypopharynx or has spread to the tissues around the hypopharynx. The cancer has spread to more than one lymph node on the same side of the neck as the cancer, to lymph nodes on one or both sides of the neck, or to any lymph node that measures more than 6 centimeters (over 2 inches).

- The cancer has spread to other parts of the body.

Recurrent

Recurrent disease means that the cancer has come back (recurred) after it has been treated. It may come back in the hypopharynx or in another part of the body.

Treatment Option Overview

How Cancer of the Hypopharynx Is Treated

There are treatments for all patients with cancer of the hypopharynx. Two kinds of treatment are used:

- surgery (taking out the cancer)
- radiation therapy (using high-dose x-rays or other high-energy rays to kill cancer cells)

Chemotherapy (using drugs to kill cancer cells) is being tested in clinical trials.

Surgery is a common treatment of cancer of the hypopharynx. A doctor may remove the larynx and part of the throat in an operation called a laryngopharyngectomy. If the cancer is in the lymph nodes, the lymph nodes may be removed (lymph node dissection).

Radiation therapy uses high-energy x-rays to kill cancer cells and shrink tumors. Radiation may come from a machine outside the body (external radiation therapy) or from putting materials that produce radiation (radioisotopes) through thin plastic tubes in the area where the cancer cells are found (internal radiation therapy). Giving drugs with the radiation therapy to make the cancer cells more sensitive to radiation (radiosensitization) is being tested in clinical trials.

If smoking is stopped before radiation therapy is started, a patient has a better chance of surviving longer. External radiation to the thyroid or the pituitary gland may change the way the thyroid gland works. The doctor may wish to test the thyroid gland before and after therapy to make sure it is working properly.

Chemotherapy uses drugs to kill cancer cells. Chemotherapy may be taken by pill, or it may be put into the body by a needle in the vein or muscle. Chemotherapy is called a systemic treatment because the drug enters the bloodstream, travels through the body, and can kill cancer cells throughout the body.

Because the hypopharynx helps people with breathing, eating, and talking, a patient may need special help adjusting to the side effects of the cancer and its treatment. The patient's doctor will consult with several kinds of doctors who can help determine the best treatment. Trained medical staff can also help the patient recover from treatment. The patient may need plastic surgery or help learning to eat and speak if all or part of the hypopharynx is taken out.

Treatment by Stage

Treatment of cancer of the hypopharynx depends on where the cancer is in the hypopharynx, the stage of the disease, and the patient's age and overall health.

Standard treatment may be considered because of its effectiveness in patients in past studies, or participation in a clinical trial may be considered. Not all patients are cured with standard therapy and some standard treatments may have more side effects than are desired. For these reasons, clinical trials are designed to find better ways to treat cancer patients and are based on the most up-to-date information. Clinical trials are ongoing in many parts of the country for patients with cancer of the hypopharynx. To learn more about clinical trials, call the Cancer Information Service at 1-800-4-CANCER (1-800-422-6237); TTY at 1-800-332-8615.

Stage I Hypopharyngeal Cancer

Treatment may be one of the following:

1. Surgery to remove the larynx and the pharynx (laryngopharyngectomy).

524

2. Surgery followed by radiation therapy.

3. Radiation therapy alone.

Stage II Hypopharyngeal Cancer

Treatment may be one of the following:

1. Surgery to remove the larynx and the pharynx (laryngopharyngectomy) and lymph nodes in the neck, followed by radiation therapy.

2. A clinical trial of chemotherapy followed by radiation therapy or surgery.

Stage III Hypopharyngeal Cancer

Treatment may be one of the following:

1. Surgery plus radiation therapy.

2. A clinical trial of chemotherapy followed by surgery or radiation therapy.

3. A clinical trial of surgery and radiation therapy followed by chemotherapy.

4. A clinical trial of chemotherapy combined with radiation therapy.

Stage IV Hypopharyngeal Cancer

If the cancer can be removed by surgery, treatment may be one of the following:

1. Surgery plus radiation therapy.

2. A clinical trial of chemotherapy followed by surgery or radiation therapy.

If the cancer cannot be removed by surgery, treatment may be one of the following:

1. Radiation therapy. Clinical trials are testing new ways of giving radiation therapy.

2. A clinical trial of chemotherapy combined with radiation therapy.

Recurrent Hypopharyngeal Cancer

Treatment may be one of the following:

1. Surgery to remove the cancer.

2. Radiation therapy.

3. A clinical trial of chemotherapy.

To Learn More..... Call 1-800-4-CANCER

To learn more about cancer of the hypopharynx, call the National Cancer Institute's Cancer Information Service at 1-800-4-CANCER (1-800-422-6237); TTY at 1-800-332-8615. By dialing this toll-free number, trained information specialists can answer your questions.

For more information from the National Cancer Institute, please write to this address:

National Cancer Institute
Office of Cancer Communications
31 Center Drive, MSC 2580
Bethesda, MD 20892-2580

Chapter 66

Cancer of the Larynx

What You Need to Know about Cancer of the Larynx

Each year, more than 12,000 people in the United States learn that they have cancer of the *larynx*. This chapter will give you some important information about the symptoms, diagnosis, and treatment of this type of cancer. This chapter also has information to help you deal with cancer of the larynx if it affects you or someone you know.

Booklets available from the National Cancer Institute are listed at the end of this chapter. Our materials cannot answer every question you may have about cancer of the larynx. They cannot take the place of talks with doctors, nurses, and other members of the health care team. We hope our information will help with those talks.

Researchers continue to look for better ways to diagnose and treat cancer of the larynx, and our knowledge keeps growing. For up-to-date information, call the NCI-supported Cancer Information Service (CIS) toll free at 1-800-4-CANCER (1-800-422-6237). The CIS is described in the "Resources" section at the end of this chapter.

The Larynx

The larynx, also called the voice box, is a 2-inch-long, tube-shaped organ in the neck. We use the larynx when we breathe, talk, or swallow.

National Cancer Institute, NIH Pub. No. 95-1568, March 1995.

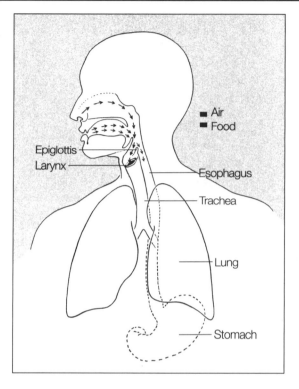

Figure 66.1. *This picture shows the larynx and the normal pathways for air and food.*

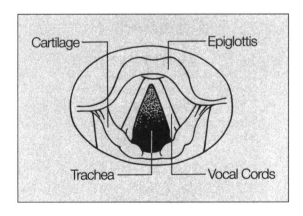

Figure 66.2. *This is how the larynx looks from above. It's what the doctor can see with a mirror.*

The larynx is at the top of the windpipe (*trachea*). Its walls are made of *cartilage*. The large cartilage that forms the front of the larynx is sometimes called the Adam's apple. The *vocal cords*, two bands of muscle, form a "V" inside the larynx.

Each time we inhale (breathe in), air goes into our nose or mouth, then through the larynx, down the trachea, and into our lungs. When we exhale (breathe out), the air goes the other way. When we breathe, the vocal cords are relaxed, and air moves through the space between them without making any sound.

When we talk, the vocal cords tighten up and move closer together. Air from the lungs is forced between them and makes them vibrate, producing the sound of our voice. The tongue, lips, and teeth form this sound into words.

The *esophagus*, a tube that carries food from the mouth to the stomach, is just behind the trachea and the larynx. The openings of the esophagus and the larynx are very close together in the throat. When we swallow, a flap called the *epiglottis* moves down over the larynx to keep food out of the windpipe.

What Is Cancer?

Cancer is a group of more than 100 different diseases. They all affect the body's basic unit, the cell. Cancer occurs when cells become abnormal and divide without control or order.

Like all other organs of the body, the larynx is made up of cells. Normally, cells divide to produce more cells only when the body needs them. This orderly process helps keep us healthy.

If cells keep dividing when new cells are not needed, a mass of extra *tissue* forms. This mass of tissue, called a growth or *tumor*, can be *benign* or *malignant*.

- Benign tumors are not cancer. They do not spread to other parts of the body and are seldom a threat to life. Benign tumors can usually be removed, but certain types may return.

- Malignant tumors are cancer. They can invade and destroy nearby healthy tissues and organs. Cancer cells can also break away from the tumor and enter the bloodstream and the *lymphatic system*. That is how cancer spreads to other parts of the body. This spread is called *metastasis*.

Cancer of the larynx is also called *laryngeal cancer*. It can develop in any region of the larynx—the *glottis* (where the vocal cords are), the *supraglottis* (the area above the cords), or the *subglottis* (the area that connects the larynx to the trachea).

If the cancer spreads outside the larynx, it usually goes first to the *lymph nodes* (sometimes called lymph glands) in the neck. It can also spread to the back of the tongue, other parts of the throat and neck, the lungs, and sometimes other parts of the body.

Cancer that spreads is the same disease and has the same name as the original (primary) cancer. When cancer of the larynx spreads, it is called metastatic laryngeal cancer.

Symptoms

The symptoms of cancer of the larynx depend mainly on the size and location of the tumor. Most cancers of the larynx begin on the vocal cords. These tumors are seldom painful, but they almost always cause hoarseness or other changes in the voice. Tumors in the area above the vocal cords may cause a lump on the neck, a sore throat, or an earache. Tumors that begin in the area below the vocal cords are rare. They can make it hard to breathe, and breathing may be noisy.

A cough that doesn't go away or the feeling of a lump in the throat may also be warning signs of cancer of the larynx. As the tumor grows, it may cause pain, weight loss, bad breath, and frequent choking on food. In some cases, a tumor in the larynx can make it hard to swallow.

Any of these symptoms may be caused by cancer or by other, less serious problems. Only a doctor can tell for sure. People with symptoms like these usually see an ear, nose, and throat specialist (*otolaryngologist*).

Diagnosis

To find the cause of any of these symptoms, the doctor asks about the patient's medical history and does a complete physical exam. In addition to checking general signs of health, the doctor carefully feels the neck to check for lumps, swelling, tenderness, or other changes. The doctor can also look inside the larynx in two ways:

* Indirect *laryngoscopy*. The doctor looks down the throat with a small, long-handled mirror to check for abnormal areas and to see whether the vocal cords move as they should. This test is painless, but a local *anesthetic* may be sprayed in the throat to prevent gagging. This exam is done in the doctor's office.

- Direct laryngoscopy. The doctor inserts a lighted tube (*laryngoscope*) through the patient's nose or mouth. As the tube goes down the throat, the doctor can look at areas that cannot be seen with a simple mirror. A local anesthetic eases discomfort and prevents gagging. Patients may also be given a mild sedative to help them relax. Sometimes the doctor uses a general anesthetic to put the person to sleep. This exam may be done in a doctor's office, an outpatient clinic, or a hospital.

If the doctor sees abnormal areas, the patient will need to have a *biopsy*. A biopsy is the only sure way to know whether cancer is present. For a biopsy, the patient is given a local or general anesthetic, and the doctor removes tissue samples through a laryngoscope. A *pathologist* then examines the tissue under a microscope to check for cancer cells. If cancer is found, the pathologist can tell what type it is. Almost all cancers of the larynx are *squamous cell carcinomas*. This type of cancer begins in the flat, scale-like cells that line the epiglottis, vocal cords, and other parts of the larynx.

If the pathologist finds cancer, the patient's doctor needs to know the stage (extent) of the disease to plan the best treatment. To find out the size of the tumor and whether the cancer has spread, the doctor usually orders more tests, such as *x-rays*, a *CT* (or *CAT*) scan, and/or an *MRI*. During a CT scan, many x-rays are taken. A computer puts them together to create detailed pictures of areas inside the body. An MRI scan produces pictures using a huge magnet linked to a computer.

Treatment Options

Treatment for cancer of the larynx depends on a number of factors. Among these are the exact location and size of the tumor and whether the cancer has spread. To develop a treatment plan to fit each patient's needs, the doctor also considers the person's age, general health, and feelings about the possible treatments.

Many patients want to learn all they can about their disease and their treatment choices so they can take an active part in decisions about their medical care. When discussing treatment options, the patient may want to talk with the doctor about taking part in a research study of new treatment methods. Such studies, called *clinical trials*, are discussed in the section titled "Clinical Trials."

The patient and the doctor should discuss the treatment choices very carefully because treatments for this disease may change the way a person looks and the way he or she breathes and talks. In many cases, the

531

patient meets with both the doctor and a *speech pathologist* to talk about treatment options and possible changes in voice and appearance.

People with cancer of the larynx have many important questions. The doctor and other members of the health care team are the best ones to answer them. Most patients want to know the extent of their cancer, how it can be treated, how successful the treatment is expected to be, and how much it is likely to cost. These are some questions patients may want to ask the doctor:

- What are my treatment choices?
- Would a clinical trial be appropriate for me?
- What are the expected benefits of each kind of treatment?
- What are the risks and possible side effects of each treatment?
- How will I speak after treatment?
- How will I look?
- Will I need to change my normal activities? If so, for how long?
- When will I be able to return to work?
- How often will I need to have checkups?

When a person is diagnosed as having cancer, shock and stress are natural reactions. These feelings may make it difficult for patients to think of everything they want to ask the doctor. Often, it helps to make a list of questions. To help remember what the doctor says, patients may take notes or ask whether they may use a tape recorder. Some people also want to have a family member or friend with them when they talk to the doctor—to take part in the discussion, to take notes, or just to listen.

Getting a Second Opinion

Treatment decisions are complex. Before starting treatment, the patient might want a second doctor to review the diagnosis and treatment plan. It may take a week or two to arrange for a second opinion. A short delay will not reduce the chance that treatment will be successful. Some insurance companies require a second opinion; others cover a second opinion if the patient requests it.

There are a number of ways to find a doctor who can give a second opinion:

- The patient's doctor may be able to suggest a specialist to consult.
- The Cancer Information Service, at 1-800-4-CANCER, can tell callers about treatment facilities, including cancer centers and other programs supported by the National Cancer Institute.

- Patients can get the names of doctors from their local medical society, a nearby hospital, or a medical school.

Treatment Methods

Cancer of the larynx is usually treated with *radiation therapy* (also called radiotherapy) or *surgery*. These are types of *local therapy*; this means they affect cancer cells only in the treated area. Some patients may receive *chemotherapy*, which is called *systemic therapy*, meaning that drugs travel through the bloodstream. They can reach cancer cells all over the body. The doctor may use just one method or combine them, depending on the patient's needs.

In some cases, the patient is referred to doctors who specialize in different kinds of cancer treatment. Often several specialists work together as a team. The medical team may include a surgeon; ear, nose, and throat specialist; cancer specialist (*oncologist*); radiation oncologist; speech pathologist; nurse; and dietitian. A dentist may also be an important member of the team, especially for patients who will have radiation therapy.

Radiation therapy uses high-energy rays to damage cancer cells and stop them from growing. The rays are aimed at the tumor and the area close to it. Whenever possible, doctors suggest this type of treatment because it can destroy the tumor and the patient does not lose his or her voice. Radiation therapy may be combined with surgery; it can be used to shrink a large tumor before surgery or to destroy cancer cells that may remain in the area after surgery. Also, radiation therapy may be used for tumors that can't be removed with surgery or for patients who cannot have surgery for other reasons. If a tumor grows back after surgery, it is generally treated with radiation.

Radiation therapy is usually given 5 days a week for 5 to 6 weeks. At the end of that time, the tumor site very often gets an extra "boost" of radiation. The National Cancer Institute book *Radiation Therapy and You* is a useful source of information about this form of treatment.

Surgery or surgery combined with radiation is suggested for some newly diagnosed patients. Also, surgery is the usual treatment if a tumor does not respond to radiation therapy or grows back after radiation therapy. When patients need surgery, the type of operation depends mainly on the size and exact location of the tumor.

If a tumor on the vocal cord is very small, the surgeon may use a laser, a powerful beam of light. The beam can remove the tumor in much the same way that a scalpel does.

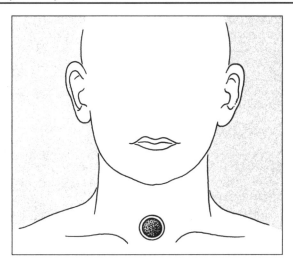

Figure 66.3. *This is a person with a stoma.*

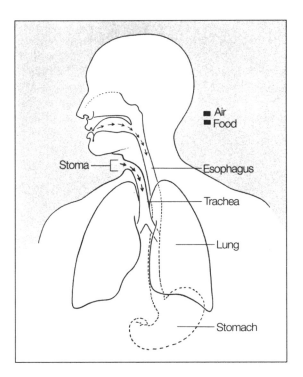

Figure 66.4. *This picture shows the pathways for air and food after a total laryngectomy.*

Surgery to remove part or all of the larynx is a partial or total *laryngectomy*. In either operation, the surgeon performs a *tracheostomy*, creating an opening called a *stoma* in the front of the neck. (The stoma may be temporary or permanent.) Air enters and leaves the trachea and lungs through this opening. A *tracheostomy tube*, also called a trach ("trake") tube, keeps the new airway open.

A partial laryngectomy preserves the voice. The surgeon removes only part of the voice box—just one vocal cord, part of a cord, or just the epiglottis—and the stoma is temporary. After a brief recovery period, the trach tube is removed, and the stoma closes up. The patient can then breathe and talk in the usual way. In some cases, however, the voice may be hoarse or weak.

In a total laryngectomy, the whole voice box is removed, and the stoma is permanent. The patient, called a *laryngectomee*, breathes through the stoma. A laryngectomee must learn to talk in a new way.

If the doctor thinks that the cancer may have started to spread, the lymph nodes in the neck and some of the tissue around them are removed. These nodes are often the first place to which laryngeal cancer spreads.

Chemotherapy is the use of drugs to kill cancer cells. The doctor may suggest one drug or a combination of drugs. In some cases, anticancer drugs are given to shrink a large tumor before the patient has radiation therapy or surgery. Also, chemotherapy may be used for cancers that have spread.

Anticancer drugs for cancer of the larynx are usually given by injection into the bloodstream. Often the drugs are given in cycles—a treatment period followed by a rest period, then another treatment and rest period, and so on. Some patients have their chemotherapy in the outpatient part of the hospital, at the doctor's office, or at home. However, depending on the drugs, the treatment plan, and the patient's general health, a hospital stay may be needed. The National Cancer Institute publication *Chemotherapy and You* has helpful information about this type of treatment.

Treatment Studies

Researchers are looking for treatment methods that are more effective against cancer of the larynx and have fewer side effects. When laboratory research shows that a new method has promise, it is used to treat cancer patients in clinical trials. These trials are designed to find out whether the new approach is both safe and effective and to answer scientific questions. Patients who take part in clinical trials make an important contribution to medical science and may have the first chance to benefit from improved treatment methods.

Many clinical trials of new treatments for cancer of the larynx are under way. Doctors are studying new types and schedules of radiation therapy, new drugs, new drug combinations, and new ways of combining various types of treatment. Scientists are trying to increase the effectiveness of radiation therapy by giving treatments twice a day instead of once. Also, they are studying drugs called "radiosensitizers." These drugs make the cancer cells more sensitive to radiation.

People who have had cancer of the larynx have an increased risk of getting a new cancer in the larynx or in the lungs, mouth, or throat. Doctors are looking for ways to prevent these new cancers. Some research has shown that a drug related to vitamin A may protect people from new cancers.

Patients who are interested in taking part in a trial should talk with their doctor. They may want to read the National Cancer Institute booklet *What Are Clinical Trials All About?*, which explains the possible benefits and risks of treatment studies.

One way to learn about clinical trials is through PDQ, a computerized resource developed by the National Cancer Institute. PDQ contains information about cancer treatment and about clinical trials in progress all over the country. The Cancer Information Service can provide PDQ information to doctors, patients, and the public.

Side Effects of Treatment

The methods used to treat cancer are very powerful. It is hard to limit the effects of therapy so that only cancer cells are removed or destroyed; healthy cells also may be damaged. That's why treatment often causes unpleasant side effects.

The side effects of cancer treatment vary. They depend mainly on the type and extent of the treatment. Also, each person reacts differently. Doctors try to plan the patient's therapy to keep problems to a minimum. Doctors, nurses, dietitians, and speech pathologists can explain the side effects of treatment and suggest ways to deal with them. It may also help to talk with another patient. In many cases, a social worker or another member of the medical team can arrange a visit with someone who has had the same treatment.

Radiation Therapy

During radiation therapy, healing after dental treatment may be a problem. That's why doctors want their patients to begin treatment with their teeth and gums as healthy as possible. They often recommend that patients have a complete dental exam and get any needed dental work done before the radiation therapy begins. It's also important to continue to see the dentist regularly because the mouth may be sensitive and easily irritated during cancer therapy.

In many cases, the mouth is tender during treatment, and some patients may get mouth sores. The doctor may suggest a special rinse to numb the mouth and reduce the discomfort.

Radiation to the larynx causes changes in the saliva and may reduce the amount of saliva. Because saliva normally protects the teeth, tooth decay can be a problem after treatment. Good mouth care can help keep the teeth and gums healthy and can make the patient feel more comfortable. Patients should do their best to keep their teeth clean. If it's hard to floss or brush the teeth in the usual way, patients can use gauze, a soft toothbrush, or a special toothbrush that has a spongy tip instead of bristles. A mouthwash made with diluted peroxide, salt water, and baking soda can keep the mouth fresh and help protect the teeth from decay. It may also be helpful to use a fluoride toothpaste and/or a fluoride rinse to reduce the risk of cavities. The dentist may suggest a special fluoride program to keep the mouth healthy.

If reduced saliva makes the mouth uncomfortably dry, drinking plenty of liquids is helpful. Some patients use a special spray (artificial saliva) to relieve the dryness.

Patients who have radiation therapy instead of surgery do not have a stoma. They breathe and talk in the usual way, although the treatment can change the way their voice sounds. Also, their voice may be weak at the end of the day, and it is not unusual for the voice to be affected by changes in the weather. Voice changes and the feeling of a lump in the throat may come from swelling in the larynx caused by the radiation. The treatment can also cause a sore throat. The doctor may suggest medicine to reduce swelling or relieve pain.

During radiation therapy, patients may become very tired, especially in the later weeks. Resting is important, but doctors usually advise their patients to try to stay as active as they can. It's also common for the skin in the treated area to become red or dry. The skin should be exposed to the air but protected from the sun, and patients should avoid wearing clothes that rub the area. During radiation therapy, hair usually does not grow in the treated area; if it does, men should not shave. Good skin care is important at this time. Patients will be shown how to keep the area clean, and they should not put anything on the skin before their radiation treatments. Also, they should not use any lotion or cream at other times without the doctor's advice.

Some patients complain that radiation therapy makes their tongue sensitive. They may lose their sense of taste or smell or may have a bitter taste in their mouth. Drinking plenty of liquids may lessen the bitter taste. Often, the doctor or nurse can suggest other ways to ease these problems. And it helps to keep in mind that, although the side effects of radiation therapy may not go away completely, most of them gradually become less troublesome and patients feel better when the treatment is over.

Surgery

Keeping the patient comfortable is an important part of routine hospital care. If pain occurs, it can be relieved with medicine. Patients should feel free to discuss pain control with the doctor.

For a few days after surgery, the patient isn't able to eat or drink. At first, an *intravenous (IV)* tube supplies fluids. Within a day or two, the digestive tract is getting back to normal, but the patient still cannot swallow because the throat has not healed. Fluids and nutrition are given through a feeding tube (put in place during surgery) that goes through the nose and throat to the stomach. As the swelling in the throat goes away and the area begins to heal, the feeding tube is removed. Swallowing may be difficult at first, and the patient may need the guidance of a nurse or speech pathologist. Little by little, the patient returns to a regular diet.

After the operation, the lungs and windpipe produce a great deal of mucus, also called *sputum*. To remove it, the nurse applies gentle suction with a small plastic tube placed in the stoma. Soon, the patient learns to cough and to suction mucus through the stoma without the nurse's help. For a short time, it may also be necessary to suction saliva from the mouth because swelling in the throat prevents swallowing.

Normally, air is moistened by the tissues of the nose and throat before it reaches the windpipe. After surgery, air enters the trachea directly through the stoma and cannot be moistened in the same way. In the hospital, patients are kept comfortable with a special device that adds moisture to the air.

For several days after a partial laryngectomy, the patient breathes through the stoma. Soon the trach tube is removed; within the next few weeks, the stoma closes. The patient then breathes and speaks in the usual way, although the voice may not sound exactly the same as before.

After a complete laryngectomy, the stoma is permanent. The patient breathes, coughs, and "sneezes" through the stoma and has to learn to talk in a new way. The trach tube stays in place for at least several weeks (until the skin around the stoma heals), and some people continue to use the tube all or part of the time. If the tube is removed, it is usually replaced by a smaller *tracheostomy button* (also called a stoma button). After a while, some laryngectomees get along without either a tube or a button.

After a laryngectomy, parts of the neck and throat may be numb because nerves have been cut. Also, following surgery to remove lymph nodes in the neck, the shoulder and neck may be weak and stiff.

Chemotherapy

The side effects of chemotherapy depend on the drugs that are given. In general, anticancer drugs affect rapidly growing cells, such as blood cells that fight infection, cells that line the digestive tract, and cells in *hair follicles*. As a result, patients may have side effects such as lower resistance to infection, loss of appetite, nausea, vomiting, or mouth sores. They may also have less energy and may lose their hair.

Effects of Treatment on Eating

Loss of appetite can be a problem for patients treated for laryngeal cancer. People may not feel hungry when they are uncomfortable or tired.

Patients who have had a laryngectomy may lose their interest in food because the operation changes the way things smell and taste. Radiation therapy also tends to affect the sense of taste. The side effects of chemotherapy can also make it hard to eat. Yet good nutrition is important. Eating well means getting enough calories and protein to prevent weight loss, regain strength, and rebuild normal tissues.

After surgery, learning to swallow again may take some practice with the help of a nurse or speech pathologist. Some patients find liquids easier to swallow; others do better with solid foods. If eating is difficult because the mouth is dry from radiation therapy, patients may want to try soft, bland foods moistened with sauces or gravies. Others enjoy thick soups, puddings, and high-protein milkshakes. The nurse and the dietitian will help the patient choose the right kinds of food. Also, many patients find that eating several small meals and snacks during the day works better than trying to have three large meals. The National Cancer Institute booklets *Radiation Therapy and You*, *Chemotherapy and You*, and *Eating Hints* suggest a variety of other ways to deal with eating problems.

Rehabilitation

Learning to live with the changes brought about by cancer of the larynx is a special challenge. Rehabilitation is a very important part of the treatment plan. The medical team makes every effort to help patients return to their normal activities as soon as possible.

Each laryngectomee must be able to care for the stoma. Before leaving the hospital, the patient learns to remove and clean the trach tube or stoma button, suction the trach, and care for the area around the stoma. The skin is less likely to become irritated if it is kept clean.

When shaving, men should keep in mind that the neck may be numb for several months after surgery. To avoid nicks and cuts, it may be best to use an electric shaver until normal feeling returns.

Most people continue to use a stoma cover after the area heals. Stoma covers—such as scarves, neckties, ascots, and special bibs—can be attractive as well as useful. They help keep moisture in and around the stoma. Also, laryngectomees may be sensitive to dust and smoke, and the cover filters the air that enters the stoma. The cover also catches any discharge from the windpipe when the person coughs or sneezes.

Whenever the air is too dry, as it may be in heated buildings in the winter, the tissues of the windpipe and lungs may react by producing extra mucus. Also, the skin around the stoma may get crusty and bleed. Using a *humidifier* at home or in the office can lessen these problems.

A person who has had neck surgery may find that the neck is somewhat smaller. Also, the neck, shoulder, and arm may not be able to move as well as before. The doctor may advise physical therapy to help the person move more normally.

After surgery, laryngectomees work in almost every type of business and can do nearly all of the things they did before. However, they cannot hold their breath, so straining and heavy lifting may be difficult. Also, laryngectomees have to give up swimming and water skiing unless they have special instruction and equipment because it would be very dangerous for water to get into the windpipe and lungs through the stoma. Wearing a special plastic stoma shield or holding a washcloth over the stoma keeps water out when showering or shaving.

Learning to Speak Again

It's natural to be fearful and upset if the voice box must be removed. Talking is part of nearly everything we do, and losing the ability to talk—even temporarily—can be frightening. Patients and their families and friends need understanding and support during this very difficult time.

Until patients learn to talk again, it's important for them to be able to communicate in other ways. In the beginning, everyone who has had a laryngectomy has to communicate by writing, gesturing, or pointing to pictures, words, or letters. Some people like to use a "magic slate" for writing notes. Others use pads of paper and pens or pencils. It's handy to have a supply of pads that fit easily in a pocket or purse. In addition, some patients use a typewriter or computer. Others carry a small dictionary or a picture book (sometimes called a picture dictionary) and point to the words they need. Patients may want to select some of these items before the operation.

Within a week or so after a partial laryngectomy, most people can talk in the usual way. After a total laryngectomy, patients must learn to speak in a new way. A speech pathologist usually meets with the patient before surgery to explain the methods that can be used. In many cases, speech lessons can begin before the person leaves the hospital.

Patients may try out various new ways of talking. One way is to use air forced into the esophagus to produce the new voice (*esophageal speech*). Or the voice can come from some type of mechanical larynx. Some people rely on a mechanical larynx only until they learn esophageal speech, some decide to use this device instead of esophageal speech, and some use both.

Even though esophageal speech may sound low-pitched and gruff, many people want to use this method instead of a mechanical larynx because it sounds more like regular speech. Also, there's nothing to carry around, and the person's hands are free. A speech pathologist teaches the laryngectomee how to force air into the top of the esophagus and then push it out again. The puff of air is like a burp. It vibrates the walls of the throat, producing sound for the new voice. The tongue, lips, and teeth form words as the sound passes through the mouth.

For some laryngectomees, air for esophageal speech comes through a *tracheoesophageal puncture*. The surgeon creates a small opening between the trachea and the esophagus. A plastic or silicone valve is inserted into this opening through the stoma. The valve keeps food out of the trachea. When the stoma is covered, air from the lungs is forced into the esophagus through the valve. This air produces sound by making the walls of the throat vibrate. Words are formed in the mouth.

It takes practice and patience to learn esophageal speech, and not everyone is successful. How quickly a person learns, how natural the new voice sounds, and how understandable the speech is depend partly on the type and extent of the surgery. Other important factors are the patient's desire to learn and the help that's available. Patience and support from loved ones are important, too.

A mechanical larynx may be used until the person learns esophageal speech or if esophageal speech is too difficult. The device may be powered by batteries (*electrolarynx*) or by air (*pneumatic larynx*). The speech pathologist can help the patient choose a device and learn to use it.

One kind of electrolarynx looks like a small flashlight. It has a disk that makes a humming sound. The device is held against the neck, and the sound travels through the neck to the mouth. (This device may not be suitable for people who have had radiation therapy.) Another type of electrolarynx has a flexible plastic tube that carries sound to the person's mouth from a hand-held device.

A pneumatic larynx is held over the stoma and uses air from the lungs instead of batteries to make it vibrate. The sound it makes travels to the mouth through a plastic tube.

Followup Care

Regular followup is very important after treatment for cancer of the larynx. The doctor will check closely to be sure that the cancer has not returned. Checkups include exams of the stoma, neck, and throat. From time to time, the doctor does a complete physical exam, blood and urine tests, and x-rays. People treated with radiation therapy or partial laryngectomy will have laryngoscopy.

People who have been treated for cancer of the larynx have a higher-than-average risk of developing a new cancer in the mouth, throat, or other areas of the head and neck. This is especially true for those who smoke. Most doctors strongly urge their patients to stop smoking to cut down the risk of a new cancer and to reduce other problems, such as coughing.

Living with Cancer

The diagnosis of cancer can change the lives of patients and the people who care about them. These changes can be hard to handle. It's natural for patients and their families and friends to have many different and sometimes confusing emotions.

At times, patients and their loved ones may feel frightened, angry, or depressed. These are normal reactions when people face a serious health problem. Most people handle their problems better if they can share their thoughts and feelings with those close to them. Sharing can help everyone feel more at ease and can open the way for people to show one another their concern and offer their support.

Worries about tests, treatments, hospital stays, learning to talk again, and medical bills are common. Doctors, nurses, speech pathologists, social workers, and other members of the health care team can help calm fears and ease confusion. They can also provide information and suggest resources.

Patients and their families are naturally concerned about what the future holds. Sometimes they use statistics to try to figure out the chance of being cured. It is important to remember, however, that statistics are averages based on large numbers of patients. They can't be used to predict what will happen to a certain patient because no two cancer patients are alike. The doctor who takes care of the patient is the best one to discuss that person's outlook (*prognosis*).

People should feel free to ask the doctor about their prognosis, but not even the doctor knows for sure what will happen. Doctors may talk about surviving cancer, or they may use the term remission rather than cure. Even though many people with cancer of the larynx recover completely, doctors use these terms because the disease can recur.

Support for Cancer Patients

Living with a serious disease isn't easy. Cancer patients and those who care about them face many problems and challenges. Finding the strength to cope with these difficulties is easier when people have helpful information and support services.

People who have cancer of the larynx may have concerns about the future, family and social relationships, and finances. Sometimes they worry that changes in how they look and talk will affect the way people feel about them. They may worry about holding a job, caring for their family, or making new friends.

The doctor can explain the disease and give advice about treatment, going back to work, or daily activities. It may also help to talk with a nurse, social worker, counselor, or member of the clergy, especially about feelings or other very personal matters.

Many patients find that it's useful to get to know other people who are facing problems like theirs. They can meet other cancer patients through self-help and support groups. Often, a social worker at the hospital or clinic can suggest local and national groups that can help with emotional support, rehabilitation, financial aid, transportation, or home care.

The American Cancer Society is one such group. This nonprofit organization has many services for patients and their families. Local offices of the American Cancer Society are listed in the white pages of the telephone book. More information about this resource is listed in the "Resources" section.

The International Association of Laryngectomees publishes educational materials and sponsors meetings and other activities for people who have lost their voice because of cancer. Many local laryngectomy clubs are members of this Association. For more information, patients may contact the national office, whose address and telephone number are listed in the "Resources" section. Information also is available from local American Cancer Society offices.

The public library is a good place to find books and articles on living with cancer. Cancer patients and their families can also find helpful suggestions in the National Cancer Institute booklets *Taking Time* and *Facing Forward*.

Information about other programs and services is available through the Cancer Information Service. The toll-free number is 1-800-4-CANCER.

Cause and Prevention

Cancer of the larynx occurs most often in people over the age of 55. In the United States, it is four times more common in men than in women and is more common among black Americans than among whites. Scientists at hospitals and medical centers all across the country are studying this disease to learn more about what causes it and how to prevent it.

Doctors cannot explain why one person gets cancer of the larynx and another does not, but we are sure that no one can "catch" cancer from another person. Cancer is **not** contagious.

One known cause of cancer of the larynx is cigarette smoking. Smokers are far more likely than nonsmokers to develop this disease. The risk is even higher for smokers who drink alcohol heavily.

People who stop smoking can greatly reduce their risk of cancer of the larynx, as well as cancer of the lung, mouth, pancreas, bladder, and esophagus. Also, by quitting, those who have already had cancer of the larynx can cut down the risk of getting a second cancer of the larynx or a new cancer in another area. Special counseling or self-help groups are useful for some people who are trying to stop smoking. Some hospitals have groups for people who want to quit. Also, the Cancer Information Service and the American Cancer Society may have information about groups in local areas to help people quit smoking.

Working with asbestos can increase the risk of getting cancer of the larynx. Asbestos workers should follow work and safety rules to avoid inhaling asbestos fibers.

People who think they might be at risk for developing cancer of the larynx should discuss this concern with their doctor. The doctor may be able to suggest ways to reduce the risk and can suggest an appropriate schedule for checkups.

Resources

Information about cancer is available from many sources. Several are listed below. You may also wish to check your local library or contact support groups in your community.

Cancer Information Service (CIS)

The Cancer Information Service, a program of the National Cancer Institute, is a nationwide telephone service for cancer patients and their families and friends, the public, and health care professionals. The staff can answer questions in English or Spanish and can send free National Cancer Institute printed materials. They also know about local resources and services. One toll-free number, 1-800-4-CANCER (1-800-422-6237), connects callers with the office that serves their area.

American Cancer Society (ACS)

The American Cancer Society is a voluntary organization with a national office and local units all over the country. It supports research, conducts educational programs, and offers many services to patients and their families. To obtain information about services and activities in local areas, including clubs for laryngectomees, call the Society's toll-free number, 1-800-ACS-2345 (1-800-227-2345), or the number listed under American Cancer Society in the white pages of the telephone book.

International Association of Laryngectomees (IAL)
1599 Clifton Road, N.E.
Atlanta, GA 30329
1-800-ACS-2345

The International Association of Laryngectomees is sponsored by the American Cancer Society. The Association supplies printed information and sponsors meetings and other activities. It publishes a directory of speech instructors and maintains a list of sources of supplies for laryngectomees. Most Lost Chord Clubs, New Voice Clubs, and other clubs for laryngectomees are members of this organization and are listed in its directory. Information about clubs is available from the American Cancer Society.

American Speech-Language-Hearing Association (ASHA)
Consumer Division
10801 Rockville Pike
Rockville, MD 20852
1-800-638-TALK; (301) 897-5700 (calls from Maryland)

The American Speech-Language-Hearing Association is a professional association. Its Consumer Division provides information on all types of communication problems and can refer patients to speech therapy programs.

The National Coalition for Cancer Survivorship (NCCS)
1010 Wayne Avenue, Suite 300
Silver Spring, MD 20910
(301) 650-8868

The National Coalition for Cancer Survivorship is a volunteer group concerned with issues faced by people with cancer and people who have recovered from cancer. It deals with legal, financial, emotional, and social matters. This group can advise people about their rights related to jobs and insurance. It has a speakers bureau and can supply printed information, including lists of cancer support groups in many areas.

Other Booklets

Cancer patients, their families and friends, and others may find the following booklets useful. They are available free of charge by calling 1-800-4-CANCER.

Booklets about Cancer Treatment

- *Chemotherapy and You: A Guide to Self-Help During Treatment*
- *Radiation Therapy and You: A Guide to Self-Help During Treatment*
- *Eating Hints for Cancer Patients*
- *Questions and Answers About Pain Control* (also available from the American Cancer Society)
- *What Are Clinical Trials All About?*

Booklets about Living With Cancer

- *Taking Time: Support for People With Cancer and the People Who Care About Them*
- *Facing Forward: A Guide for Cancer Survivors*
- *When Someone in Your Family Has Cancer*
- *When Cancer Recurs: Meeting the Challenge Again*
- *Advanced Cancer: Living Each Day*

Chapter 67

Obtaining Cancer Updates from the National Cancer Institute

What Is PDQ?

PDQ is a computer system that gives up-to-date information on cancer and its prevention, detection, treatment, and supportive care. It is a service of the National Cancer Institute (NCI) for people with cancer and their families and for doctors, nurses, and other health care professionals.

To ensure that it remains current, the information in PDQ is reviewed and updated each month by experts in the fields of cancer treatment, prevention, screening, and supportive care. PDQ also provides information about research on new treatments (clinical trials), doctors who treat cancer, and hospitals with cancer programs. The treatment information in this chapter is based on information in the PDQ summary for health professionals on this cancer.

How to Use PDQ

PDQ can be used to learn more about current treatment of different kinds of cancer. You may find it helpful to discuss this information with your doctor, who knows you and has the facts about your disease. PDQ can also provide the names of additional health care professionals who specialize in treating patients with cancer.

National Cancer Institute PDQ Database, http://rex.nci.nih.gov/PA-TIENTS/INFO_PEOPL_Doc.html; last modified February 1998.

Before you start treatment, you also may want to think about taking part in a clinical trial. PDQ can be used to learn more about these trials. A clinical trial is a research study that attempts to improve current treatments or finds information on new treatments for patients with cancer. Clinical trials are based on past studies and information discovered in the laboratory. Each trial answers certain scientific questions in order to find new and better ways to help patients with cancer. Information is collected about new treatments, their risks, and how well they do or do not work. When clinical trials show that a new treatment is better than the treatment currently used as "standard" treatment, the new treatment may become the standard treatment. Listings of current clinical trials are available on PDQ. Many cancer doctors who take part in clinical trials are listed in PDQ.

To learn more about cancer and how it is treated, or to learn more about clinical trials for your kind of cancer, call the National Cancer Institute's Cancer Information Service. The number is 1-800-4-CAN-CER (1-800-422-6237); TTY at 1-800-332-8615. The call is free and a trained information specialist will be available to answer cancer-related questions.

PDQ is updated whenever there is new information. Check with the Cancer Information Service to be sure that you have the most up-to-date information.

To Learn More

To Learn More..... Call 1-800-4-CANCER
TTY at 1-800-332-8615

The Cancer Information Service also has booklets about cancer that are available to the public and can be sent on request. The following general booklets on questions related to cancer may be helpful:

- What You Need To Know About Cancer

- Taking Time: Support for People with Cancer and the People Who Care About Them

- What Are Clinical Trials All About?

- Chemotherapy and You: A Guide to Self-Help During Treatment

- Radiation Therapy and You: A Guide to Self-Help During Treatment

- Eating Hints for Cancer Patients

- Advanced Cancer: Living Each Day

- When Cancer Recurs: Meeting the Challenge Again

There are other places where people can get material and information about cancer treatment and services. The social service office at a hospital can be checked for local and national agencies that can help with getting information about finances, getting to and from treatment, getting care at home, and dealing with problems.

For more information from the National Cancer Institute, please write to this address:

National Cancer Institute
Office of Cancer Communications
31 Center Drive, MSC 2580
Bethesda, MD 20892-2580

Index

Index

555